I0089545

Metabolically Healthy Obesity

Special Issue Editor
Catherine M. Phillips

MDPI • Basel • Beijing • Wuhan • Barcelona • Belgrade

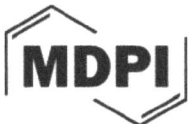

MDPI

Special Issue Editor
Catherine M. Phillips
HRB Centre for Diet and Health Research
University College Cork
University College Dublin
Ireland

Editorial Office
MDPI AG
St. Alban-Anlage 66
Basel, Switzerland

This edition is a reprint of the Special Issue published online in the open access journal *Nutrients* (ISSN 2072-6643) in 2016 (available at: http://www.mdpi.com/journal/nutrients/special_issues/ metabolically_healthy_obesity).

For citation purposes, cite each article independently as indicated on the article page online and as indicated below:

Lastname, F.M.; Lastname, F.M. Article title. *Journal Name*. **Year**. *Article number*, page range.

First Edition 2018

ISBN 978-3-03842-686-8 (Pbk)
ISBN 978-3-03842-687-5 (PDF)

Articles in this volume are Open Access and distributed under the Creative Commons Attribution (CC BY) license, which allows users to download, copy and build upon published articles even for commercial purposes, as long as the author and publisher are properly credited, which ensures maximum dissemination and a wider impact of our publications. The book taken as a whole is © 2018 MDPI, Basel, Switzerland, distributed under the terms and conditions of the Creative Commons license CC BY-NC-ND (http://creativecommons.org/licenses/by-nc-nd/4.0/).

Table of Contents

About the Special Issue Editor

Catherine M. Phillips is a Senior Research Fellow and Principal Investigator in the HRB funded Centre for Health and Diet Research, with joint appointments at University College Dublin and University College Cork, Ireland. Following a BSc. (Hons) in Biochemistry from University College Dublin and a Ph.D. in Clinical Medicine from Trinity College Dublin Dr. Phillips research interests have spanned investigation of the genetic and lifestyle determinants of both metabolic and mental health. Her current research interests focus on the role of circulating biomarkers, diet and body composition in the context of intergenerational and lifecourse health.

Preface to "Metabolically Healthy Obesity"

This book, compiled from a Special Issue of the journal Nutrients, demonstrates the wide spectrum of current research efforts underway internationally which aim to advance our understanding of the role of biological, genetic, dietary and lifestyle factors as determinants of metabolically healthy obese (MHO) phenotypes. Included are 15 articles, with contributions from South Africa, Canada, China, Colombia, Lebanon as well as several countries of the European Union. Comprising original research articles based on observational and intervention studies in humans and animal models, narrative reviews and a systematic review and meta-analysis these contributions describe the current state of the art and illustrate the breadth of cutting edge research underway in this field.

The evidence suggests that MHO is a transient phenotype. While transitions between phenotypes over time may account for disparities in both their reported prevalence and risk of developing cardiometabolic disease or mortality, characterisation of the factors which distinguish those who progress to or maintain MHO from those who transition from MHO to metabolically unhealthy obesity is important as it may uncover potential intervention targets. Both Zheng et al., and Muoz-Garach et al., examine MHO stability, the former in the context of investigating the impact of weight change, whereas in the latter paper they analyze responsiveness to traditional lifestyle recommendations and bariatric surgery.

The use of biomarkers to improve our understanding of the biological mechanisms underpinning MHO is highlighted. Allam-Ndoul et al. employ a metabolomics approach to investigate differences in plasma metabolomic profiles between normal weight and overweight/obese individuals, with or without metabolic syndrome (MetS). Bermdez-Cardona and colleagues determine fatty acid profiles in obese youth with and without MetS. The role of gut microbiota as a determinant of MHO and how dietary medium chain triglycerides can ameliorate metabolic health via their capacity to improve both the intestinal ecosystem and permeability is discussed by Rial et al. Pujia et al., investigate whether a difference in fasting fat utilization exists between overweight/obese individuals with a favorable cardiovascular risk profile and those with MetS and Type 2 diabetes (T2DM). Two studies focus on blood pressure. Yang et al., explore associations between BMI and mortality in hypertensive adults. Zhang and colleagues investigate fasting ghrelin concentrations during a high-salt diet among non-obese and normotensive subjects. Nguyen and co-workers focus on MHO in combination with human immunodeficiency virus (HIV). In a sample of HIV infected people recruited across primary care facilities in South Africa they assess the distribution of body size phenotypes in people with HIV infection overall and according to antiretroviral therapy, diagnosed duration of the infection and CD4 count.

Animal studies may be particularly useful in mechanistic research. Zubira and colleagues examine the balance of hypertrophic/hyperplastic adipose tissue expansion and the metabolic profile in a high glucocorticoids mouse model. Using a mouse model of diet-induced obesity, Soni et al., examine the effect of high fat diet supplemented with marine fatty acids (eicosapentaenoic acid and docosahexaenoic acid) on skeletal muscle function.

Limited and inconsistent data regards the impact of dietary interventions in human MHO exist. In a systematic review and meta-analysis Stelmach-Mardas et al., assess the effect of dietary intervention on changes in metabolic health profiles of MHO subjects. Matta et al., examine the socio-demographic correlates of MHO and investigate the independent effect of dietary patterns. Scant data regards genetic predisposition to MHO is available. Gajewska et al., investigate whether certain genetic backgrounds (selected functional single nucleotide polymorphisms in LEP, LEPR and ADIPOQ) are associated with changes in serum levels of their corresponding adipocytokines and weight loss in prepubertal obese children undergoing lifestyle intervention. In further analysis of the role of adipocytokines Savino et al., investigate correlations between mother and infant BMI, their serum leptin values and breast milk leptin concentration in early infancy. This is important as increasing evidence suggests that early life exposure to a range of environmental factors, including nutrition for example, plays a critical role in defining offspring health, both in childhood and in later life. According to the Developmental Origins of Health and Disease (DOHaD) hypothesis, transient environmental exposures during critical periods of development (such as the pre-conceptional, fetal and early infant phases of life) can alter normal physiology and have a persistent impact on metabolism and gene expression thereby influencing offspring phenotype and disease risk in later life.

The contributions presented here illustrate that a great body of research regarding obesity-associated metabolic health phenotypes has been performed to date. However it is clear that much remains to be done. These contributions also serve to identify gaps and new avenues which warrant further investigation, particularly with respect to life course epidemiology based on the DOHaD hypothesis and whether risk stratification of obese individuals based on their metabolic health status may offer new opportunities for more personalised approaches in diagnosis, intervention and treatment.

Finally I would like to acknowledge the excellent work of the authors and reviewers, their time and contributions have made this book possible.

Catherine Phillips
Special Issue Editor

nutrients

MDPI

Article

Individuals with Metabolically Healthy Overweight/Obesity Have Higher Fat Utilization than Metabolically Unhealthy Individuals

Arturo Pujia [1], Carmine Gazzaruso [2], Yvelise Ferro [1], Elisa Mazza [1], Samantha Maurotti [1], Cristina Russo [1], Veronica Lazzaro [3], Stefano Romeo [1,4] and Tiziana Montalcini [1,*]

[1] Department of Medical and Surgical Science, University Magna Grecia, Catanzaro 88100, Italy; pujia@unicz.it (A.P.); yferro@unicz.it (Y.F.); elisamazza@inwind.it (E.M.); samabiotec@yahoo.it (S.M.); cristina_russo_cr@libero.it (C.R.); romeo@unicz.it (S.R.)
[2] Clinical Institute "Beato Matteo", Vigevano 27029, Italy; c.gazzaruso@gmail.com
[3] Department of Health Science, University Magna Grecia, Catanzaro 88100, Italy; veronicalazzaro09@gmail.com
[4] Department of Molecular and Clinical Medicine, University of Gothenburg, Gothenburg 40530, Sweden
* Correspondence: tmontalcini@unicz.it; Tel.: +39-961-369-5172; Fax: +39-961-369-7223

Received: 29 September 2015; Accepted: 8 December 2015; Published: 4 January 2016

Abstract: The mechanisms underlying the change in phenotype from metabolically healthy to metabolically unhealthy obesity are still unclear. The aim of this study is to investigate whether a difference in fasting fat utilization exists between overweight/obese individuals with a favorable cardiovascular risk profile and those with Metabolic Syndrome and Type 2 diabetes. Furthermore, we sought to explore whether there is an association between fasting fat utilization and insulin resistance. In this cross-sectional study, 172 overweight/obese individuals underwent a nutritional assessment. Those with fasting glucose $\geqslant$126 mg/dL or antidiabetic treatment were considered to be diabetics. If at least three of the NCEP criteria were present, they had Metabolic Syndrome, while those with less criteria were considered to be healthy overweight/obese. An indirect calorimetry was performed to estimate Respiratory Quotient, an index of nutrient utilization. A lower Respiratory Quotient (*i.e.*, higher fat utilization) was found in healthy overweight/obese individuals than in those with Metabolic Syndrome and Type 2 diabetes (0.85 ± 0.05; 0.87 ± 0.06; 0.88 ± 0.05 respectively, $p = 0.04$). The univariate and multivariable analysis showed a positive association between the Respiratory Quotient and HOMA-IR (slope in statistic (B) = 0.004; $\beta = 0.42$; $p = 0.005$; 95% Confidence interval = 0.001–0.006). In this study, we find, for the first time, that the fasting Respiratory Quotient is significantly lower (fat utilization is higher) in individuals who are metabolically healthy overweight/obese than in those with metabolically unhealthy obesity. In addition, we demonstrated the association between fat utilization and HOMA-IR, an insulin resistance index.

Keywords: obesity; nutrition assessment; fat utilization; Metabolic Syndrome; metabolically unhealthy Obesity; diabetes

1. Introduction

Epidemiological research established that overweight and obese individuals do not always show high rates of cardiovascular diseases (CVD) and mortality [1,2]. Those without dyslipidemia, insulin resistance, and hypertension are characterized by a low risk, despite the presence of an elevated body mass index (BMI) [3]. However, this phenotype seems to be a transient state [4,5] since a high risk of developing Type 2 diabetes mellitus (T2DM) has been demonstrated in those who maintain an unhealthy lifestyle over time [5]. The mechanism underlying the switch in phenotype from the metabolically healthy status to T2DM is still unclear. Obesity, inflammation, and worsening of insulin resistance are recognized as important risk factor in the pathogenesis of diabetes [6,7] but other mechanisms could play a role. A high fat (HF) diet results in an increase in β-oxidation [8]. However, other investigations demonstrated a reduction in β-oxidation [9–16]. These studies are not conflicting because the mechanisms described above could be sequential (first it increases and then, it decreases), leading to the switch from a metabolically healthy but overweight/obesity status to T2DM. In this regard, it is well known that nutrient utilization can be assessed with Indirect Calorimetry by measuring the ratio between carbon dioxide production and oxygen consumption (Respiratory Quotient (RQ)) [17]. Some investigations have demonstrated that subjects who tend to burn less fat have an increased RQ value [18,19]. High RQ is associated with a high rate of subsequent weight gain [20]. Recently, a high post-absorptive RQ was associated with hypertension [21] and increased Carotid Intima-Media Thickness (CIMT), a well-known predictor of cardiovascular events [22,23] in individuals with obesity [24]. Furthermore, fasting RQ is higher in individuals with obesity and hypertriglyceridemia [25] and in overweight/obese individuals with cardiac remodelling than in those who are just obese [26]. In this study, we sought to investigate whether a difference in RQ (and thus, in fat utilization) exists between overweight/obese individuals with a favorable cardiovascular risk profile and those with Metabolic Syndrome (MS) and T2DM, and whether RQ is associated with insulin resistance. This investigation could be useful to hypothesize the mechanisms underlying the progression from a metabolically healthy but overweight/obese phenotype towards metabolically unhealthy obesity and T2DM, and probably to distinguish subjects who will be at a high risk for T2DM and cardiovascular diseases.

2. Methods

In this cross-sectional study, the population consisted of white overweight/obese subjects who were undergoing health-screening tests at our outpatient nutrition clinic. All the participants were over 45 years old with a BMI of more than 24.9. Participants underwent a medical interview and the nutritional assessment to verify if there had been any changes in their food habits or if they followed a special diet or used any dietary supplements in the three months prior to our tests. We enrolled consecutively only those who had not performed these actions. All enrolled individuals had the same diet, determined by nutritional intake assessment, *i.e.*, a solid-food diet that supplied 50%–55% of the calories as carbohydrate, 18%–20% as protein, and no more than 30% as fat.

All patients included in the study were not suffering from any diseases (like chronic obstructive pulmonary disease, thyroid dysfunction, cancer, congestive heart failure, myocardial infarction, stroke) and did not take any drug (anti-obesity medications, psychotropic drugs and chronotropic agents)which could affect respiratory gas exchange or had debilitating diseases known to affect blood pressure or plasma glucose or lipid concentrations (like stage 2–5 chronic kidney disease and end stage liver failure) as determined by medical history, a physical examination, and laboratory tests.

Furthermore, we assessed the presence of the known classical cardiovascular (CV) risk factors, MS presence and anthropometric characteristics. The following criteria were used to define the distinct CV risk factors: diabetes: fasting blood glucose $\geqslant$126 mg/dL or antidiabetic treatment; hyperlipidemia: total cholesterol >200 mg/dL and/or triglycerides >200 mg/dL or lipid lowering drugs use; hypertension: systolic blood pressure $\geqslant$130 mmHg and/or diastolic blood pressure $\geqslant$85 mmHg or antihypertensive treatment; overweight: 25 kg/m^2 $\leqslant$ BMI < 30 kg/m^2; obesity: body mass index (BMI) $\geqslant$30 kg/m^2; smoking: a current smoker who has smoked more than 100 cigarettes in their lifetime and smokes cigarettes every day or some days [27,28].

The selection criteria for MS individuals were based on the National Cholesterol Education Program's (NCEP) Adult Treatment Panel III report (ATP III). Individuals with 0–2 cardiometabolic abnormalities were identified as having a metabolically healthy but overweight/obese phenotype, while those with at least three or more abnormalies were identified as having MS [29]. Furthermore, all participants underwent the instrumental evaluation of the carotid intima-media thickness (CIMT).

Therefore, in this study we enrolled 172 overweight/obese subjects, categorized into the following three groups: healthy overweight/obese (with maximum two NCEP abnormalities and without T2DM); MS (with three or more NCEP abnormality and without T2DM) and T2DM (only those with fasting glucose $\geqslant$126 mg/dL or antidiabetic treatment). Written informed consent was obtained. The protocol was approved by local ethic committee at the University Hospital (projects codes 2013-1/CE). The investigation conforms to the principles outlined in the Declaration of Helsinki.

2.1. Blood Pressure Measurement

The measurement of the systemic blood pressure (systolic blood pressure (SBP) and diastolic blood pressure (DBP)) of both arms was obtained by an auscultatory blood pressure technique with aneroid sphygmomanometer. Clinic BP was obtained in supine patients, after 5 min of quiet rest. A minimum of three BP readings were taken using an appropriate BP cuff size (the inflatable part of the BP cuff covered about 80 percent of the circumference of upper arm) as previously described [30].

2.2. Biochemical Evaluation

Venous blood was collected after fasting overnight into vacutainer tubes (Becton & Dickinson, Plymouth, UK) and centrifuged within 4 h. Serum glucose, total cholesterol, high density lipoprotein (HDL)-cholesterol, and triglycerides were measured with enzymatic colorimetric test. Low-density lipoprotein (LDL) cholesterol level was calculated by the Friedewald formula: total cholesterol—HDL cholesterol—(triglycerides/5). Plasma insulin concentration was determined by radioimmunoassay. We calculated Homeostasis Model Assessment of Insulin Resistance (HOMA-IR) by the following formula:

$$HOMA\text{-}IR = Fasting\,blood\,glucose\,(mg/dL) \times insulin\,(U/mL)/405$$

Quality control was assessed daily for all determinations.

2.3. Anthropometric Measurements

All tests were performed after a 12 h overnight fast. Body weight was measured with a calibrated scale with the subjects lightly dressed, subtracting the weight of clothes. Height was measured with a wall-mounted stadiometer (TANITA, Middlesex, UK). BMI was calculated with the following formula: weight (kg)/height (m)^2. Waist circumferences and hip circumferences (WC and HC) were measured with a nonstretchable tape over the unclothed abdomen at the narrowest point between costal margin and iliac crest at the level of the widest diameter around the buttocks, respectively [31]. Bioelectrical impedance analysis (BIA) (BIA-101, Akernsrl, Florence, Italy) was performed to estimate the percentage of Total Body Water (TBW), Fat Mass (FM), Muscle Mass (MM), total Fat-Free Mass (FFM) [32].

2.4. Dietary Intake Assessment

The participant's nutritional intake was calculated using nutritional software MetaDieta 3.0.1 (Metedasrl, San Benedetto del Tronto, Italy). Dietary intake data comprised a 24-h recall and a seven-day diet record. The 24-h recall was collected via an interview by a dietitian who used images associated with a comprehensive food list in the program. All participants were also given a food diary, measuring sheet with life-size images of a spoon, cup and bottle sizes for food diaries. The INRAN (National Institute of Food Research) 2000 and IEO (European Institute of Oncology) 2008 database serves as the source of food composition information in the program. The data was entered by dietitians into the program. All foods are assigned a unique code which allows categorization of foods into food groups. The resulting database was exported into SPSS (IBM Corporation, New York, NY, USA) for analysis.

2.5. RQ Assessment—Indirect Calorimetry

RQ and the Resting Energy Expenditure (REE) were measured by Indirect Calorimetry using the open circuit technique (Viasys Healthcare, Hoechberg, Germany). All tests were performed after fasting overnigh, between hours of 7 a.m. and 8:30 a.m. after 48 h abstention from exercise, in a sedentary position. The participant rested quietly for 30 min in an isolated room at a controlled temperature (21–24 °C). Respiratory gas exchange was measured within a canopy circuit for at least 30 min, until steady state was achieved. The calorimeter quantifies the volume of O_2 inspired and CO_2 expired by the subject. Resting Energy Expenditure is calculated by the Weir formula. RQ was calculated as CO_2 production/O_2 consumption. Criteria for a valid measurement was at least 15 min of steady state, with less than 10% fluctuation in minute ventilation and oxygen consumption and less than 5% fluctuation in RQ [26,33].

2.6. Carotid Arteries Assessment

The participants underwent B-mode ultrasonography of the extracranial carotid arteries by use of a high-resolution ultrasound instrument (Toshiba Medical Systems Corporation, model TUS-A500, 1385, Shimoishigami, Otawara-Shi, Tochigi, Japan). We used a 5- to 12-MHz linear array multifrequency transducer. All the examinations were performed by the same ultrasonographer blinded to clinical information with patients in the supine position. ECG leads were attached to the ultrasound recorder for on-line continuous heart rate monitoring. The right and left common (CCA) and internal carotid arteries (including bifurcations) were evaluated with the head of the subjects turned away from the sonographer and the neck extended with mild rotation. The IMT, defined as the distance between intimal-luminal interface and medial—adventitial interface, was measured as previously described [24]. In posterior approach and with the sound beam set perpendicular to the arterial surface, 1 cm from the bifurcation, three longitudinal measurements of IMT were completed on the right and left common carotid arteries far-wall, at sites free of any discrete plaques. The mean of the three right and left longitudinal measurements was then calculated. Then, we calculated and used for statistical analysis the mean CIMT between right and left CCA. The coefficient variation of the methods was 3.3%.

3. Statistical Analysis

Data is reported as mean $\pm$ SD. Thirty subjects for each group are required to detect a significant difference of RQ greater than 2% (21–26) with 80% power on a two-sided level of significance of 0.05. A chi-square test was performed to analyze the prevalence of the cardiovascular risk factors and medications. ANOVA was performed to compare the means between groups with a Fisher's LSD test as a post-hoc analysis. REE and RQ values were eventually adjusted according to the difference in FFM between groups or if RQ and REE correlated with FFM.

The Pearson's correlation was used to identify the variables correlated with RQ given that the continuous variables were normally distributed. We analyzed the correlation with the following variables: REE, FFM, age, BMI, WC, glucose, LDL, HDL, triglycerides, PAS, PAD, HOMA-IR. Stepwise multivariable linear regression analysis was used to test the association between RQ and the variables selected among those correlated with RQ in the univariate analysis, with $p < 0.1$. When we tested the association with HOMA-IR and cardiometabolic risk factors, glucose was excluded since it was considered as part of HOMA-IR. Significant differences were assumed to be present at $p < 0.05$ (two-tailed). All comparisons were performed using SPSS 20.0 for Windows (IBM Corporation, New York, NY, USA).

4. Results

Among the participants, we enrolled 80, 58, and 34 individuals who were overweight/obese, with MS and Type 2 Diabetes, respectively. Since we did not find any difference of RQ between gender and between individuals taking medications or not (data not shown) we presented the data altogether.

The demographic and anthropometric characteristics, the prevalence of cardiovascular risk factors, and medications use of the population are indicated in Table 1. Healthy overweight/obese had a lower RQ than those with MS and Type 2 diabetes ($p = 0.04$; ANOVA, Table 2). In particular, healthy overweight/obese had a lower RQ than MS ($p = 0.04$; post-hoc analysis) and a lower RQ than T2DM ($p = 0.03$; *post-hoc* analysis; Table 2), respectively. FFM did not differ between groups ($p = 0.92$). Furthermore, RQ and FFM (as absolute value) did not correlate ($r = 0.11$ and $p = 0.27$). As expected, CIMT were significantly higher in T2DM than in MS ($p = 0.03$; post-hoc analysis) and the healthy overweight/obese ($p = 0.02$; post-hoc analysis).

Table 3 shows the factors significantly associated with RQ in the univariate analysis, which were the following: HOMA-IR, glucose, triglycerides, SBP. In the multivariable analysis, RQ remained still associated with HOMA-IR, while triglycerides and SBP were not associated (Table 4).

5. Discussion

In this investigation, we find that fasting RQ, an index of nutrient utilization assessed by indirect calorimetry, is significantly lower in individuals with metabolically healthy overweight/obesity than in those with MS and T2DM. This suggests that individuals who are healthy overweight/obese are still able, to some extent, to utilize fat in the fasting state while fat utilization is significantly reduced in individuals with unhealthy obesity (Table 2). These results could help to hypothesize that new factors are involved in the pathogenesis of T2DM and potential new therapeutic goals exist. Furthermore, in this population, we demonstrated the association between RQ and HOMA-IR, which is widely utilized as an insulin resistance index (Table 4). This result could have important implications in predicting diabetes, which must be confirmed by longitudinal studies. The mechanisms underlying the switch in phenotype from healthy overweight/obese to T2DM are still unknown and our study was not designed to investigate these mechanisms. However, our study may be useful in generating intriguing hypotheses. Whether [34,35] or not [36–39] increase in fatty acid β-oxidation leads to insulin resistance is still a subject of debate. There is evidence that obesity-associated glucose intolerance might develop from an overload of fatty acid in muscle mitochondria [40]. It has been demonstrated that the excessive availability of fatty acids may exert an insulin-desensitizing action in muscle mitochondria [8]. Furthermore, it has been demonstrated that a HF diet and/or obesity can increase the expression of several β-oxidative enzymes [41] and reduce RQ [8]. It is interesting that these events precede the onset of insulin resistance [8]. Our findings are in line with these studies since we find that individuals who are metabolically healthy overweight/obese have, to some extent, a greater ability to burn fat (lower RQ) in comparison to those with MS and T2DM. However, it has also been demonstrated that an unhealthy lifestyle, including HF feeding and the absence of physical activity, favors incomplete β-oxidation caused by the mismatch between β-oxidation and tricarboxylic acid cycle activity, contributing to mitochondrial damage [41,42]. Incomplete fatty acid oxidation also facilitates the production of reactive oxygen species (ROS) which can cause damage to mitochondrial enzymes [42]. Furthermore, the production of ROS represents a common pathway in the cascade of events that finally results in β-cell failure [43]. Consequently, as confirmed by other investigations, both glucose-tolerance and fat oxidation are decreased [9–11,44–46]. Together these studies lead us to hypothesize that a reduction in fatty acid oxidation is achieved over time, probably in the context of an unhealthy lifestyle. The significant difference of RQ (of fasting fat utilization) between metabolically healthy but overweight/obese phenotype, with MS and T2DM individuals may confirm this mechanism.

Table 1. Demographic, anthropometric and clinical characteristics of the population.

Variables	Overweight/Obese (OO) (n = 80)	Metabolic Syndrome (MS) (n = 58)	T2 Diabetes (T2DM) (n = 34)	P ANOVA	p Post-Hoc Analysis
Females (%)	31.3	34.5	35.3	0.63	/
Age (years)	56 ± 10	58 ± 9	62 ± 10	0.016	OO *vs.* T2DM 0.004
Weight (Kg)	83 ± 17	87 ± 21	85 ± 20	0.505	/
BMI (Kg/m^2)	33 ± 6	34 ± 7	34 ± 6	0.514	/
WC (cm)	102 ± 14	106 ± 15	108 ± 13	0.120	/
HC (cm)	109 ± 15	110 ± 12	110 ± 11	0.905	/
SBP (mmHg)	122 ± 11	133 ± 15	130 ± 13	<0.001	OO *vs.* MS < 0.001, OO *vs.* T2DM 0.003
DBP (mmHg)	78 ± 8	80 ± 11	77 ± 9	0.161	/
Glucose-mg/dL (mmol/L)	91 ± 9 (5.06 ± 0.5)	100 ± 10 (5.56 ± 0.5)	130 ± 45 (7.22 ± 2.5)	<0.001	OO *vs.* MS 0.019, OO *vs.* T2DM < 0.001, MS *vs.* T2DM < 0.001
Insulin-mU/L (pmol/L)	16 ± 8 (114.7 ± 57)	23 ± 20 (164.9 ± 143)	35 ± 26 (250.9 ± 186)	0.039	OO *vs.* T2D 0.012
HOMA-IR	3.7 ± 2	6 ± 5	12 ± 11	0.004	OO *vs.* T2DM 0.001, MS *vs.* T2DM 0.017
TotCholesterol-mg/dL (mmol/L)	199 ± 38 (5.14 ± 0.98)	213 ± 42 (5.5 ± 1.09)	195 ± 47 (5.04 ± 1.2)	0.055	OO *vs.* MS 0.042, MS *vs.* T2DM 0.037
HDL (mmol/L)	1.52 ± 0.41	1.16 ± 0.36	1.37 ± 0.44	<0.001	OO *vs.* MS < 0.001, OO *vs.* T2DM 0.017, MS *vs.* T2DM 0.046
LDL (mmol/L)	3.18 ± 0.83	3.39 ± 0.96	2.97 ± 1.06	0.141	/
Triglycerides (mmol/L)	91 ± 28 (1.03 ± 0.32)	201 ± 81 (2.27 ± 0.91)	151 ± 85 (1.70 ± 0.96)	<0.001	OO *vs.* MS < 0.001, OO *vs.* T2D < 0.001, MS *vs.* T2D < 0.001
Prevalence					
Hypertension (%)	12	26	52	0.001	/
Dyslipidemia (%)	19	29	30	0.129	/
Smokers (%)	38	46	24	0.390	/
Antidiabetic agents (%)	0	0	56	<0.001	/
Antihypertensive agents (%)	0	0	56	<0.001	/
Lipid lowering agents (%)	0	0	44	<0.001	/

Legend: BMI, body mass index; DBP, diastolic blood pressure; HC, hip circumferences; HDL, high density lipoprotein; HOMA IR, Homeostasis Model Assessment of Insulin Resistance; LDL, low density lipoprotein; SBP, systolic blood pressure; Tot Cholesterol, total cholesterol; WC, Waist circumferences.

Table 2. Respiratory quotient, resting energy expenditure, body composition, and carotid intima-media thickness according to groups (Overweight/Obese, with Metabolic Syndrome, with Type 2 Diabetes Mellitus).

Variables	Overweight/Obese (OO) ($n = 80$)	Metabolic Syndrome (MS) ($n = 58$)	T2 Diabetes (T2DM) ($n = 34$)	P ANOVA	p Post-Hoc Analysis
REE (FFM adjusted; kcal)	1371 ± 33	1392 ± 42	1383 ± 45	0.93	/
RQ	0.85 ± 0.05	0.87 ± 0.06	0.88 ± 0.05	0.042	OO *vs.* MS 0.044 OO *vs.* T2DM 0.033
TBW (%)	45 ± 10	47 ± 9	47 ± 8	0.596	/
ECW (%)	31 ± 15	32 ± 14	37 ± 14	0.272	/
FFM (%)	59 ± 12	61 ± 12	61 ± 10	0.707	/
MM (%)	38 ± 8	40 ± 8	39 ± 9	0.665	/
FM (%)	36 ± 9	36 ± 8	36 ± 8	0.943	/
FFM (%)	59 ± 12	61 ± 12	61 ± 10	0.707	/
FFM (kg)	50.4 ± 18	52.4 ± 25	51.8 ± 18	0.92	/
CIMT (mm)	0.7 ± 0.2	0.7 ± 0.2	0.8 ± 0.2	0.054	OO *vs.* T2D 0.024 MS *vs.* T2D 0.038

Legend: CIMT, carotid intima-media thickness; ECW, extracellular water; FFM, free fat mass; FM, fat mass; MM, muscle mass; REE, resting energy expenditure; RQ, respiratory quotient; TBW, total body water.

Table 3. Pearson correlation-factors correlated to respiratory quotient.

Variable	Correlation Parameters	Age	REE	BMI	WC	FFM	HOMA-IR	Glucose	LDL	Triglycerides	HDL	SBP	DBP
RQ	r	0.07	0.04	−0.03	0.02	0.92	0.42	0.16	−0.03	0.19	−0.11	0.18	0.08
	p	0.35	0.53	0.65	0.79	0.27	0.005	0.03	0.62	0.01	0.13	0.01	0.25

Legend: BMI, body mass index; DBP, diastolic blood pressure; FFM, free fat mass; HDL, high density lipoprotein; HOMA IR, Homeostasis Model Assessment of Insulin Resistance; LDL, low density lipoprotein; REE, resting energy expenditure; RQ, respiratory quotient; SBP, systolic blood pressure; WC, Waist circumference.

Table 4. Multivariate linear regression analysis—factors associated with respiratory quotient.

Dependent Variable RQ	B	SE	β	t	P	95% C.I.	
						Lower Limit	Upper Limit
HOMA-IR	0.004	0.001	0.42	2.98	0.005	0.001	0.006
Triglycerides	0.001	0.001	0.20	1.37	0.17	−0.002	0.002
SBP	0.001	0.001	0.05	0.34	0.73	−0.001	0.001

Legend: RQ, respiratory quotients; HOMA-IR, Homeostasis Model Assessment of Insulin Resistance; SBP, systolic blood pressure.

Furthermore, it is well recognized that despite the substantial research efforts in the last 10–15 years, many individuals unavoidably progress to T2DM [47] thus, longitudinal studies are needed to clarify the eventual role of RQ in predicting the risk of diabetes. Additional studies are also needed to find appropriate intervention (dietetic, pharmacological) to maintain the healthy phenotype by increasing fat oxidation [48].

In this study, some strengths and weaknesses must be pointed out. For some researchers, it is important to consider HOMA-IR to define metabolically healthy obese individuals [49]. However, at present there is a lack of consensus on this definition [50–52]. According to previous investigations, we used the NCEP ATP III criteria to define individual who were "metabolically healthy" [53,54], taking the CVD risk into account [55]. Our study was limited by cross-sectional design, thus, it is impossible to infer causality. Nevertheless, cross-sectional studies indicate associations that may exist and are therefore useful in generating hypotheses for future research. In addition, in our study the statistical analysis is robust and adequate. Our results were not purely random as established by previous investigations [9–16,20–26] and were confirmed by multiple statistical analyses. The investigation was carried out on representative samples of the population which originates from a Mediterranean context, potentially increasing knowledge on this issue from a geographical perspective. Finally, our results are in line with those of other authors who demonstrated the association between metabolic inflexibility, which is independently associated with fasting RQ, and insulin resistance [56]. However, to our knowledge, this is the first time that a difference in fasting RQ has been found between individuals who are metabolically healthy but overweight/obese who have MS and T2DM.

6. Conclusions

We find that fasting fat utilization is significantly lower in individuals who are metabolically healthy overweight/obese than in those who are metabolically unhealthy. These results can help to hypothesize the factors involved in the pathogenesis of T2DM.

Acknowledgments: Acknowledgments: This research did not receive any specific grant from any funding agency in the public, commercial or not-for-profit sector.

Author Contributions: Author Contributions: Tiziana Montalcini, Arturo Pujia and Carmine Gazzaruso were responsible for study design, data analysis, for writing manuscript and approved the final version. Yvelise Ferro and Samantha Maurotti were responsible for enrollment and integrity of data. Elisa Mazza performed instrumental assessment; Stefano Romeo, Cristina Russo and Veronica Lazzaro contributed to interpretation of the data. All authors gave their final approval of the submitted version.

Conflicts of Interest: Conflicts of Interest: The authors declare no conflict of interest.

References

1. Calori, G.; Lattuada, G.; Piemonti, L.; Garancini, M.P.; Ragogna, F.; Villa, M.; Mannino, S.; Crosignani, P.; Bosi, E.; Luzi, L.; *et al.* Prevalence, metabolic features, and prognosis of metabolically healthy obese Italian individuals: The cremona study. *Diabetes Care* **2011**, *34*, 210–215. [CrossRef] [PubMed]
2. Kip, K.E.; Marroquin, O.C.; Kelley, D.E.; Johnson, B.D.; Kelsey, S.F.; Shaw, L.J.; Rogers, W.J.; Reis, S.E. Clinical importance of obesity *versus* the metabolic syndrome in cardiovascular risk in women: A report from the Women's Ischemia Syndrome Evaluation (WISE) study. *Circulation* **2004**, *109*, 706–713. [CrossRef] [PubMed]

3. Stefan, N.; Haring, H.U.; Hu, F.B.; Schulze, M.B. Metabolically healthy obesity: Epidemiology, mechanisms, and clinical implications. *Lancet Diabetes Endocrinol.* **2013**, *1*, 152–162. [CrossRef]

4. Meigs, J.B.; Wilson, P.W.F.; Fox, C.S.; Vasan, R.S.; Nathan, D.M.; Sullivan, L.M.; D'Agostino, R.B. Body mass index, metabolic syndrome, and risk of type 2 diabetes or cardiovascular disease. *J. Clin. Endocrinol. Metab.* **2006**, *91*, 2906–2912. [CrossRef] [PubMed]

5. Appleton, S.L.; Seaborn, C.J.; Visvanathan, R.; Hill, C.L.; Gill, T.K.; Taylor, A.W.; Adams, R.J. North West Adelaide Health Study Team. Diabetes and cardiovascular disease outcomes in the metabolically healthy obese phenotype: A cohort study. *Diabetes Care* **2013**, *36*, 2388–2394. [CrossRef] [PubMed]

6. DeBoer, M.D. Obesity, systemic inflammation, and increased risk for cardiovascular disease and diabetes among adolescents: A need for screening tools to target interventions. *Nutrition* **2013**, *29*, 379–386. [CrossRef] [PubMed]

7. Arner, P. Regional differences in protein production by human adipose tissue. *Biochem. Soc. Trans.* **2001**, *29*, 72–75. [CrossRef] [PubMed]

8. Koves, T.R.; Ussher, J.R.; Noland, R.C.; Slentz, D.; Mosedale, M.; Ilkayeva, O.; Bain, J.; Stevens, R.; Dyck, J.R.; Newgard, C.B.; *et al.* Mitochondrial overload and incomplete fatty acid oxidation contribute to skeletal muscle insulin resistance. *Cell Metab.* **2008**, *7*, 45–56. [CrossRef] [PubMed]

9. Bandyopadhyay, G.K.; Yu, J.G.; Ofrecio, J.; Olefsky, J.M. Increased malonyl-CoA levels in muscle from obese and type 2 diabetic subjects lead to decreased fatty acid oxidation and increased lipogenesis; thiazolidinedione treatment reverses these defects. *Diabetes* **2006**, *55*, 2277–2285. [CrossRef] [PubMed]

10. Kelley, D.E.; Goodpaster, B.; Wing, R.R.; Simoneau, J.A. Skeletal muscle fatty acid metabolism in association with insulin resistance, obesity, and weight loss. *Am. J. Physiol.* **1999**, *277*, E1130–E1141. [PubMed]

11. Blaak, E.E. Basic disturbances in skeletal muscle fatty acid metabolism in obesity and type 2 diabetes mellitus. *Proc. Nutr. Soc.* **2004**, *63*, 323–330. [CrossRef] [PubMed]

12. Toft-Nielsen, M.B.; Damholt, M.B.; Madsbad, S.; Hilsted, L.M.; Hughes, T.E.; Michelsen, B.K.; Holst, J.J. Determinants of the impaired secretion of glucagon-like peptide-1 in type 2 diabetic patients. *J. Clin. Endocrinol. Metab.* **2001**, *86*, 3717–3723. [CrossRef] [PubMed]

13. Vilsbøll, T.; Krarup, T.; Deacon, C.F.; Madsbad, S.; Holst, J.J. Reduced postprandial concentrations of intact biologically active glucagon-like peptide 1 in type 2 diabetic patients. *Diabetes* **2001**, *50*, 609–613. [CrossRef] [PubMed]

14. De León, D.D.; Crutchlow, M.F.; Ham, J.Y.; Stoffers, D.A. Role of glucagon-like peptide-1 in the pathogenesis and treatment of diabetes mellitus. *Int. J. Biochem. Cell Biol.* **2006**, *38*, 845–859. [CrossRef] [PubMed]

15. Pannacciulli, N.; Bunt, J.C.; Koska, J.; Bogardus, C.; Krakoff, J. Higher fasting plasma concentrations of glucagon-like peptide 1 are associated with higher resting energy expenditure and fat oxidation rates in humans. *Am. J. Clin. Nutr.* **2006**, *84*, 556–560. [PubMed]

16. Conarello, S.L.; Li, Z.; Ronan, J.; Roy, R.S.; Zhu, L.; Jiang, G.; Liu, F.; Woods, J.; Zycband, E.; Moller, D.E.; *et al.* Mice lacking dipeptidyl peptidase IV are protected against obesity and insulin resistance. *Proc. Natl. Acad. Sci. USA* **2003**, *100*, 6825–6830. [CrossRef] [PubMed]

17. McNeill, G.; Bruce, A.C.; Ralph, A.; James, W.P. Inter-individual differences in fasting nutrient oxidation and the influence of diet composition. *Int. J. Obes.* **1988**, *12*, 455–463. [PubMed]

18. Schutz, Y. Abnormalities of fuel utilization as predisposing to the development of obesity in humans. *Obes. Res.* **1995**, *3* (Suppl. 2), S173–S178. [CrossRef]

19. Schutz, Y.; Flatt, J.P.; Jéquier, E. Failure of dietary fat intake to promote fat oxidation: A factor favoring the development of obesity. *Am. J. Clin. Nutr.* **1989**, *50*, 307–314. [PubMed]

20. Zurlo, F.; Lillioja, S.; Esposito-Del Puente, A.; Nyomba, B.L.; Raz, I.; Saad, M.F.; Swinburn, B.A.; Knowler, W.C.; Bogardus, C.; Ravussin, E. Low ratio of fat to carbohydrate oxidation as predictor of weight gain: Study of 24-h RQ. *Am. J. Physiol.* **1990**, *259*, E650–E657. [PubMed]

21. Ferro, Y.; Gazzaruso, C.; Coppola, A.; Romeo, S.; Migliaccio, V.; Giustina, A.; Pujia, A.; Montalcini, T. Fat utilization and arterial hypertension in overweight/obese subjects. *J. Transl. Med.* **2013**, *11*, 159. [CrossRef] [PubMed]

22. Lorenz, M.W.; Markus, H.S.; Bots, M.L.; Rosvall, M.; Sitzer, M. Prediction of clinical cardiovascular events with carotid intima-media thickness: A systematic review and meta-analysis. *Circulation* **2007**, *115*, 459–467. [CrossRef] [PubMed]

23. Di Bello, V.; Carerj, S.; Perticone, F.; Benedetto, F.; Palombo, C.; Talini, E.; Giannini, D.; la Carrubba, S.; Antonini-Canterin, F.; di Salvo, G.; *et al.* Carotid intima-media thickness in asymptomatic patients with arterial hypertension without clinical cardiovascular disease: Relation with left ventricular geometry and mass and coexisting risk factors. *Angiology* **2009**, *60*, 705–713. [CrossRef] [PubMed]

24. Montalcini, T.; Gazzaruso, C.; Ferro, Y.; Migliaccio, V.; Rotundo, S.; Castagna, A.; Pujia, A. Metabolic fuel utilization and subclinical atherosclerosis in overweight/obese subjects. *Endocrine* **2013**, *44*, 380–385. [CrossRef] [PubMed]

25. Montalcini, T.; Lamprinoudi, T.; Morrone, A.; Mazza, E.; Gazzaruso, C.; Romeo, S.; Pujia, A. Nutrients utilization in obese individuals with and without hypertriglyceridemia. *Nutrients* **2014**, *21*, 790–798. [CrossRef] [PubMed]

26. Montalcini, T.; Lamprinoudi, T.; Gorgone, G.; Ferro, Y.; Romeo, S.; Pujia, A. Subclinical cardiovascular damage and fat utilization in overweight/obese individuals receiving the same dietary and pharmacological interventions. *Nutrients* **2014**, *6*, 5560–5571. [CrossRef] [PubMed]

27. Centers for Disease Control and Prevention. Tobacco use among adults—United States. *MMWR* **2006**, *55*, 1145–1148.

28. Psaty, B.M.; Furberg, C.D.; Kuller, L.H.; Bild, D.E.; Rautaharju, P.M.; Polak, J.F.; Bovill, E.; Gottdiener, J.S. Traditional risk factors and subclinical disease measures as predictors of first myocardial infarction in older adults: The cardiovascular health study. *Arch. Intern. Med.* **1999**, *59*, 1339–1347. [CrossRef]

29. Expert Panel on Detection, Evaluation, and Treatment of High Blood Cholesterol in Adults. Executive summary of The Third Report of The National Cholesterol Education Program (NCEP) Expert Panel on Detection, Evaluation, and Treatment of High Blood Cholesterol in Adults (Adult Treatment Panel III). *JAMA* **2001**, *285*, 2486–2497.

30. Montalcini, T.; Gorgone, G.; Fava, A.; Romeo, S.; Gazzaruso, C.; Pujia, A. Carotid and brachial arterial enlargement in postmenopausal women with hypertension. *Menopause* **2012**, *9*, 145–149. [CrossRef] [PubMed]

31. Montalcini, T.; Gorgone, G.; Garzaniti, A.; Gazzaruso, C.; Pujia, A. Artery remodelling and abdominal adiposity in nonobese postmenopausal women. *Eur. J. Clin. Nutr.* **2010**, *64*, 1022–1024. [CrossRef] [PubMed]

32. Talluri, T.; Lietdke, R.J.; Evangelisti, A.; Talluri, J.; Maggia, G. Fat-free mass qualitative assessment with bioelectric impedance analysis (BIA). *Ann. N. Y. Acad. Sci.* **1999**, *873*, 94–98. [CrossRef] [PubMed]

33. Zemel, M.B.; Bruckbauer, A. Effects of a leucine and pyridoxine-containing nutraceutical on fat oxidation, and oxidative and inflammatory stress in overweight and obese subjects. *Nutrients* **2012**, *4*, 529–541. [CrossRef] [PubMed]

34. Mazumder, P.K.; O'Neill, B.T.; Roberts, M.W.; Buchanan, J.; Yun, U.J.; Cooksey, R.C.; Boudina, S.; Abel, E.D. Impaired cardiac efficiency and increased fatty acid oxidation in insulin-resistant *ob/ob* mouse hearts. *Diabetes* **2004**, *53*, 2366–2374. [CrossRef] [PubMed]

35. Young, M.E.; Guthrie, P.H.; Razeghi, P.; Leighton, B.; Abbasi, S.; Patil, S.; Youker, K.A.; Taegtmeyer, H. Impaired long-chain fatty acid oxidation and contractile dysfunction in the obese Zucker rat heart. *Diabetes* **2002**, *51*, 2587–2595. [CrossRef] [PubMed]

36. Choi, C.S.; Savage, D.B.; Abu-Elheiga, L.; Liu, Z.X.; Kim, S.; Kulkarni, A.; Distefano, A.; Hwang, Y.J.; Reznick, R.M.; Codella, R.; *et al.* Continuous fat oxidation in acetyl-CoA carboxylase 2 knockout mice increases total energy expenditure, reduces fat mass, and improves insulin sensitivity. *Proc. Natl. Acad. Sci. USA* **2007**, *104*, 16480–16485. [CrossRef] [PubMed]

37. Turner, N.; Bruce, C.R.; Beale, S.M.; Hoehn, K.L.; So, T.; Rolph, M.S.; Cooney, G.J. Excess lipid availability increases mitochondrial fatty acid oxidative capacity in muscle: Evidence against a role for reduced fatty acid oxidation in lipid-induced insulin resistance in rodents. *Diabetes* **2007**, *56*, 2085–2092. [CrossRef] [PubMed]

38. Aasum, E.; Belke, D.D.; Severson, D.L.; Riemersma, R.A.; Cooper, M.; Andreassen, M.; Larsen, T.S. Cardiac function and metabolism in Type 2 diabetic mice after treatment with BM 17.0744, a novel PPAR-alpha activator. *Am. J. Physiol. Heart Circ. Physiol.* **2002**, *283*, H949–H957. [CrossRef] [PubMed]

39. Belke, D.D.; Larsen, T.S.; Gibbs, E.M.; Severson, D.L. Altered metabolism causes cardiac dysfunction in perfused hearts from diabetic (*db/db*) mice. *Am. J. Physiol. Endocrinol. Metab.* **2000**, *279*, E1104–E1113. [PubMed]

40. An, J.; Muoio, D.M.; Shiota, M.; Fujimoto, Y.; Cline, G.W.; Shulman, G.I.; Koves, T.R.; Stevens, R.; Millington, D.; Newgard, C.B. Hepatic expression of malonyl-CoA decarboxylase reverses muscle, liver and whole-animal insulin resistance. *Nat. Med.* **2004**, *10*, 268–274. [CrossRef] [PubMed]

41. Yechoor, V.K.; Patti, M.E.; Saccone, R.; Kahn, C.R. Coordinated patterns of gene expression for substrate and energy metabolism in skeletal muscle of diabetic mice. *Proc. Natl. Acad. Sci. USA* **2002**, *99*, 10587–10592. [CrossRef] [PubMed]

42. Roden, M. Muscle triglycerides and mitochondrial function: Possible mechanisms for the development of type 2 diabetes. *Int. J. Obes. (Lond.)* **2005**, *2* (Suppl. 2), S111–S115. [CrossRef]

43. Ma, Z.A.; Zhao, Z.; Turk, J. Mitochondrial dysfunction and β-cell failure in type 2 diabetes mellitus. *Exp. Diabetes Res.* **2012**, *2012*. [CrossRef] [PubMed]

44. Robitaille, J.; Houde, A.; Lemieux, S.; Pérusse, L.; Gaudet, D. Variants within the muscle and liver isoforms of the carnitine palmitoyltransferase I (CPT$_1$) gene interact with fat intake to modulate indices of obesity in French-Canadians. *J. Mol. Med.* **2007**, *85*, 129–137. [PubMed]

45. Wolfgang, M.J.; Kurama, T.; Dai, Y.; Suwa, A.; Asaumi, M.; Matsumoto, S.I.; Cha, S.H.; Shimokawa, T.; Lane, M.D. The brain-specific carnitine palmitoyltransferase-1c regulates energy homeostasis. *Proc. Natl. Acad. Sci. USA* **2006**, *103*, 7282–7287. [PubMed]

46. Kim, T.; Moore, J.F.; Sharer, J.D.; Yang, K.; Wood, P.A.; Yang, Q. Carnitine Palmitoyltransferase 1b Deficient Mice Develop Severe Insulin Resistance after Prolonged High Fat Diet Feeding. *J. Diabetes Metab.* **2014**, *5*, 1000401. [CrossRef] [PubMed]

47. Bergman, M. Inadequacies of current approaches to prediabetes and diabetes prevention. *Endocrine* **2013**, *44*, 623–633. [PubMed]

48. Den Besten, G.; Bleeker, A.; Gerding, A.; van Eunen, K.; Havinga, R.; van Dijk, T.H.; Oosterveer, M.H.; Jonker, J.W.; Groen, A.K.; Reijngoud, D.J.; *et al.* Short-Chain Fatty Acids Protect against High-Fat Diet-Induced Obesity via a PPARγ-Dependent Switch from Lipogenesis to Fat Oxidation. *Diabetes* **2015**, *64*, 2398–2408. [CrossRef] [PubMed]

49. Hinnouho, G.M.; Czernichow, S.; Dugravot, A.; Batty, G.D.; Kivimaki, M.; Singh-Manoux, A. Metabolically healthy obesity and risk of mortality: Does the definition of metabolic health matter? *Diabetes Care* **2013**, *36*, 2294–2300. [PubMed]

50. Rey-López, J.P.; de Rezende, L.F.; Pastor-Valero, M.; Tess, B.H. The prevalence of metabolically healthy obesity: A systematic review and critical evaluation of the definitions used. *Obes. Rev.* **2014**, *15*, 781–790. [CrossRef] [PubMed]

51. Phillips, C.M. Metabolically healthy obesity: Definitions, determinants and clinical implications. *Rev. Endocr. Metab. Disord.* **2013**, *14*, 219–227. [PubMed]

52. Blüher, M. Are there still healthy obese patients? *Curr. Opin. Endocrinol. Diabetes Obes.* **2012**, *19*, 341–346. [CrossRef] [PubMed]

53. Katzmarzyk, P.T.; Church, T.S.; Janssen, I.; Ross, R.; Blair, S.N. Metabolic syndrome, obesity, and mortality: Impact of cardiorespiratory fitness. *Diabetes Care* **2005**, *28*, 391–397. [CrossRef] [PubMed]

54. Voulgari, C.; Tentolouris, N.; Dilaveris, P.; Tousoulis, D.; Katsilambros, N.; Stefanadis, C. Increased heart failure risk in normal-weight people with metabolic syndrome compared with metabolically healthy obese individuals. *J. Am. Coll. Cardiol.* **2011**, *58*, 1343–1350. [CrossRef] [PubMed]

55. Song, Y.; Manson, J.E.; Meigs, J.B.; Ridker, P.M.; Buring, J.E.; Liu, S. Comparison of usefulness of body mass index *versus* metabolic risk factors in predicting 10-year risk of cardiovascular events in women. *Am. J. Cardiol.* **2007**, *100*, 1654–1658. [CrossRef] [PubMed]

56. Di Sarra, D.; Tosi, F.; Bonin, C.; Fiers, T.; Kaufman, J.M.; Signori, C.; Zambotti, F.; Dall'Alda, M.; Caruso, B.; Zanolin, M.E.; *et al.* Metabolic inflexibility is a feature of women with polycystic ovary syndrome and is associated with both insulin resistance and hyperandrogenism. *J. Clin. Endocrinol. Metab.* **2013**, *98*, 2581–2588. [CrossRef] [PubMed]

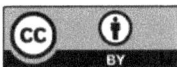

© 2016 by the authors. Licensee MDPI, Basel, Switzerland. This article is an open access article distributed under the terms and conditions of the Creative Commons Attribution (CC BY) license (http://creativecommons.org/licenses/by/4.0/).

nutrients

Article

Profile of Free Fatty Acids and Fractions of Phospholipids, Cholesterol Esters and Triglycerides in Serum of Obese Youth with and without Metabolic Syndrome

Juliana Bermúdez-Cardona and Claudia Velásquez-Rodríguez *

Research Group in Food and Human Nutrition, Universidad de Antioquia (UdeA),
Calle 70 No. 52-21 Medellín 050010238, Colombia; juliana.bermudez@udea.edu.co
* Correspondence: claudia.velasquez@udea.edu.co; Tel.: +057-4-219-6497

Received: 11 November 2015; Accepted: 11 January 2016; Published: 15 February 2016

Abstract: The study evaluated the profile of circulating fatty acids (FA) in obese youth with and without metabolic syndrome (MetS) to determine its association with nutritional status, lifestyle and metabolic variables. A cross-sectional study was conducted in 96 young people, divided into three groups: obese with MetS (OBMS), obese (OB) and appropriate weight (AW). FA profiles were quantified by gas chromatography; waist circumference (WC), fat folds, lipid profile, high-sensitivity C-reactive protein, glucose, insulin, the homeostasis model assessment (HOMA index), food intake and physical activity (PA) were assessed. The OBMS group had significantly greater total free fatty acids (FFAs), palmitic-16:0 in triglyceride (TG), palmitoleic-16:1n-7 in TG and phospholipid (PL); in the OB group, these FAs were higher than in the AW group. Dihomo-gamma-linolenic (DHGL-20:3n-6) was higher in the OBMS than the AW in PL and FFAs. Linoleic-18:2n-6 in TG and PL had the lowest proportion in the OBMS group. WC, PA, total FFA, linoleic-18:2n-6 in TG and DHGL-20:3n-6 in FFAs explained 62% of the HOMA value. The OB group presented some higher proportions of FA and biochemical values than the AW group. The OBMS had proportions of some FA in the TG, PL and FFA fractions that correlated with disturbances of MetS.

Keywords: obesity; metabolic syndrome; fatty acids; serum; youth

1. Introduction

Obesity is a pandemic that affects 34.3% of the adult population, generating an increase in the prevalence of chronic diseases [1]. Obesity is also present in youth; in 2013, the prevalence of overweight reached 22.6% in girls and 23.9% in boys in industrialized countries [2]. In Latin America, it is estimated that there are between 16.5 and 22.1 million obese adolescents, with a prevalence of overweight of 17% in Colombia, 20% in Brazil, and 35% in Mexico and Chile [3].

Obesity, mainly abdominal, induces metabolic disturbances, such as insulin resistance (IR), glucose intolerance, decreased high-density lipoproteins (HDL-C), elevated triglycerides (TG) and increased blood pressure, which together make up Metabolic Syndrome (MetS) [4].

In states of chronic excess energy, both subcutaneous and visceral adipocytes undergo hypertrophy and saturation of their storage capacity, along with infiltration and activation of macrophages; these events result in an increased release of fatty acids (FAs) and pro-inflammatory substances, such as tumor necrosis factor (TNF)α and interleukin (IL)-6, which generates tissue dysfunction and metabolic damage [5,6].

The release of pro-inflammatory substances and free FAs (FFAs) could be the connection between central obesity and metabolic disturbances. Once released into the portal circulation, FAs invade organs, such as the liver, where the excessive deposit of triglycerides affects lipoprotein synthesis and may induce simple steatosis or fatty liver (FL), which may be complicated by liver inflammation (non-alcoholic steatohepatitis, NASH), alterations that induce the development of non-alcoholic fatty liver disease (NAFLD), which is widely considered to be the liver expression of metabolic syndrome [7,8]. The FFAs also affect the pancreas where they impair insulin production (lipotoxicity); in addition, they simultaneously generate IR in muscle and adipose tissue through the activation of pathways such as protein kinase C (PKCθ) [6,9].

The FA profile can be modulated with food, as some FAs, such as linoleic-18:2n-6 and αlinolenic-18:3n-3, are not synthesized by humans and reflect dietary intake. Thus, circulating FA levels and cell membrane compositions depend on this intake. In serum, the FA profile specifically reflects the intake of the last two to six weeks, and tissue FAs represent the dietary patterns of months or years [10]. Blood levels of FAs, such as palmitoleic-16:1n-7 and DHGL-20:3n-6, are less dependent on intake and could reflect endogenous metabolism (lipogenesis) [11,12].

Research in adults has demonstrated the relationship between an altered FA profile, obesity, IR and MetS [13,14]. This profile is characterized by high percentages of saturated fatty acids (SFAs), such as palmitic-16:0 and stearic-18:0, and monounsaturated FAs (MUFAs), such as palmitoleic-16:1n-7, and decreased percentages of polyunsaturated fatty acids (PUFAs), including arachidonic acid (ARA-20:4n-6) and docosahexaenoic acid (DHA-22:6n-3) [14,15].

In obese individuals, a decrease in PUFAs may be due to a deficit in the synthesis and elongation of essential FAs, caused by metabolic disturbances arising from obesity, such as hyperinsulinemia; a high SFA intake and a low PUFA intake, especially omega-3 [16]. However, the FA profile in adults is affected by intervening variables, such as atheromatous disease, advanced metabolic disorders and long-term exposure to unfavorable lifestyle factors (*i.e.*, a sedentary lifestyle, overeating, and alcohol and tobacco consumption) [17].

In youth, describing the circulating FA profile could contribute to a better understanding of the obesity-IR-MetS relationship, given that confounding factors are less involved in metabolic analyses at early ages. However, the results in youth are also conflicting, possibly because fractions from which circulating FAs are recovered are different and not comparable among studies. Some obtain FA from cholesterol esters (CE) and others from phospholipids (PL), fractions in which FAs are mainly recovered from HDL-C and low-density lipoprotein (LDL-C), respectively, which are influenced by consumption [18]. Other studies recover FAs from TG, which is the fraction of highest proportion in circulation and mainly reflects endogenous synthesis of FAs produced from energetic nutrients (carbohydrates and fats) that travel in very-low-density lipoproteins (VLDL) [19]. Finally, others report FFAs released from adipose tissue and carried by albumin, which could be an indirect marker of the FA composition of adipose tissue in states of obesity if recovered after a 10- to 12-h fast [18,20]. Given the differences between fractions and modulations of the FA profile by diet, comparisons of results and the establishment of a consensus on FA profiles are complex. Therefore, the objective of this study is to evaluate the profile of circulating FAs in obese youth with and without MetS between 10 and 18 years old and to determine its association with nutritional status, lifestyle and components of MetS.

2. Materials and Methods

Study design: A cross-sectional study was developed that included 96 youth, boys and girls, 10 to 18 years old, selected from a previous population study [21].

The sample size necessary to form three groups was defined with the software Primer®, considering an alpha error of 0.05, a power of 85% and an expected minimum difference between the case and control groups in the concentrations of different FAs according to reports from other studies: Palmitic-16:0 in CE [22] and FFAs [23]; Palmitoleic-16:1n-7 in PL, CE and TG [22,24]; Stearic-18:0 in PL [22] and FFAs [23]; and DHGL-20:3n-6 in PL [24,25] and CE [22], which indicated a number of 32 youth per group.

The groups were formed as follows: (1) obese with MetS (OBMS): body mass index (BMI) >98 percentile [26] and diagnosis of MetS; (2) obese (OB): BMI >98 percentile and without MetS; and (3) appropriate weight (AW): BMI between the 15–85 percentile and none of the components of MetS. Groups were matched one to one by age, gender, pubertal maturation and socioeconomic stratum.

MetS was diagnosed when the affected youth had three or more of the following criteria: TG $\geqslant$110 mg/dL, HDL-C $\leqslant$40 mg/dL, fasting blood glucose $\geqslant$100 mg/dL, blood pressure $\geqslant$90 percentile and waist circumference (WC) $\geqslant$90 percentile [27].

Youth who consumed drugs for metabolic disturbances of MetS or nutritional supplements, who had diabetes mellitus (DM) II, who were elite athletes or who were pregnant or lactating were excluded from the study.

Anthropometric evaluation: weight and height were measured; BMI was calculated (kg/m^2) and was classified according to the 2007 World Health Organization (WHO) standard [26]; fat fold measurements were taken at the triceps and subscapular areas, % of body fat was calculated and classified according to Lohman [28]; and WC was taken and classified according to Fernández [29]. Measurements were performed with equipment and techniques for international use [28].

Food consumption: The 24-h recall was distributed on different weekdays. A second recall was consequently distributed among a random subsample constituted by 20% of the study population (19 adolescents) to calculate intra-individual variation [30,31]. The Evaluation Program of Dietary Intake (EVINDI-v4) was used [32]. The nutrient report was processed using the PC version of the Software for Intake Distribution Estimation (SIDE) program, Iowa State University, version 1.0, June 2004.

Physical activity (PA): The 3-day Physical Activity Recall (3DPAR) method was applied [33]. Metabolic equivalent (METs) values of each activity were obtained from the Compendium of Physical Activities of the American College of Sports Medicine [34]. The PA of 3–6 METs was classified as moderate to vigorous intensity (MVPA), and vigorous PA (VPA) was classified as >6 METs [35].

Time dedicated to watching television and playing video games: The reported times were converted into hours/day and were classified into two categories: less than three hours and three or more hours per day [36].

Clinical and biochemical tests: Pubertal maturation was evaluated and classified by self-report according to Tanner's methodology [37,38].

Blood pressure was taken with a mercury sphygmomanometer (Riester®) and was classified according to Fourth Task Force methodology [39].

An antecubital venous blood sample was taken following a 10- to 12-h fast, and serum was obtained and stored at -80 °C. Total cholesterol (TC), HDL-C, LDL-C and TG were determined by spectrophotometry in an RA-50 photocolorimeter (Bayer, series 71663, Dublin, Ireland) using specific enzymatic colorimetric kits (BioSystems Reagents and Instruments, Barcelona, Spain). Blood glucose and insulin were determined by micro-particle enzyme immunoassay (MEIA) [40]. IR was estimated by the mathematical model of the HOMA (Homeostasis Model Assessment) index using the HOMA Calculator Version 2.2.2 software, copyrighted by the Diabetes Trials Unit of the University of Oxford. IR was defined as a HOMA $\geqslant$3.1, based on three criteria: 3.1 was the HOMA in the 95 percentile in the population under study [21], 3.1 was the cutoff point established by others authors [41,42]. hsCRP was determined by immunoturbidimetry and was classified as low cardiovascular risk <1 mg/L, average risk 1-3 mg/L and high risk >3 mg/L [43].

Profile of circulating FFAs: Lipid extraction from serum was performed according to the Folch method [44]. For separation of CE, TG and PL fractions, the methodology by solid-phase extraction (SPE) of Agren J [45] and Kaluzny M [46] was used. To the dry extract of each fraction, hexane and boron trifluoride (BF$_3$) in 20% methanol were added, and the mixture was heated between 80 °C and 90 °C for one hour. [47]. Chromatographic analysis was performed in an Agilent 6890N gas chromatograph with a flame ionization detector (FID), TR-CN100 column, 60 m $\times$ 0.25 mm $\times$ 0.2 µm ID, oven temperature program beginning at 90 °C $\times$ 7 min, increased at a rate of 5 °C/min to 240 °C for

15 min, detector temperature of 300 °C, and He carrier gas at a flow of 1.1 mL/min. FA identification was performed by comparisons of retention times with the standard FAME Mix of 37 components (Supelco, Bellefonte, PA). The results are presented as relative amounts of each FA.

Total concentrations of SFA, MUFA and PUFA were calculated from the sum of each FA from 14 to 22 carbons of each family, in each fraction. The product/precursor ratios were calculated as an indirect indicator of the activity of the desaturase enzymes. These ratios were as follows: stearoyl CoA desaturase = Palmitoleic-16:$1n$-7/Palmitic-16:0 and Oleic-18:$1n$-9/Stearic-18:0, delta-5 desaturase = ARA-20:$4n$-6/DHGL-20:$3n$-6 and delta-6 desaturase = DHGL-20:$3n$-6/Linoleic-18:$2n$-6, as previously reported [10,13,48].

Ethical management: The investigation was classified as having a minimum risk according to the Colombian Ministry of Health, Resolution 008439, Article 11 of October 1993. The study was approved by the University of Antioquia Bioethics Committee. Informed consent was signed by the youth and their parents and included the Helsinki declaration.

Statistical analysis: Normality was established with the Shapiro-Wilk test. The difference among groups was performed by analysis of variance (ANOVA) or Kruskall-Wallis. For comparisons between two groups, Scheffe or Mann-Whitney U tests were performed. Qualitative variables were expressed with frequencies; quantitative variables, with means and standard deviations or medians and interquartile ranges. For associations of qualitative variables Chi^2 and Odds Ratium were used, while Pearson *R* or Spearman *Rho* were used for quantitative variables. A stepwise multiple linear regression model was applied to explain the HOMA (dependent variable in logarithmic units) with WC, average METs, linoleic-18:$2n$-6 in TG, DHGL-20:$3n$-6 in FFAs and total FFAs as independent variables; the model was adjusted by food intake variables: daily intake of calories, simple carbohydrates, saturated fat, monounsaturated fat and polyunsaturated fat. R^2 and ANOVA determined the fit of the model, and fulfillment of assumptions (Durbin Watson, normality of residuals, inflation factor of the variance and independence) was checked. Finally, the β values of the crude and the adjusted model were transformed with antilogarithm to express in units of the dependent variable: HOMA, in Table 5. A $p < 0.05$ was considered significant. Statistical analysis was performed using the program Statistical Package for the Social Sciences (SPSS®) V 21.0.

3. Results

Matched variables between groups did not show significant differences (Table 1).

Table 1. Matched characteristics of the study groups.

		OBMS $n = 32$	OB $n = 32$	AW $n = 32$	p *,†
Age (Me, IQR)		13.9 (4.8)	14.2 (4.1)	14.0 (4.2)	0.93 *
Gender (%)	Boys	56.3	56.3	56.3	1.00 †
	Girls	43.8	43.8	43.8	
Pubertal Maturation (%)	Prepubescent	12.5	12.5	12.5	0.99 †
	Pubescent	25.0	21.9	25.0	
	Post-pubescent	62.5	65.6	62.5	
Socioeconomic Stratum (%)	Low	53.1	53.1	50.0	0.84 †
	Medium	37.5	31.3	38.5	
	High	9.4	15.6	11.5	

OBMS: obesity with metabolic syndrome; OB: obesity; AW: Appropriate weight; Me: medians; IQR: interquartile ranges; * Kruskal Wallis; † Pearson Chi squared.

Both obese groups showed similar behaviors for fat percentage and inflammation. The risk of mild chronic inflammation (high-sensitivity C-reactive protein (hsCRP > 1 mg/dL)) in obese youth was 2.6 times greater than in the appropriate weight (AW) group (odds ratio 2.6; confidence interval 1.27–5.54; $p = 0.001$), only this risk was significant; hsCRP correlated with fat percentage ($r = 0.51$

$p = 0.001$). The obese with MetS (OBMS) group had higher BMI, WC, blood glucose, insulin, HOMA and TG and lower HDL-C compared to the other two groups ($p = 0.001$). A total of 97.3% of the OBMS group simultaneously had high TG and low HDL-C, according to the criteria used in the diagnosis of MetS in this study. Of the OBMS, 53.1% simultaneously had high WC and HOMA; both variables were correlated ($Rho = 0.71$; $p < 0.001$) (Table 2).

Table 2. Anthropometric, biochemical, food intake and physical activity variables of the study groups [1].

	OBMS n = 32	OB n = 32	AW n = 32	p [*,†]
Anthropometric				
BMI kg/m^2	31.1 ± 5.0 [a, 2]	27.1 ± 2.9 [b]	20.2 ± 2.3 [c]	<0.001 [*]
Waist circumference cm	91.2 ± 10.9 [a]	80.5 ± 5.6 [b]	67.6 ± 5.4 [c]	<0.001 [*]
Subscapular fold mm	29.9 ± 10.9 [a]	25.5 ± 8.1 [a]	11.5 ± 3.5 [b]	<0.001 [*]
Triceps fold mm	25.2 ± 6.7 [a]	23.6 ± 6.2 [a]	12.9 ± 4.1 [b]	<0.001 [*]
% fat	38.1 (18.7) [a]	34.7 (15.8) [a]	22.2 (14.2) [b]	<0.001 [†]
Biochemical				
Blood glucose mg/dL	90.3 ± 8.2 [a]	83.7 ± 7.5 [b]	83.3 ± 6.9 [b]	<0.001 [*]
Insulin mU/L	25.7 (12.4) [a]	11.5 (7.8) [b]	7.1(4.1) [c]	<0.001 [†]
HOMA	3.2 (1.7) [a]	1.5 (1.0) [b]	0.9(0.5) [c]	<0.001 [†]
Cholesterol (mg/dL)	192.6 ± 50.3 [a]	172.3 ± 34.5	162.1 ± 27.9 [b]	<0.001 [*]
Triglycerides (mg/dL)	162 (94) [a]	92 (37) [b]	71 (32) [c]	<0.001 [†]
HDL-C (mg/dL)	38 (6) [a]	45 (15) [b]	54 (15) [c]	<0.001 [†]
LDL-C (mg/dL)	99 (61) [a]	88 (37) [a]	79 (31) [b]	<0.001 [†]
hsCRP (mg/dL)	1.7 (2.9) [a]	0.9 (2.5) [a]	0.4 (0.7) [b]	<0.001 [†]
Nutrient consumption/day				
Kilocalories	2238 (436) [a]	2007 (264) [a]	2442 (229) [b]	<0.001 [†]
Total fat (g)	79.5 (14.6) [a]	70.3 (12.5) [b]	96.9 (44.0) [c]	<0.001 [†]
Saturated fat (g)	31.3 (9.2)	28.5 (8.3) [a]	36.4 (20.1) [b]	0.015 [†]
Monounsaturated fat (g)	26.7 (5.1) [a]	25.5 (3.5) [a]	30.0 (1.7) [b]	<0.001 [†]
Polyunsaturated fat (g)	16.3 (1.6) [a]	15.4 (1.5) [b]	15.7 (1.8) [c]	0.004 [†]
Total carbohydrates (g)	294 (50) [a]	276 (57) [a]	329 (36) [b]	<0.001 [†]
Complex carbohydrates (g)	232 (58) [a]	222 (51) [a]	263 (28) [b]	<0.001 [†]
Fiber (g)	14 ± 2 [a]	14 ± 3 [a]	16 ± 1 [b]	0.001 [*]
Physical activity				
METs/day	61.5 (15.4)	61.1 (10.0)	62.8 (14.7)	0.88 [†]
MVPA Blocks	1.3 (3.60)	1.3 (2.3)	1.0 (2.5)	0.317 [†]
VPA Blocks	0.1 (1.0)	0.3 (1.0)	0.0 (1.3)	0.991 [†]
Hours of TV/day	3.6 ± 1.7	3.8 ± 2.7	3.3 ± 3.1	0.57 [*]

OBMS: obesity with metabolic syndrome; OB: obesity; AW: Appropriate weight; BMI: Body Mass Index; HOMA: Homeostasis Model Assessment; HDL-C: high-density lipoprotein; LDL-C: low-density lipoprotein; hsCRP: high-sensitivity C-reactive protein; MET: Metabolic equivalent; MVPA: moderate to vigorous physical activity; VPA: vigorous physical activity; [1] Averages ± standard deviations and medians (interquartile ranges); [2] Different letters between lines show significant differences between groups; [*] ANOVA with Scheffé or [†] Kruskal-Wallis with Mann–Whitney U post-test.

In the TG fraction, the OBMS group has a significantly higher proportion of SFAs compared to the other groups ($p = 0.001$); additionally, the OB group had a higher proportion of SFAs compared to the AW ($p = 0.028$). Total MUFAs was significantly greater in the OBMS group compared to the AW group ($p = 0.003$). The proportion of palmitoleic-16:1n-9 for OBMS and OB was higher than AW ($p = 0.009$). Of the total PUFAs represented in this case by linoleic-18:2n-6, the OBMS group had the lowest proportion among the three groups ($p = 0.001$), followed by the OB group, with the highest being AW ($p = 0.042$) (Table 3). In this fraction, palmitic-16:0 correlated directly with the HOMA ($Rho = 0.55$ $p = 0.001$) and serum TG ($Rho = 0.66$ $p = 0.001$) and inversely with HDL-C ($Rho = -0.52$ $p = 0.001$). Linoleic-18:2n-6 was correlated inversely with the HOMA (*Rho* = −0.56 *p* = 0.001) and serum TG (*Rho* = −0.70 *p* = 0.001) and directly with HDL-C (*Rho* = 0.49 *p* = 0.001) (Table S1).

Table 3. Major fatty acids in lipid fractions of youth according to the study groups [1].

FA (% Total FA)	OBMS n = 32	OB n = 32	AW n = 32	p [*,†]
Triglycerides				
SFA sum	38.3 (7.1) [a, 2]	34.6 (8.9) [b]	30.8 (7.6) [c]	<0.001 [†]
Palmitic-16:0	29.7 ± 4.0 [a]	26.4 ± 3.7 [b]	23.6 ± 3.3 [c]	<0.001 [*]
Stearic-18:0	6.2 (3.8)	7.4 (4.1)	7.2 (3.8)	0.42 [†]
MUFA sum	36.1 ± 5.2 [a]	33.5 ± 5.0	31.7 ± 5.0 [b]	0.003 [*]
Palmitoleic-16:1n-7 [3]	4.5 (2.0) [a]	4.1 (1.4) [a]	3.0 (1.6) [b]	0.009 [†]
Oleic-18:1n-9	32.1 ± 4.3	30.7 ± 3.9	30.1 ± 4.3	0.14 [*]
PUFA sum	-	-	-	-
Linoleic-18:2n-6	25.6 ± 5.8 [a]	32.2 ± 6.3 [b]	36.4 ± 7.5 [c]	<0.001 [†]
Phospholipids				
SFA sum	52.8 (11.3) [a]	54.1 (11.3)	56.4 (5.9) [b]	0.017 [†]
Palmitic-16:0	30.6 ± 3.4 [a]	31.7 ± 3.0	33.2 ± 3.0 [b]	0.006 [*]
Stearic-18:0	19.8 (4.9)	20.1 (6.0)	21.2 (2.1)	0.34 [†]
Behenic-22:0	0.5 (0.2) [a]	0.6 (0.2) [b,c]	0.8 (0.2) [b,c]	0.015 [†]
MUFA sum	17.5 (7.3) [a]	15.1 (8.3) [b,c]	13.8 (3.5) [b,c]	<0.001 [†]
Palmitoleic-16:1n-7 [4]	0.9 (0.4) [a]	0.8 (0.2) [b]	0.5 (0.2) [c]	<0.001 [†]
Oleic-18:1n-9	16.7 (7.3) [a]	14.1 (8.1) [b,c]	13.5 (3.4) [b,c]	<0.001 [†]
PUFA sum	30.0 (4.8)	31.1 (3.8)	29.9 (4.1)	0.74 [†]
Linoleic-18:2n-6	18.0 ± 2.2 [a]	19.2 ± 2.6 [a]	21.0 ± 2.8 [b]	<0.001 [*]
DHGL-20:3n-6	2.8 ± 0.7 [a]	2.5 ± 0.4	2.1 ± 0.5 [b]	<0.001 [*]
Eicosatrienoic-20:3n-3 [5]	8.2 ± 2.2	7.7 ± 2.0	5.6 ± 2.7	0.063 [*]
Arachidonic-20:4n6	5.0 (1.2)	5.3 (1.5)	4.8 (2.3)	0.77 [*]
Cholesterol Esters				
SFA sum	35.7 (15.5)	35.1 (16.0)	35.7 (13.2)	0.92 [†]
Palmitic-16:0	33.2 ± 7.7	31.0 ± 7.1	31.2 ± 5.2	0.35 [*]
Stearic-18:0 [6]	10.4 (12.1)	11.3 (7.0)	12.3 (9.3)	0.96 [†]
MUFA sum	-	-	-	-
Oleic-18:1n-9	28.4 (4.1)	26.3 (8.2)	26.2 (5.7)	0.44 [†]
PUFA sum	-	-	-	-
Linoleic-18:2n-6	35.9 ± 9.5	34.5 ± 10.7	35.2 ± 10.4	0.84 [*]
Free Fatty Acids				
SFA sum	44.7 (4.1)	46.1 (6.4)	43.2 (6.7)	0.59 [†]
Myristic-14:0	1.1 (0.2)	1.4 (0.1)	1.1 (0.5)	0.47 [*]
Palmitic-16:0	30.0 (2.4)	30.0 (3.7)	30.8 (4.5)	0.93 [†]
Stearic-18:0	14.4 (2.2)	15.4 (2.7)	14.5 (3.4)	0.45 [†]
MUFA sum	20.9 (4.1)	19.1 (4.6)	19.1 (5.6)	0.22 [†]
Palmitoleic-16:1n-7 [7]	1.7 (0.7)	1.7 (0.5)	1.5 (0.6)	0.46 [†]
Oleic-18:1n-9	19.3 (4.0)	17.9 (3.3)	18.4 (3.4)	0.31 [†]
PUFA sum	33.5 (3.4)	34.0 (4.1)	34.4 (4.9)	0.68 [†]
Linoleic-18:2n-6	21.7 (3.3)	22.6 (3.3)	24.5 (5.3)	0.14 [†]
DHGL-20:3n-6	3.0 ± 0.6 [a]	2.8 ± 0.6	2.4 ± 2.5 [b]	<0.001 [*]
Arachidonic-20:4n6	6.6 (1.1)	6.5 (3.1)	5.8 (2.0)	0.25 [†]
DHA-22:6n-3	1.9 ± 0.4	1.9 ± 0.5	1.8 ± 0.5	0.51 [*]
Total FFA (mg/dL)	199.5 (40.0) [a]	100.8 (24.1) [b]	98.8 (29.9) [b]	0.014 [†]

OBMS: obesity with metabolic syndrome; OB: obesity; AW: Appropriate weight; SFA: saturated fatty acid; MUFA: monounsaturated fatty acid; PUFA: polyunsaturated fatty acid; FFA: free fatty acid; DHGL: Dihomo-gamma-linolenic; DHA: docosahexaenoic acid; * ANOVA; [†] Kruskal-Wallis test; [1] Data expressed as Averages±standard deviations or medians (interquartile ranges); [2] Different letters between lines show significant differences between groups, according to the Scheffé post-test for parametric variables or the Mann–Whitney U test for nonparametric variables; [3] OBMS *n* = 28, OB *n* = 20, AW *n* = 16; [4] OBMS *n* = 28 OB *n* = 25, AW *n* = 8; [5] OBMS *n* = 15, OB *n* = 13, AW *n* = 6; [6] OBMS *n* = 15, OB *n* = 13, AW *n* = 6; [7] OBMS *n* = 27, OB *n* = 19; AW *n* = 8.

In the PL fraction, total SFAs were present in significantly lower amounts in the OBMS group compared to the AW group. The OBMS group had higher total MUFAs compared to the other two groups ($p = 0.001$), with no difference between the OB and AW groups ($p = 0.05$). In particular, palmitoleic-16:1n-7 was higher in OBMS compared to the other two groups ($p = 0.001$), and time was higher in OB than AW ($p = 0.004$). With respect to linoleic-18:2n-6, a significantly lower proportion was found in the OBMS and the OB group compared to the AW group ($p = 0.001$, $p = 0.021$, respectively). DHGL-20:3n-6 had a significantly higher proportion in the OBMS group compared to the AW group ($p = 0.001$), with no differences between OB and AW ($p = 0.079$) (Table 3). In the PL fraction, palmitoleic-16:1n-7 was directly associated with serum TG ($Rho = 0.54$ $p = 0.001$) and inversely associated with HDL-C ($Rho = -0.43$ $p = 0.001$). DHGL-20:3n-6 correlated directly with the HOMA ($Rho = 0.36$ $p = 0.000$) and serum TG ($Rho = 0.33$ $p = 0.001$), while linoleic-18:2n-6 correlated inversely with the HOMA ($Rho = -0.31$ $p = 0.002$) and serum TG ($Rho = -0.29$ $p = 0.004$) and directly with HDL-C ($Rho = 0.30$ $p = 0.003$) (Table S1).

In the FFA fraction, total circulating FFAs were significantly greater in the OBMS group, with double the concentration compared to the other groups ($p = 0.014$). The OB group had the same concentration of total FFAs as the AW group (Table 3). Among PUFAs, DHGL-20:3n-6 was significantly higher in the OBMS group than in the AW group ($p = 0.001$); with no differences between OB and AW. The DHGL-20:3n-6/linoleic-18:2n-6 ratio was significantly greater in the OBMS and OB groups compared to the AW group ($p = 0.001$) (Table 4). DHGL-20:3n-6 correlated directly with the HOMA ($Rho = 0.36$ $p = 0.001$) and TG ($Rho = 0.33$ $p = 0.001$) (Table S1).

Table 4. Ratios of fatty acids in lipid fractions of youth according to the study groups [1].

Ratio of Fatty Acids	OBSM $n = 32$	OB $n = 32$	AW $n = 32$	p [*,†]
Triglycerides				
16:1/16:0 [3]	0.1 (0.1) [a, 2]	0.1 (0.2)	0.1 (0.1) [b]	0.005 [†]
18:1/18:0	5.1 ± 1.9	4.4 ± 1.9	4.4 ± 1.8	0.30 [†]
Phospholipids				
16:1n-7/16:0 [4]	0.03 (0.01) [a]	0.02 (0.01) [b]	0.01 (0.01) [c]	<0.001 [†]
18:1n-9/18:0	0.8 (0.7) [a]	0.7 (0.7)	0.6 (0.2) [b]	<0.001 [†]
20:3n-6/18:2n-6	0.2 (0.1) [a]	0.1 (0.0) [b]	0.1 (0.0) [c]	<0.001 [†]
20:4n6/20:3n6	1.9 (0.7)	2.0 (1.2)	2.3 (1.4)	0,059 [†]
Cholesterol Esters				
18:1n-9/18:0 [5]	2.3 (2.6)	2.4 (1.7)	2.1 (1.6)	0.94 [*]
Free Fatty Acids				
16:1/16:0 [6]	0.5 (0.0)	0.6 (0.0)	0.5 (0.0)	0.57 [†]
18:1n-9/18:0	1.3 (0.4)	1.2 (0.4)	1.3 (0.4)	0.47 [†]
20:3n-6/18:2n-6	0.1 ± 0.0 [a]	0.1 ± 0.0 [a]	0.1 ± 0.0 [b]	<0.001 [*]
20:4n6/20:3n6	2.2 (0.8)	2.3 (0.8)	2.5 (1.5)	0.22 [†]

OBMS: obesity with metabolic syndrome; OB: obesity; AW: Appropriate weight; * ANOVA; [†] Kruskal-Wallis test; [1] Data expressed as Averages±standard deviations, medians (interquartile ranges); [2] Different letters between lines show significant differences between groups, according to the Scheffé post-test for parametric variables or the Mann–Whitney U test for nonparametric variables; [3] OBMS $n = 28$, OB $n = 20$, AW $n = 16$; [4] OBMS $n = 28$, OB $n = 25$, AW $n = 18$; [5] OBMS $n = 15$, OB $n = 13$, AW $n = 6$; [6] OBMS $n = 27$, OB $n = 19$, AW $n = 8$.

A descriptive multivariate analysis of the HOMA revealed that WC increased the average HOMA by 1.025, total FFAs increased average HOMA by 1.004, and each unit of DHGL-20:3n-6 in FFAs increased the average HOMA by 1.258, while physical activity (METs) and linoleic-18:2n-6 in TG decreased average HOMA by -1.018 and -1.016, respectively. The independent variables explained 62% of the behavior of the HOMA. All relationships observed were significant and remained the same after making adjustments for food consumption variables (Table 5).

Table 5. Multiple linear regression model with explanatory variables of the HOMA index.

Variables	β *	β †	IC †	p †	IFV †
Waist circumference	1.025	1.025	0.008; 0.015	0.000	1.543
Average METs/d	−1.018	−1.018	−0.012; −0.003	0.001	1.278
Linoleic-18:2n-6 in TG	−1.016	−1.016	−0.013; −0.001	0.024	1.606
DHGL-20:3n-6 in FFA	1.276	1.258	0.028; 0.172	0.007	1.767
Total FFA in mg/dL	1.004	1.004	0.000; 0.003	0.028	1.379

HOMA: The Homeostatic model assessment.* Raw model: R^2: 0.637, ANOVA: $p = 0.0001$, Normality: $p = 0.200$, Colinearity: Inflation factor of the variance (IFV) <5, Durbin Watson: 0.930. Values expressed in HOMA units. † Adjusted for total calories, saturated fat, monounsaturated fat, polyunsaturated fat and simple carbohydrates. Values expressed in HOMA units. Adjusted model: R^2: 0.620, ANOVA: 0.0001, Normality: $p = 0.050$, Colinearity: IFV < 5, Durbin Watson: 0.987.

4. Discussion

This study detected proportions of some FA for youth with OBMS in the TG, PL and FFA fractions that correlated with disturbances of MetS.

In OBMS the TG fraction showed significantly higher concentrations of total SFAs and MUFAs, but a lower concentration of PUFAs. This pattern could be due to accelerated hepatic lipogenesis that results in the incorporation of FAs, such as palmitic-16:0, palmitoleic-16:1n-7 and oleic-18:1n-9 in VLDL, with a simultaneous decrease in the amount of linoleic-18:2n-6 [19].

This study, consistent with that detected previously by others, found high proportions of MUFAs in the OBMS and OB groups [23,24,49]. Palmitoleic-16:1n-7 was directly and significantly associated with serum TG. The palmitoleic-16:1n-7/palmitic-16:0 and oleic-18:1n-9/stearic-18:0 ratios that could indirectly indicate enzyme activity of delta-9 desaturase were higher in the OBMS group, consistent with other studies [10–12,24] where they have been associated with obesity [10], IR and MetS [12]. The increase in the activity levels of desaturase enzymes in obesity could be related to hyperinsulinemia arising from excess states, as insulin is a potent activator and regulator of delta-6 and delta-9 desaturases [50].

This study found low proportions of PUFAs in the OBMS group. The concentrations of linoleic-18:2n-6 in both the TG and PL fractions were correlated directly with HDL-C and inversely with serum TG and the HOMA. These inverse relationships could be explained because reduced availability of PUFAs in cell membranes has been associated with lower fluidity and changes in insulin sensitivity [51].

DHGL-20:3n-6, a product of desaturation and elongation of linoleic-18:2n-6, appears at significantly higher percentages in the PL and FFA fractions in the OBMS group than in the AW group; consistent with this finding, the DHGL-20:3n-6/linoleic-18:n-6 ratio was higher in the OBMS group in both fractions, with similar results as those reported by Okada [11]. DHGL-20:3n-6 in the PL and FFA fractions correlated positively and significantly with WC, HOMA and TG, which agrees with other studies that conclude that this FA is associated with greater IR, cardiovascular risk [10,22,24,25] and inflammation [22]. In adults, Kurotani et al. also associated this FA and the DHGL-20:3n-6/linoleic-18:2n-6 ratio with early markers of IR and DM, such as high levels of C peptide [52]. DHGL-20:3n-6 is a precursor of thromboxanes and series 1 prostanoids (anti-inflammatory) via cyclooxygenase; its increase in these young people, without a simultaneous increase in ARA-20:4n-6, could indicate a compensatory mechanism associated with increased activity of delta-6 desaturase, which would enhance the anti-inflammatory activity helping to maintain the balance between pro- and anti-inflammatory substances [53].

The main finding in the FFA fraction was that the OBMS group had double the circulating total FFAs of other groups. This finding has been reported by other authors [54,55], in addition to its positive correlations with WC, insulin, HOMA [55], CT and serum TG [54]. The increase in total FFAs suggests that in those who present central obesity, adipocytes increase FA release due to saturation of the storage capacity and stress to the endoplasmic reticulum of visceral adipocytes. This effect diminishes the anti-lipolytic signal of insulin, perpetuating the release of FAs from visceral adipose tissue, which, once in circulation, are lipotoxic and are associated with the development of lipid alterations, IR and MetS [6,55,56].

Given the aforementioned associations, it was investigated whether FAs could explain the link between visceral obesity and insulin resistance in these youth using a multiple linear regression model. It was found that 62% of the HOMA was explained by the increases in total FFAs, DHGL-20:3*n*-6 in FFA and WC, in addition to decreases in linoleic-18:2*n*-6 in TG and the average METs/d.

The OB group presented proportions similar to those of the AW group in DHGL-20:4*n*-6 and in the total amount of circulating FFAs, variables – which in the OBMS group – has been associated with metabolic alterations, especially with IR. However, the OB group, compared to the AW group, presented a greater proportion of SFAs and MUFAs, a lower proportion of PUFAs in the TG fraction, higher values of WC, HOMA and TG and lower proportions of HDL-C, which is consistent with increased lipogenesis and confirms that obesity itself is a disorder that leads to future metabolic abnormalities and probably to NAFLD, if weight gain continues; consequently, the OB youth group should not be considered metabolically healthy. In these obese youth, therapeutic measures necessary to avoid or diminish MetS and NAFLD should be considered, especially in stimulating weight reduction with an increase in physical activity and the adoption of healthy eating habits, among others, as well as encouraging a greater consumption of polyunsaturated fat, a source of Omega 3 FA; if necessary, prescribe the consumption of lipid-lowering agents [57].

Like Waresnjo, this study found no association between circulating FAs and the PA level [12]; however, PA was incorporated as an explanatory variable of the HOMA in the multiple regression model, indicating that certain FAs in the profile and environmental factors influence its value.

In this study, the AW group consumed more calories and fats than the obese groups, results that have been reported by other authors [58,59]; these findings may be due to underestimations in evaluations of self-reported consumption, especially in obese individuals, or, when excess weight is evident, obese individuals decrease food intake. Therefore, current consumption cannot be correlated with nutritional status.

We did not detect a consumption pattern that could explain the differences in the FA profiles among the groups. Qualitative analysis of diets allowed us to establish that these youth did not consume significant omega-3 food sources, such as fish or seed oils, which could explain to some degree the low proportions of these FAs in the different fractions. In any event, to eliminate the effect of consumption on the descriptive model of the HOMA index, an adjustment was made for these variables, and the model was not modified.

This study has some limitations: the 24-h recall does not allow establishing individual associations with biochemical variables because of intra-individual variations in food intake; estimation of desaturase enzymes was performed using an indirect method due to technical difficulties involving their measurement *in vivo*. The diagnostic criteria for NAFLD in youth were not evaluated, which prevents establishing some degree of association with the profile of the fatty acids of the different fractions.

Finally, it is expected that there will be further research involving more complex lipids, such as waxes and eicosanoids, and methodological designs that establish causal relationships between the FA profile and metabolic disturbances that make up MetS, especially in children and youths.

5. Conclusions

This study detected proportions of some FA for youth with OBMS in the TG, PL and FFA fractions that correlated with disturbances of MetS, principally IR. High concentrations of total FFAs, high proportions of palmitic-16:0 in TG, high palmitoleic-16:1*n*-7 and low linoleic-18:2*n*-6 in TG and PL, and high DHGL-20:2*n*-6 in PL and FFAs could all be early markers of IR in youths. The findings further suggest that the connection between FA profiles and metabolic disturbances is associated more with high WC than BMI. The OB group presented greater proportions of SFA and MUFA and lower proportions of PUFA, as well as some higher biochemical values than those youth with AW, suggesting the possibility of developing future metabolic abnormalities if weight gain continues.

Supplementary Materials: Supplementary Materials: The following are available online at http://www.mdpi.com/2072-6643/8/2/54/s1, Table S1 Correlations between fatty acids of triglycerides, phospholipids, free fatty acids fractions, and cardiovascular risk factors in adolescents.

Acknowledgments: Acknowledgments: Resources were received from *Colciencias* Contract 487 (2012) and from the Universidad de Antioquia 2013–2014 through funds from the Committee for Research Development.

Author Contributions: Author Contributions: Claudia Velásquez-Rodríguez designed the study and directed the statistical analysis. Juliana Bermúdez-Cardona conducted the research and performed the statistical analysis. Claudia Velásquez-Rodríguez and Juliana Bermúdez-Cardona wrote the manuscript and are responsible for final content of the article.

Conflicts of Interest: Conflicts of Interest: The authors declare no conflict of interest.

Abbreviations

ARA	arachidonic acid
AW	appropriate weight
BMI	Body Mass Index
CE	cholesterol ester
HDL-C	high-density lipoprotein
LDL-C	low-density lipoprotein
DHA	docosahexaenoic acid
DHGL	dihomo-γ-linolenic acid
DM	diabetes mellitus
FA	fatty acid
FFA	free fatty acid
HOMA	Homeostasis Model Assessment
hsCRP	high-sensitivity C-reactive protein
HT	hypertension
IR	insulin resistance
MET	Metabolic equivalent
MetS	metabolic syndrome
MUFA	monounsaturated fatty acid
MVPA	moderate to vigorous physical activity
OBMS	obese with metabolic syndrome
OB	obese
PA	physical activity
PL	phospholipid
PUFA	polyunsaturated fatty acid
SFA	saturated fatty acid
TG	triglyceride
VLDL	very-low-density lipoprotein
VPA	vigorous physical activity
WC	waist circumference

References

1. World Health Organization. *Global Status Report on Noncommunicable Diseases*; Publisher: World Health Organization (WHO), Geneve, Switzerland, 2011.

2. Ng, M.; Fleming, T.; Robinson, M.; Thomson, B.; Graetz, N.; Margono, C.; Mullany, E.C. Global, regional, and national prevalence of overweight and obesity in children and adults during 1980–2013: A systematic analysis for the Global Burden of Disease Study 2013. *Lancet* **2014**, *384*, 766–781. [CrossRef]
3. Rivera, J.Á.; de Cossío, T.G.; Pedraza, L.S.; Aburto, T.C.; Sánchez, T.G.; Martorell, R. Childhood and adolescent overweight and obesity in Latin America: A systematic review. *Lancet. Diabetes Endocrinol.* **2014**, *2*, 321–332. [CrossRef]
4. Eckel, R.H.; Grundy, S.M.; Zimmet, P.Z. The metabolic syndrome. *Lancet* **2005**, *365*, 1415–1428. [CrossRef]
5. Lafontan, M. Adipose tissue and adipocyte dysregulation. *Diabetes Metab.* **2014**, *40*, 16–28. [CrossRef] [PubMed]
6. Shulman, G.I. Ectopic fat in insulin resistance, dyslipidemia, and cardiometabolic disease. *N. Engl. J. Med.* **2014**, *371*, 1131–1141. [CrossRef] [PubMed]
7. Tarantino, G. Spleen: A new role for an old player? *World J. Gastroenterol.* **2011**, *17*, 3776–3784. [CrossRef] [PubMed]
8. Takahashi, Y.; Fukusato, T.; Inui, A.; Fujisawa, T. Nonalcoholic fatty liver disease and nonalcoholic steatohepatitis. *Nihon Rinsho* **2012**, *70*, 1827–1834. [CrossRef] [PubMed]
9. Aguilera, C.M.; Gil-Campos, M.; Cañete, R.; Gil, A. Alterations in plasma and tissue lipids associated with obesity and metabolic syndrome. *Clin. Sci.* **2008**, *114*, 183–193. [CrossRef] [PubMed]
10. Steffen, L.M.; Vessby, B.; Jacobs, D.R.; Steinberger, J.; Moran, A.; Hong, C.-P.; Sinaiko, A.R. Serum phospholipid and cholesteryl ester fatty acids and estimated desaturase activities are related to overweight and cardiovascular risk factors in adolescents. *Int. J. Obes.* **2008**, *32*, 1297–1304. [CrossRef] [PubMed]
11. Okada, T.; Furuhashi, N.; Kuromori, Y.; Miyashita, M.; Iwata, F.; Harada, K. Plasma palmitoleic acid content and obesity in children. *Am. J. Clin. Nutr.* **2005**, *82*, 747–750. [PubMed]
12. Warensjö, E.; Ohrvall, M.; Vessby, B. Fatty acid composition and estimated desaturase activities are associated with obesity and lifestyle variables in men and women. *Nutr. Metab. Cardiovasc. Dis.* **2006**, *16*, 128–136. [CrossRef] [PubMed]
13. Warensjö, E.; Risérus, U.; Vessby, B. Fatty acid composition of serum lipids predicts the development of the metabolic syndrome in men. *Diabetologia* **2005**, *48*, 1999–2005. [CrossRef] [PubMed]
14. Paillard, F.; Catheline, D.; Duff, F.; le Bouriel, M.; Deugnier, Y.; Pouchard, M.; Daubert, J.-C.; Legrand, P. Plasma palmitoleic acid, a product of stearoyl-coA desaturase activity, is an independent marker of triglyceridemia and abdominal adiposity. *Nutr. Metab. Cardiovasc. Dis.* **2008**, *18*, 436–440. [CrossRef] [PubMed]
15. Warensjö, E.; Sundström, J.; Lind, L.; Vessby, B. Factor analysis of fatty acids in serum lipids as a measure of dietary fat quality in relation to the metabolic syndrome in men. *Am. J. Clin. Nutr.* **2006**, *84*, 442–448. [PubMed]
16. Araya, J.; Rodrigo, R.; Pettinelli, P.; Araya, A.V.; Poniachik, J.; Videla, L.A. Decreased liver fatty acid delta-6 and delta-5 desaturase activity in obese patients. *Obesity* **2010**, *18*, 1460–1463. [CrossRef] [PubMed]
17. Nikolaidis, M.G.; Mougios, V. Effects of Exercise on the Fatty-Acid Composition of Blood and Tissue Lipids. *Sport Med.* **2004**, *34*, 1051–1076. [CrossRef]
18. Hodson, L.; Skeaff, C.M.; Fielding, B.A. Fatty acid composition of adipose tissue and blood in humans and its use as a biomarker of dietary intake. *Prog. Lipid Res.* **2008**, *47*, 348–380. [CrossRef] [PubMed]
19. Kotronen, A.; Velagapudi, V.; Yetukuri, L.; Westerbacka, J.; Bergholm, R.; Ekroos, K.; Makkonen, J.; Taskinen, M.-R.; Oresic, M.; Yki-Järvinen, H. Serum saturated fatty acids containing triacylglycerols are better markers of insulin resistance than total serum triacylglycerol concentrations. *Diabetologia* **2009**, *52*, 684–690. [CrossRef] [PubMed]
20. Kishino, T.; Watanabe, K.; Urata, T.; Takano, M.; Uemura, T.; Nishikawa, K.; Mine, Y.; Matsumoto, M.; Ohtsuka, K.; Ohnishi, H.; *et al.* Visceral fat thickness in overweight men correlates with alterations in serum fatty acid composition. *Clin. Chim. Acta* **2008**, *398*, 57–62. [CrossRef] [PubMed]
21. Agudelo, G.; Velásquez, C.; Bedoya, G.; Estrada, A.; Manjarrés, L.M.; Patiño, F. Variations in the prevalence of metabolic syndrome in adolescents according to different criteria used for diagnosis: which definition should be chosen for this age group? *Metab. Syndr. Relat. Disord.* **2014**, *12*, 202–209. [CrossRef] [PubMed]
22. Klein-platat, C.; Drai, J.; Oujaa, M.; Schlienger, J.; Simon, C. Plasma fatty acid composition is associated with the metabolic syndrome and low-grade inflammation in overweight adolescents. *Am. J. Clin. Nutr.* **2005**, *82*, 1178–1184. [PubMed]

23. Gil-Campos, M.; del Carmen Ramírez-Tortosa, M.; Larqué, E.; Linde, J.; Aguilera, C.M.; Cañete, R.; Gil, A. Metabolic syndrome affects fatty acid composition of plasma lipids in obese prepubertal children. *Lipids* **2008**, *43*, 723–732. [CrossRef] [PubMed]

24. Decsi, T.; Csábi, G.; Török, K.; Erhardt, É.; Minda, H.; Burus, I.; Molnár, S.; Molnár, D. Polyunsaturated Fatty Acids in Plasma Lipids of Obese Children With and Without Metabolic Cardiovascular Syndrome. *Lipids* **2000**, *35*, 1179–1184. [CrossRef] [PubMed]

25. Elizondo, L.; Serrano, M.; Ugalde, P.; Cuello, C.; Borbolla, J. Plasma phospholipid fatty acids in obese male and female Mexican children. *Ann. Nutr. Metab.* **2010**, *57*, 234–241. [CrossRef] [PubMed]

26. De Onis, M.; Onyango, A.W.; Borghi, E.; Siyam, A.; Siekmann, J. Development of a WHO growth reference for school-aged children and adolescents. *Bull. World Health Organ.* **2007**, *85*, 660–667. [CrossRef] [PubMed]

27. Ford, E.S.; Li, C.; Cook, S.; Choi, H.K. Serum concentrations of uric acid and the metabolic syndrome among US children and adolescents. *Circulation* **2007**, *115*, 2526–2532. [CrossRef] [PubMed]

28. Lohman, T.; Roche, A.; Martorell, F. *Anthropometric standardization reference manual.*; Human Kinetics Books: Champaign, IL, USA, 1988.

29. Fernandez, J.; Redden, D.; Pietrobelli, A.; Allison, D. Waist circumference percentiles in nationally representative samples of African-American, European-American, and Mexican-American children and adolescents. *J. Pediatr.* **2004**, *145*, 439–444. [CrossRef] [PubMed]

30. Food and Nutrition Board; Institute of Medicine. *Dietary Reference Intakes. Application in Dietary Assessment*; National Academy Press: Washington DC, 2000.

31. Manjarrés, L. Métodos para precisar la recolección de la ingesta dietética en estudios poblacionales. *Perspect. Nutr. Humana* **2007**, *9*, 155–163.

32. Manjarrés, L.; Manjarrés, S. *Programa de Evaluación de Ingesta Dietética EVINDI v4*; Colombia Universidad de Antioquia. Escuela de Nutrición y Dietética: Medellín, Colombia, 2008.

33. Pate, R.R.; Ross, R.; Trost, S.G.; Sirard, J.R.; Dowda, M. Validation of a 3-Day Physical Activity Recall Instrument in Female Youth Recall Instrument in Female Youth. *Pediatr. Exerc. Sci.* **2003**, *15*, 257–265.

34. Dowda, M.; Saunders, R.; Hastings, L.; Gay, J.; Evans, A. Physical activity and sedentary pursuits of children living in residential children's homes. *J. Phys. Act. Health* **2009**, *6*, 195–202. [PubMed]

35. Ainsworth, B.E.; Haskell, W.L.; Whitt, M.C.; Irwin, M.L.; Swartz, A.N.N.M.; Strath, S.J.; Brien, W.L.O.; Bassett, D.R.; Schmitz, K.H.; Emplaincourt, P.O.; *et al.* Compendium of Physical Activities: An MET intensities. *Med. Sci. Sport. Exerc.* **2000**, *32*, S498–S504. [CrossRef]

36. Gomez, L.F.; Parra, D.C.; Lobelo, F.; Samper, B.; Moreno, J.; Jacoby, E.; Lucumi, D.I.; Matsudo, S.; Borda, C. Television viewing and its association with overweight in Colombian children: results from the 2005 National Nutrition Survey: A cross sectional study. *Int. J. Behav. Nutr. Phys. Act.* **2007**, *4*. [CrossRef] [PubMed]

37. Marshall, W.; Tanner, J. Variations in pattern of pubertal changes in girls. *Arch. Dis. Child.* **1969**, *44*, 291–303. [CrossRef] [PubMed]

38. Marshall, W.; Tanner, J. Variations in the pattern of pubertal changes in boys. *Arch. Dis. Child.* **1970**, *45*, 13–23. [CrossRef] [PubMed]

39. National High Blood Pressure Education Program Working Group on High Blood Pressure in Children and Adolescents The fourth report on the diagnosis, evaluation, and treatment of high blood pressure in children and adolescents. *Pediatrics* **2004**, *114*, 555–577.

40. National Cholesterol Education Program Third Report of the National Cholesterol Education Program (NCEP) Expert Panel on Detection, Evaluation, and Treatment of High Blood Cholesterol in Adults (Adult Treatment Panel III) final report. *Circulation* **2002**, *106*, 3143–3421.

41. Lee, J.M.; Okumura, M.J.; Davis, M.M.; Herman, W.H.; Gurney, J.G. Prevalence and determinants of insulin resistance among U.S. adolescents: a population-based study. *Diabetes Care* **2006**, *29*, 2427–2432. [CrossRef] [PubMed]

42. Yin, J.; Li, M.; Xu, L.; Wang, Y.; Cheng, H.; Zhao, X.; Mi, J. Insulin resistance determined by Homeostasis Model Assessment (HOMA) and associations with metabolic syndrome among Chinese children and teenagers. *Diabetol. Metab. Syndr.* **2013**, *5*, 71. [CrossRef] [PubMed]

43. Myers, G.L.; Rifai, N.; Tracy, R.P.; Roberts, W.L.; Alexander, R.W.; Biasucci, L.M.; Catravas, J.D.; Cole, T.G.; Cooper, G.R.; Khan, B.V.; *et al.* CDC/AHA Workshop on Markers of Inflammation and Cardiovascular Disease: Application to Clinical and Public Health Practice: report from the laboratory science discussion group. *Circulation* **2004**, *110*, e545–e549. [CrossRef] [PubMed]

44. Folch, J.; Lees, M.; Stannley, S. A simple method for the isolation and purification of total lipid from animal tissues. *J. Biol. Chem.* **1957**, *226*, 497–509. [PubMed]

45. Agren, J.; Julkunen, A.; Penttila, I. Rapid separation of serum lipids for fatty acid analysis by a single aminopropyl column. *J. Lipid Res.* **1992**, *33*, 1871–1876. [PubMed]

46. Kaluzny, M.; Duncan, L.; Merrit, M.; Epps, D. Rapid separation of lipid classes in high yield and purity using bonded phase columns. *J. Lipid Res.* **1985**, *26*, 135–140. [PubMed]

47. Kang, J.X.; Wang, J. A simplified method for analysis of polyunsaturated fatty acids. *BMC Biochem.* **2005**, *6*, 5. [CrossRef] [PubMed]

48. Ntambi, J. Regulation of stearoyl-CoA desaturases and role in metabolism. *Prog. Lipid Res.* **2004**, *43*, 91–104. [CrossRef]

49. Zong, G.; Zhu, J.; Sun, L.; Ye, X.; Lu, L.; Jin, Q.; Zheng, H.; Yu, Z.; Zhu, Z.; Li, H.; Sun, Q.; Lin, X. Associations of erythrocyte fatty acids in the de novo lipogenesis pathway with risk of metabolic syndrome in a cohort study of middle-aged and older Chinese. *Am. J. Clin. Nutr.* **2013**, *98*, 319–326. [CrossRef] [PubMed]

50. Nakamura, M.T.; Nara, T.Y. Structure, function, and dietary regulation of delta6, delta5, and delta9 desaturases. *Annu. Rev. Nutr.* **2004**, *24*, 345–376. [CrossRef] [PubMed]

51. Tremblay, A.J.; Després, J.-P.; Piché, M.-È.; Nadeau, A.; Bergeron, J.; Alméras, N.; Tremblay, A.; Lemieux, S. Associations between the fatty acid content of triglyceride, visceral adipose tissue accumulation, and components of the insulin resistance syndrome. *Metabolism* **2004**, *53*, 310–317. [CrossRef] [PubMed]

52. Kurotani, K.; Sato, M.; Ejima, Y.; Nanri, A.; Yi, S.; Pham, N.M.; Akter, S.; Poudel-Tandukar, K.; Kimura, Y.; Imaizumi, K.; Mizoue, T. High levels of stearic acid, palmitoleic acid, and dihomo-γ-linolenic acid and low levels of linoleic acid in serum cholesterol ester are associated with high insulin resistance. *Nutr. Res.* **2012**, *32*, 669–675. [CrossRef] [PubMed]

53. Roke, K.; Ralston, J.C.; Abdelmagid, S.; Nielsen, D.E.; Badawi, A.; El-Sohemy, A.; Ma, D.W.L.; Mutch, D.M. Variation in the *FADS1/2* gene cluster alters plasma *n-6* PUFA and is weakly associated with hsCRP levels in healthy young adults. *Prostaglandins Leukot. Essent. Fatty Acids* **2013**, *89*, 257–263. [CrossRef] [PubMed]

54. Sabin, M.A.; de Hora, M.; Holly, J.M.; Hunt, L.P.; Ford, A.L.; Williams, S.R.; Baker, J.S.; Retallick, C.J.; Crowne, E.C.; Shield, J.P.H. Fasting nonesterified fatty acid profiles in childhood and their relationship with adiposity, insulin sensitivity, and lipid levels. *Pediatrics* **2007**, *120*, e1426–e1433. [CrossRef] [PubMed]

55. Reinehr, T.; Kiess, W.; Andler, W. Insulin sensitivity indices of glucose and free fatty acid metabolism in obese children and adolescents in relation to serum lipids. *Metabolism* **2005**, *54*, 397–402. [CrossRef] [PubMed]

56. Deng, J.; Liu, S.; Zou, L.; Xu, C.; Geng, B.; Xu, G. Lipolysis response to endoplasmic reticulum stress in adipose cells. *J. Biol. Chem.* **2012**, *287*, 6240–6249. [CrossRef] [PubMed]

57. Finelli, C.; Tarantino, G. Is there any consensus as to what diet or lifestyle approach is the right one for NAFLD patients? *J. Gastrointest. Liver Dis.* **2012**, *21*, 293–302.

58. Telford, R.D.; Cunningham, R.B.; Telford, R.M.; Riley, M.; Abhayaratna, W.P. Determinants of childhood adiposity: evidence from the Australian LOOK study. *PLoS ONE* **2012**, *7*, e50014. [CrossRef] [PubMed]

59. Martín-Calvo, N.; Ochoa, M.C.; Marti, A.; Martínez-González, M.Á. Asociación entre los macronutrientes de la dieta y la obesidad en la infancia y adolescencia; un estudio de casos y controles. *Nutr. Hosp.* **2013**, *28*, 1515–1522. [PubMed]

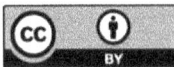

© 2016 by the authors. Licensee MDPI, Basel, Switzerland. This article is an open access article distributed under the terms and conditions of the Creative Commons Attribution (CC BY) license (http://creativecommons.org/licenses/by/4.0/).

nutrients

MDPI

Review

Gut Microbiota and Metabolic Health: The Potential Beneficial Effects of a Medium Chain Triglyceride Diet in Obese Individuals

Sabri Ahmed Rial [1], Antony D. Karelis [2], Karl-F. Bergeron [1] and Catherine Mounier [1,*]

[1]   BioMed Research Center, Biological Sciences Department, University of Quebec at Montreal, Montreal, QC H2X 1Y4, Canada; rial.ahmed_sabri@courrier.uqam.ca (S.A.R.); bergeron.karl-frederik@uqam.ca (K.-F.B.)

[2]   Department of Exercise Science, University of Quebec at Montreal, Montreal, QC H2X 1Y4, Canada; karelis.antony@uqam.ca

*   Correspondence: mounier.catherine@uqam.ca; Tel.: +1-514-987-3092

Received: 31 March 2016; Accepted: 9 May 2016; Published: 12 May 2016

Abstract: Obesity and associated metabolic complications, such as non-alcoholic fatty liver disease (NAFLD) and type 2 diabetes (T2D), are in constant increase around the world. While most obese patients show several metabolic and biometric abnormalities and comorbidities, a subgroup of patients representing 3% to 57% of obese adults, depending on the diagnosis criteria, remains metabolically healthy. Among many other factors, the gut microbiota is now identified as a determining factor in the pathogenesis of metabolically unhealthy obese (MUHO) individuals and in obesity-related diseases such as endotoxemia, intestinal and systemic inflammation, as well as insulin resistance. Interestingly, recent studies suggest that an optimal healthy-like gut microbiota structure may contribute to the metabolically healthy obese (MHO) phenotype. Here, we describe how dietary medium chain triglycerides (MCT), previously found to promote lipid catabolism, energy expenditure and weight loss, can ameliorate metabolic health via their capacity to improve both intestinal ecosystem and permeability. MCT-enriched diets could therefore be used to manage metabolic diseases through modification of gut microbiota.

Keywords: obesity; metabolically unhealthy obese; metabolically healthy obese; metabolic syndrome; non-alcoholic fatty liver disease; gut microbiota; *Bacteroidetes*; *Firmicutes*; endotoxemia; lipopolysaccharide; medium chain triglycerides; medium chain fatty acids

---

1. Introduction

Obesity has become an international public health problem with 2.1 billion people worldwide being overweight (body mass index (BMI) $\geqslant$ 25.0) and more than half a billion among them being obese (BMI $\geqslant$ 30.0) [1,2]. Obesity is now described as a pandemic with increased prevalence in both adult and child populations. Since the 1980s, the combined prevalence of obesity and overweight increased by 28% in adults and 47% in children [1,2]. Obesity is a multifactorial affection with broad etiology, and multiple comorbidities. Most of these comorbidities are thought to be the result of aberrant body fat distribution leading to the metabolic syndrome [3–5]. This pathology is associated with an elevated waist circumference, a progressive state of non-alcoholic fatty liver disease (NAFLD) [3,4], insulin resistance, type 2 diabetes (T2D), some types of cancers (especially in women), hypertension, cardiovascular diseases, reproductive abnormalities, dyslipidemias, psychological affections [6], and a severely reduced life expectancy [3,7,8]. Obesity is also considered a risk factor for several other diseases such as chronic respiratory diseases [9] and arthritis [3].

Some contributing factors for obesity progression are: unfavorable genetic determinants [10], lack of physical activity [11], socio-economic status [1], circadian cycle disturbance [12], sleep deprivation [13], hormonal dysregulation [14], persistent organic pollutants [15] and alteration of the gut microbiota [16,17]. However, the most powerful inducer of obesity and its associated adverse metabolic effects remains, by far, inappropriate food intake [18]. The modern prevalence of obesity and metabolic syndrome is likely due to the rise in consumption of energy-dense food, containing high amounts of fat and carbohydrates [18], especially in Western countries. In these countries, fats typically account for 33% to 42% of dietary energy intake, with a rich proportion of long chain saturated fat [18]. When the energy intake exceeds both the caloric needs of the body and its glycogen storage capacity, dietary carbohydrates and fats are first converted and stored as triglycerides (TG) in white adipose tissue (WAT) and, later on, in other tissues such as the liver [19,20]. Sustained and abusive accumulation of lipids in the liver induces NAFLD (highly concurrent with obesity) which may result in lipotoxicity, steatohepatitis, hepatocyte cell death, fibrosis and eventually liver cirrhosis as well as hepatocarcinoma [21].

We aim here to overview the underlying causes of obesity and its associated metabolic abnormalities while paying special attention to a unique subset of the obese population: the metabolically healthy but obese (MHO) individuals. We will highlight the potential involvement of the gut microbiome as one of several contributors to the MHO status. We will finally introduce the idea of a medium chain triglycerides (MCT)-based dietary intervention with the aim of improving the metabolic state of metabolically unhealthy obese (MUHO) patients, either through modification of their intestinal health or by directly influencing lipid metabolism.

2. Etiology of Obesity and Associated Metabolic Complications

The current paradigm posits that fat accumulation leading to obesity results from an imbalance between energy intake and energy expenditure. Post-World War II food processing and marketing practices (quickly available energy-dense foods) and reductions in physical activity are the two main factors often blamed for the contemporary prevalence of obesity. As such, most treatment options involve creation of a negative energy balance, achieved by consuming fewer calories than energy expended. Alternatively, pharmacological and surgical therapies also exist [22]. Nevertheless, complex interactions among heredity [23], epigenetic imprinting [24], lifestyle, feeding behavior [25], as well as environmental [26] and physiologic inflammatory factors [27,28] also contribute to the etiology of obesity.

2.1. Comorbidities Related to Obesity

Most obese individuals fall into the MUHO category and are at increased risk for several diseases. They suffer from a severely reduced life expectancy: a 5.8 years average decrease for men and 7 years for women [29]. The visceral adipose tissue (typically abundant in obese individuals) secretes pro-inflammatory cytokines [27,28] that are, in part, responsible for obesity-associated pathogenesis [27,28]. The resulting metabolic syndrome defines a group of metabolic risk factors linked to health problems associated with overweight and obesity such as elevated visceral adiposity, larger waist circumference (>102 cm in men and >88 cm in women), hyper-triglyceridemia (>150 mg/dL) [5], reduced HDL (high density lipoprotein) cholesterol levels (<40 mg/dL in men and <50 mg/dL in women), elevated blood pressure (systolic > 130 mmHg and/or diastolic > 85 mmHg) and high fasting glucose levels [30]. A patient with at least three of these risk factors is currently diagnosed with the metabolic syndrome.

High levels of glycemia, associated with insulin resistance, are a hallmark of prediabetes and T2D, common diseases occurring in obese individuals suffering from the metabolic syndrome [5]. According to the most recent criteria, prediabetes is defined by a fasting glucose ranging between 100 and 125 mg/dL or between 140 and 199 mg/dL 2 h *post-prandium*, while these two values often exceed 126 mg/dL and 200 mg/dL in T2D, respectively [5]. In addition, the latest medical updates indicate that 50%–90% of patients with TD2 have a BMI > 25.0 (the overweight threshold) while those with a BMI > 35 have a 20-fold higher risk of developing T2D than healthy lean patients [31].

Risk of cardiovascular diseases, including atherosclerosis, coronary artery disease, stroke and pulmonary embolism, is higher in obese patients [32]. Obesity is also associated with a large spectrum of liver abnormalities including NAFLD [33]. Several additional comorbid disease risks are associated with obesity such as cholelithias, pancreatic failure sleep apnea, gynecological abnormalities, osteoarthritis, psychiatric illness as well as some types of cancer (breast, endometrial, prostate and colon) [22].

2.2. Metabolically Healthy but Obese Individuals (MHO)

There is a large body of evidence suggesting that not all obese individuals develop such important metabolic complications [34]. A unique subtype of obese individuals has been identified as MHO [35]. Despite excessive levels of body fat mass, MHO patients present higher levels of insulin sensitivity, a normal circulating lipid profile, no pronounced hepatic steatosis nor associated inflammatory state, no hypertension, and a lower visceral, muscle and hepatic fat content compared to MUHO subjects [36]. Since there is no standard definition for the identification of the MHO phenotype, the true prevalence of MHO individuals in the obese population is currently unclear. Depending on the method and the cut-off point used for certain metabolic risk factors, the prevalence of MHO subjects may range from approximately 3% to 57% of obese adults [37,38].

The favorable metabolic profile of MHO individuals has been associated with a lower risk of developing T2D or cardiovascular disease (CVD), and having a lower mortality risk compared to MUHO individuals [39]. There is also evidence refuting the notion that MHO subjects are totally protected from metabolic diseases [40]. The fundamental mechanisms underlying the different metabolic profiles of MHO and MUHO individuals remain poorly understood [41]. However, Berezina *et al.* showed that among patients with abdominal obesity, MHO phenotype was associated with a G45G Adiponectin genotype, while the T45T genotype for Adiponectin increased metabolic disorders risks [42]. This observation is all the more interesting since Adiponectin is a potent modulator of insulin sensitivity [43]. Also, in the latter decade, a consensus has emerged, which make the gut microbial population (also called the gut microbiota) a key determinant in the host metabolic profile [17,44]. The gut microbiota should therefore be taken into consideration in dietary and clinical approaches, for both MUHO and MHO treatments.

3. The Gut Microbiota: A Determining Factor for Metabolic State

3.1. Gut Microbiota Dysbiosis in Obesity

Current estimations indicate that the human intestine is colonized by a large population of above 100 trillion microbial cells organized in several taxa and constituting the gut microbiota [45]. The total biomass of the gut microbiota exceeds 1kg and is mainly concentrated in the large intestine, where about 10^{12} bacteria per gram of colonic tissue are found [46]. Such an important quantity of "foreign" cells implies a tightly regulated acceptance by the immune system of the host [46]. The gut microbiota plays a symbiotic role, ensuring several metabolic functions essential to the host. It is involved in the degradation of polysaccharides and oligosaccharides into simple metabolites such as short chain fatty acids (SCFA). These SCFA were recently found to promote intestinal impermeability [47] as well as hepatic sugar and lipid anabolism [48–50]. The gut microbiota is also an indispensable source of essential vitamins B and K [51]. Gut microbiota composition and diversity are subjected to important variations between individuals but also within the same individual under the influence of several physiologic and environmental factors such as antibiotic consumption, lifestyle and diet [52].

The alteration of gut microbiota is closely linked to tissue inflammation and to a broad range of metabolic abnormalities, including obesity and insulin resistance [52,53]. First observations suggested a link between the gut microbiota and the metabolic state of the host [54,55]. Several studies have since confirmed a direct implication of gut microbiota in obesity progression [17].

Backhed and colleagues first demonstrated that germ-free mice were protected against high fat and high sugar diet-induced obesity, via enhanced expression of hepatic and muscular Pgc-1α (a PPAR coactivator) and activation of lipid catabolism via AMPK activity [56]. Subsequently, Cani and collaborators established a close link between gut microbiota-induced "metabolic endotoxemia" and obesity-related insulin resistance in mice. They established the paradigm of gut microbiota-mediated metabolic endotoxemia inducing chronic low-grade of inflammation in the host. In obese mice, a dramatic change in caecum-resident bacteria characterized by a decrease in low lipopolysaccharide (LPS)-expressing bacterial taxa (such as *Bifidobacteria*) and concomitant elevation in high LPS-expressing taxa (gram-negative bacteria) was observed. This lead to increased concentration of circulating pro-inflammatory LPS [55]. A prolonged high fat diet was also reported to induce physiologic high-grade inflammation, weight gain and T2D progression by an LPS-dependent gut microbiota-associated endotoxemia mechanism in mice [56]. In addition, it was shown that genetically obese *ob/ob* mice display a lower endotoxemia and caecal LPS content following the inactivation of CD14, a cell receptor involved in inflammation [55,57]. Concomitantly, in a randomly recruited human male cohort, a link has been observed between circulating LPS and food intake [58].

In mice fed a high-fat diet, and in genetically obese *ob/ob* mice, suppression of gut microbiota via administration of a broad range of antibiotics resulted in a significant decrease of LPS caecal content. Consequently, fat accumulation and body weight were diminished, endotoxemia and inflammation at both systemic- and tissue-specific levels were blunted, and insulin sensitivity was improved [57]. Intriguingly, administration of antibiotics to livestock trough water and food is typically used to promote cattle and swine growth and weight-gain [59,60]. The mechanisms underlying this opposite effect are not known yet support a link between enteric bacteria and host metabolism, suggesting variable responses between animal species [59,61,62].

A dysbiosis induced by obesogenic factors adversely enhances intestinal permeability by modulating the expression of epithelial junction genes *zo-1* and *occludin* [63,64]. An optimal gut microbiota helps maintain intestinal barrier impermeability via the production of SCFA, which serve as metabolic precursors for colonocytes in normal physiologic hypoxia conditions [47–49]. Colonocytes require the catabolism of SCFA to potentiate the Hypoxia-inducible factor 1-dependent expression of key genes involved in biosynthesis [47–49]. This may explain why, in metabolic diseases such as obesity, an inappropriate microbiota adversely impacts intestinal permeability, leading to infiltration of bacterial LPS from gut lumen into intestinal epithelia, bloodstream and tissue (such as the liver) contributing to metabolic endotoxemia [47–49,65]. In fact, administration of antibacterial agents targeting caecal aerobic and anaerobic bacteria with high efficiency (namely norfloxacin and ampicillin) to mice fed a high-fat diet and *ob/ob* mice significantly enhanced their global glucose tolerance, decreased their fasting glycaemia and circulating LPS levels, and improved the secretion of Adiponectin [66], known for its positive effects on insulin sensitivity [43]. The current model of obesity-associated endotoxemia posits that gut-derived LPS and free fatty acids activate M1 macrophages which, together with other immune cells, create a hepatic and physiologic inflammatory process sustaining the above-mentioned obesity-related comorbidities [67].

Gut microbiota is now considered as a key factor of metabolic health [44,64]. The relative abundance of some bacterial phyla within the gut microbiota are associated with specific metabolic states, and subjected to the influence of diets [54]. In fact, quantitative identification of bacteria using the 16S ribosomal RNA gene showed that obesity is associated to a notable decrease in the relative abundance of *Bacteroidetes vs. Firmicutes* (from a proportion of 40:60 in lean patients or non-obese mice down to a proportion of 20:80) [54,68,69]. Interestingly, this ratio is similarly decreased in *ob/ob* mice, in mice subjected to obesogenic and diabetogenic diets, as well as in obese human subjects [68,70,71]. Moreover, within these two superkingdoms, bacterial subpopulations are themselves submitted to specific changes reflecting metabolic health, diet and antiobesity medical interventions such as bariatric surgery-induced weight loss [72–74]. These changes are diverse and still not well established (see Delzenne and Cani for a detailed review [69]).

While these observations established a definitive link between gut microbiota disturbance and metabolic diseases progression, it is still unclear which one of the two events induces the other. This question was addressed by several microbiota transplantation experiments [44,75]. The transplantation of fecal microbiota from obese mice and obese patients into germ-free lean mice transformed the lean mice into obese mice, while the germ-free mice receiving microbiota from lean mice did not show any metabolic symptoms related to obesity or insulin resistance [54,75–77]. These findings revealed a microbiota-mediated transmissible effect of diets and metabolic status, demonstrating that gut microbiota is not simply a collateral unit modulated by metabolic diseases but an active and potent modulator of metabolism. The gut microbiota may therefore play a role in the determination of metabolic status.

3.2. Correlation of MHO Metabolic Status with Gut Microbiota Profile

To date, very few animal studies described a clear role for gut microbiota in the establishment of the MHO phenotype. Serino *et al.* showed that different cohorts of mice issued from the same C57BL6 genetic background became either diabetic or resistant to diabetes and metabolic disorders despite being fed the same obesogenic high-fat diet. Compared to diabetic mice, resistant mice showed higher insulin sensitivity, lower inflammation, improved intestinal impermeability (in the ileum, caecum and colon) and lower adipogenesis [78]. Moreover, the metabolic profile of resistant mice was similar to the metabolic profile observed in mice fed a high fat diet supplemented with gluco-oligosaccharidic fibers. Oligosaccharidic fibers are commonly used to prevent high fat diet-induced endotoxemia, dysbiosis and obesity [79]. Interestingly, the resistant mice harbored a distinctive gut microbiota. The gut microbiota of the diabetic mice, in comparison with resistant mice, was characterized by a 20% decrease in the abundance of *Firmicutes* to the benefit of *Bacteriodetes*, mainly resulting from a dramatic decrease of the *lachnospiraceae* bacterial family. Within the *Bacteroidetes* phylum, the family of S24-7 bacteria was specifically increased (3-fold). In addition, compared to the diabetic mice, the microbiota of resistant mice presented an important decrease of the *helicobacter* genus, while *actinobacteria* remained stable [78]. The authors suggested that the gut microbiota could represent a "signature of the metabolic phenotype independent of differences in host genetic background and diets". This suggestion is consistent with the results of a recent study performed in the brown bear (*Ursus arctos*) [80]. The bear is a mammal well known to accumulate very large amounts of adipose fat during the summer; developing hyperlipidemia while remaining metabolically healthy and resistant to atherosclerosis [81]. Sommer and colleagues showed that, during summer, bears harbored a different gut microbiota composition than during winter. Summer microbiota was enriched in *Firmicutes*, *Actinobacteria* and, in a lower proportion, enriched in proteobacteria while being depleted in *Bacteroidetes* [80]. Moreover, the abundance of several other bacterial families was also seasonally modulated. Interestingly, the transplantation of summer or winter microbiota from bear intestines to germ-free mice revealed a microbiota-dependent transmissible seasonal metabolic status as mice receiving summer microbiota showed a significant elevation of adiposity and body weight gain but a better glucose tolerance and a lower circulating TG level, suggesting an improved cardiometabolic state [80].

Completely ignored previously, the fungal subdivision of the gut microbiota (or "mycobiota") has recently been revealed as a determinant of human metabolic state. As for bacteria, its specific composition seems to distinguish MHO from MUHO [82]. For example, Rodriguez and collaborators showed that obese patients with relative abundance of *Eurotiomycetes* > 1% in their gut, showed improved fasting insulinemia, insulin resistance index and circulating LDL-cholesterol levels [82].

There is a definite correlation between MHO status and intestinal flora. Gut microbiota remodelling could therefore be considered as a strategy to ameliorate metabolic health. Hence, we believe that a switch from MUHO into MHO metabolic state may be possible following gut microbiota remodelling, and that dietary interventions (such as those using prebiotic or bioactive nutrients) may help in this process.

4. MHO and MUHO: From Classical Dietary Interventions to a MCT-Based One?

Obese individuals have a lower success rate of maintaining weight loss after one year compared to non-obese individuals [83]. This high risk of weight regain may lead to a pattern of weight cycling [83], and this may be associated with metabolic complications as well as CVD and mortality [84,85]. In addition, significant weight loss can increase the levels of persistent organic pollutants (POPs) in the bloodstream [86,87] and may offset the beneficial effects of weight loss. In support of this idea, a recent study showed that obese subjects with the highest POP blood levels after weight loss suffered from a delay in the improvement of lipid and liver toxicity markers [88]. Therefore, health professionals may want to favor a metabolically healthy state instead of focusing on weight loss.

4.1. Weight Management in MHO Subjects

Several studies have examined the effect of lifestyle interventions, including diet and/or exercise training in MHO individuals. These have led to contradictory findings. Some have shown that, compared to MUHO, the metabolic profile of MHO individuals after weight loss did not improve following weight loss [89–91] while other studies have reported an improvement of several metabolic risk factors [92–95]. For example, a 9-month intensive lifestyle intervention program that consisted of Mediterranean diet nutritional counselling and high intensity interval training was associated with a reduction of metabolic risk factors (e.g., blood pressure, fasting glucose level) [94]. Furthermore, weight loss following laparoscopic adjustable gastric banding in MHO patients was associated with an improvement of insulin sensitivity levels after 6 months [96]. However, a significant decrease in insulin sensitivity was observed after weight loss in a different cohort of MHO individuals [97,98]. Finally, MHO women may lose less weight than MUHO subjects after 3 months on a low fat diet [99]. Based on the current evidence, it appears difficult to prescribe an optimal lifestyle intervention program to both MUHO and MHO individuals.

4.2. The Metabolic Protective Potential of Medium Chain Triglycerides (MCTs)

4.2.1. MCTs as Bioactive Lipids

One angle of attack against metabolic diseases is the modification of the quality of dietary lipids. Such a nutritional strategy may be based on the consumption of "bioactive lipids", such as mono-unsaturated or poly-unsaturated lipids, phytosterols, and free or esterified medium chain lipids [100,101]. We will emphasize our review on the metabolic benefits of medium chain free fatty acids (MCFA) and medium chain triglycerides (MCT).

Dietary medium chain fatty acids (MCFA) range between 6 and 10 carbon-chain lengths, including hexanoate (C6:0), octanoate (C8:0) and decanoate (C10:0). Large amounts of MCFA are found, in the form of MCT, in coconut and palm kernel oils where they account for more than 50% of total lipids [102,103]. They are also found in smaller amounts in bovine milk, where they can reach 14%–15% of the total lipid mass depending on cow breeds, types of pasture and seasonal conditions [104]. MCT differ from long chain triglycerides (LCT) by several physicochemical characteristics such as their smaller molecular size. MCT are hydrolyzed both faster and more extensively during digestion. Most of the remaining non-hydrolyzed MCT are readily absorbed by intestinal cells [103]. In addition, MCFA show greater solubility in aqueous media while remaining capable of passive, non-rate-limiting diffusion across cell membranes as a result of their relative short chains [100–103,105,106]. MCFA show a low affinity for anabolic enzymes (such as diglyceride acyltransferase) therefore undergoing minimal re-esterification, a process necessary for *de novo* synthesis of TG. Once absorbed during digestion, most of MCFA and MCT are transported through the portal system directly to the liver with minimal mobilization of chylomicrons while long chain fatty acids (LCFA) are packed in chylomicrons prior to their shipment to the periphery mainly via the lymphatic system [100–103,105]. Finally, in the liver, MCFA are preferentially metabolized to generate energy [107]. In fact, MCFA are known to enter cells passively before crossing mitochondria membranes, independently of the availability of the rate-limiting carnitine palmitoyltransferase 1 (CPT-1) transport system, to fuel the β-oxidation and ATP-generating pathways [105,106], induce thermogenesis and reduce *de novo* lipogenesis [108].

Because of these properties, MCT have been used for decades to overcome many metabolic and digestive abnormalities such as pancreatic insufficiency, fat malabsorption, impaired lymphatic chylomicron transport, severe hyperchylomicronemia, and total parenteral nutrition. MCTs are also used in preterm infant formulas [106].

4.2.2. MCT-Supplemented Diets Prevent Obesity

(i) MCT and MCFA Exert Antilipogenic Effects

Using chick embryo hepatocytes, we have previously demonstrated, that free non-esterified hexanoate and octanoate significantly decrease insulin and T3 (triiodothyronine)-induced fatty acid synthase (FAS) expression and activity [108]. Activity of FAS, a key enzyme of *de novo* lipogenesis, is positively regulated in the post-prandial state by several hormones (such as insulin, ghrelin and T3) and nutrients (dietary lipid and carbohydrate derivatives) [109,110], and is an important contributor to obesity and NAFLD [20,111]. We and others have demonstrated that MCFA inhibit binding of transactivating receptors on the T3 response elements of FAS and Acetyl-CoA carboxylase (ACC) promoters [108,112–114]. Using LO2 hepatocytes, Wang and collaborators showed that the induction of cellular steatosis by LCT (esterified oleate and palmitate) is reversed by addition of either octanoate or decanoate. MCFA treatment shifts cells from global lipid anabolism to lipid catabolism and downregulates main *de novo* lipogenesis-activating transcription factors (Liver-X-receptor alpha and Sterol regulatory element binding protein-1), the lipogenic enzymes (ACC and FAS) and enzymes involved in fatty acid-uptake (Cluster of differentiation-36 and Lipoprotein lipase) [115].

(ii) The Cardiometabolic Protective Effects of Dietary MCT

The propensity of MCFA to be catabolized rather than esterified, highlights their metabolically beneficial potential. Several years ago, it was shown in rats that replacement of dietary LCT by octanoate-based MCT led to a significant attenuation of alcoholic steatosis associated with a decrease in *de novo* TG synthesis an adiposity, as well as elevated lipid oxidation [116]. Therefore, MCT-supplemented diets constitute a promising tool against adipogenic and steatogenic diseases. Feeding healthy rats with MCT-containing diets *vs.* diets containing LCT greatly decreases fat deposition without affecting whole-body protein content and assimilation [117]. Consumption of MCT is safe in regards to toxicological considerations and has been sanctioned by the FDA (Food and Drug Administration) for over 20 years [106,118]. Interestingly, dietary MCT promote post-prandial energy production. A single dose of MCT ranging between 5 and 50 g or a weeklong diet containing 40% MCT-fat systematically leads to elevated post-prandial oxygen consumption and thermogenesis, increased total lipid oxidation, higher energy expenditure and diminished energy storage in comparison with LCT administered under identical conditions [101,119–123]. Importantly, the propensity of MCT/MCFA to be degraded by oxidation is also observed in obese individuals [120,124].

Long-term replacement of LCT with TG composed of esterified MCFA and LCFA induces a measurable body fat loss without any impact on energy intake and global metabolism [101,125,126]. These specific TG, produced from the transesterification of MCT and LCT (S-MLCT) are interesting compounds because of their higher smoking temperature making them more appropriate for cooking purposes than simple mixtures of MCT and LCT. S-MLCT display a "L-M-L"-type structure (TG with LCFA in sn-1 position, MCFA in sn-2 and LCFA in sn-3), are preferable substrates for pancreatic enzymes and are therefore highly digestible [101,125,126]. Feeding healthy young volunteers for 3 months with either S-MLCT or LCT-enriched liquid formulas (1040 kJ/day) led to a bodyweight increase from the baseline in both groups [127]. Interestingly, diets supplemented with S-MLCT induced a lower increase in body fat mass compared to the LCT supplemented diets (+10% for

S-MLCT *vs.* +30% for LCT) [127]. The general metabolic profiles between the two groups were not different, with the exception of glycemia (S-MLCT = 924 *vs.* LCT = 853 mg/100 mL) [127]. A clear link was concurrently established between the propensity of MCT to increase thermogenesis and their previously reported capacity to reduce diet-induced adiposity and body weight-gain [107,128]. Wistar rats submitted to a single oral gavage of 1 g MCT or LCT showed significant elevation in oxygen consumption concomitantly with elevated thermogenesis (1.5 kcal/6 h for MCT *vs.* 0.8 kcal/6 h for LCT) [107]. Another study showed that feeding rats with a diet containing 10% MCT during 6 weeks diminished body fat mass by decreasing subcutaneous and intra-abdominal adiposity compared to a diet containing 10% LCT, suggesting that dietary-MCT lowered body fat mass by inducing thermogenesis [107]. Interestingly, MCT also lower caloric intake, compared to LCT, by improving satiety [129,130]. Octanoate, which constitutes most of the MCT used in dietary interventions, was suggested to be the main co-substrate of the Ghrelin *O*-acetyltransferase enzyme, involved in the activation of the powerful orexigenic peptide hormone Ghrelin [131–133]. However, an acute diminution of food intake induced by the consumption of MCT oil is associated with an elevation of Leptin, a hormone with a well-known anti-orexigenic effect [129]. These unsolved discrepancies between different studies highlights the necessity to better understand the molecular effects of MCT and their physiologic implications [132].

Consistent observations related to anti-obesity effects of MCT were generated through animal and human clinical studies. Daily consumption (for 12 weeks at breakfast) of bread supplemented with 14 g S-MLCT (produced by a transesterification of MCT and LCT) led, in comparison with control LCT, to a mild but significant decrease in body weight, and a decrease in subcutaneous and visceral adiposity as well as in total cholesterol level. However, the other metabolic and anthropometric parameters did not significantly vary [134]. The impact of MCT consumption on body-weight is noticeably variable depending on studies and diet protocol designs. Women on a one-month diet where 30% of total energy was supplied by MCT displayed improved fat oxidation and energy expenditure compared to women on LCT-containing meals, and showed a tendency towards decreasing body weight [135]. Interestingly, studies suggested that the catabolic effects induced by the dietary MCT may depend on BMI. In humans, MCT consumption for 4 weeks induced energy expenditure, fat oxidation and body weight loss inversely proportional to BMI [136]. A recent observation has been also made on the impact of MCFA diets on cardiac functions [137]. Compared to LCFA, a 2-week administration of a 38% fat diet containing mostly MCFA positively altered plasma lipids and potentially improved cardiac function as well as insulinemia in adult type 2 diabetics. However, this diet did not significantly impact cardiac TG load or cardiac steatosis [137].

Nevertheless, the consumption of MCT is systematically associated with higher energy expenditure compared to LCT. Solid evidences support the feasibility of using MCT preparations for nutritional trials against obesity, considering their sources, their flexible use and their safety. Compared to soybean oil (providing high amounts of LCT), coconut oil, which is the most easily obtained source of MCT, improves (in synergy with exercise) the cardiometabolic and anthropometric profiles (including waist circumference) of women presenting unhealthy abdominal obesity [138]. However, coconut oil contains other compounds such as antioxidant polyphenols also known to improve metabolic profile by lowering LDL and VLDL while increasing HDL [138,139]. St-Onge and collaborators demonstrated that consumption of a combination of MCT, phytosterols and omega-3-enriched flaxseed oil for 1 month compared to olive oil or beef tallow-based diets, led to improvement in plasma lipid profile in both healthy and overweight women as well as in MHO men [140,141]. In addition, MCT oils can be incorporated into a weight loss program without any adverse effects on metabolic health [142]. Table 1 summarizes the main studies that have revealed the antiobesity potential of MCT.

Consistent with these observations, a recent meta-analysis of randomized controlled trials, combining a broad spectrum of publication resources, showed that MCT administered for 3 weeks or more reduced body weight (−0.51 kg average), waist circumference (−1.46 cm average), hip circumference (−0.79 cm average), total body fat, total subcutaneous fat and visceral fat in comparison with LCT and despite high heterogeneity [143]. Such observations strongly support the relevance of using MCT to modulate body weight and metabolic profile in MUHO patients.

Table 1. Antiobesity effects of MCT and MCFA.

Model	Main Reported Effects for MCT or MCFA	References
Hepatocyte	Downregulated expression of genes involved in DNL and fatty acid uptake; promoted lipid catabolism; reduced steatosis; prevented deleterious lipid accumulation	[108,113,115]
Rat	Lowered TG accumulation in the liver; reduced alcoholic steatosis	[116]
Rat	Decreased body weight gain and body fat mass; lowered fat accumulation and visceral adiposity; did not affect protein assimilation nor metabolism	[107,117]
Rat	Resulted in a higher induction of oxygen consumption and thermogenesis	[107]
Human	Significantly increased postprandial oxygen consumption, energy expenditure, and fat oxidation, in a MCT dose-dependent manner and at a greater extend for lower BMIs	[119–122,135,136,142,144]
Human	Decreased global adiposity, body fat, and whole-body subcutaneous adipose tissue loss, waist circumference; significantly lowered rate of variation of body fat percentage	[127,130,134]
Human	Did not improve global adiposity	[135]
Human	Did not elevate postprandial circulating TG; did not modulate glucose response, insulinemia and circulating TG levels; lowered LDL/HDL ratio, total and HDL-cholesterol; improved cardiometabolic profile	[129,134,136,138,141]
Human	Promoted rise in leptin and peptide YY	[129]

MCT: medium chain triglyceride; MCFA: medium chain fatty acid; DNL: *de novo* lipogenesis; TG: triglyceride; BMI: body mass index; LDL: low density lipoprotein; HDL: high density lipoprotein; Peptide YY: peptide tyrosine tyrosine.

4.2.3. MCT-Supplemented Diets Improve Gut Microbiota and Intestinal Health

MCT are known for their antimicrobial properties. MCT, as well as their constituent MCFA, when provided by maternal milk (along with endogenous long chain unsaturated monoglycerides), exerted antimicrobial effects on the gastro-intestinal tract of suckling neonates and contributed to reduce pathogen transmission [145–147]. Moreover, MCT and MCFA were also shown to reduce proliferation of certain species of *Malassezia*, an infectious fungus widespread in hospitals [148].

Kono and collaborators demonstrated that MCT could prevent LPS-mediated endotoxemia. Rats were fed MCT or corn oil (a source of LCT) by daily gavage for 1 week, prior to an intravenously acute dose of endotoxic LPS. Interestingly, while LPS injection led to mortality in corn oil-fed animals, this mortality was prevented in MCT-fed rats [149]. Furthermore, in contrast with the corn oil/LPS group, the MCT/LPS group showed a lower liver injury and inflammation as revealed by a significant decrease in CD14 and tumor necrosis factor alpha (TNF-α) expression in Kupffer cells. In parallel with this, while the corn oil/LPS combination induced a significant increase of intestinal permeability compared to corn oil without LPS, the MCT/LPS combination was associated with a significant improvement of intestinal permeability [149]. In addition, MCT gavage prevented intestinal atrophy (a current problem occurring during parenteral nutrition) and massively reduced (10-fold) the bacterial fecal content [149]. This study showed that MCT administration prevented CD14-activation dependent endotoxemia mediated by LPS, a model consensually associated to obesity and metabolic syndrome.

Most studies on juvenile models use piglets because of their similarities with humans during intestinal development [150–153]. MCT supplements can be used as alternatives to antibiotics against certain types of porcine colitis [152,154,155]. MCT-fed piglets had a better gastro-intestinal health, with improved intestinal apoptotic index and mucosal turnover, and lowered intraepithelial lymphocyte infiltration (reflecting reduced local inflammation and diminished immune response) compared to controls [152,153]. Furthermore, piglets fed with MCT supplements display a marked modulation of microbial gastric and intestinal populations [152,153,156]. This contributed to a decrease in intestinal inflammation and to an improvement of gut health and integrity [157] with a direct impact on the gut bacteria from Gram-positive (low LPS) and Gram-negative (high LPS) subdivisions [156]. Another study showed that dietary organic acids (OA) and MCFA changed the gut microbiota of weaning piglets [151]. MCFA were shown to reduce the pH of the digesta because of diminished bacterial acid production. OA and MCFA altered the population distribution of *Bacteroidetes / Porphyromonas / Prevotella* phyla and *Clostridia / Streptococcus* genus in a tissue specific manner (stomach, jejunum, ileum and colon). MCFA specifically modulated the bacterial populations in specific regions such as jejunum and colon by promoting the growth of *Escherichia / Hafnia / Shigella* bacteria and *Clostridia* genus [151]. Combining SCFA and MCFA may constitute a potent tool for the management of optimal gut microbiota. This combination as well as other sources of MCT including coconuts oils, functional mixed oils, or purified MCT oils may be therefore useful for remodelling MUHO gut microbiota and improving metabolically unhealthy obesity. Table 2 summarizes these advances.

Table 2. Antimicrobial and gut-managing effects of MCT.

Model	Main Reported Effects	References
Malassezia	Supressed growth of *M. sympodialis* and *M. furfur*	[148]
Rats	Prevented acute LPS administration-induced mortality, liver injury, liver inflammation, gut impermeability and injury; blunted LPS-induced endotoxemia	[149]
Rats	Significantly blunted TNBS-induced colitis; improved both colonic MPO activity and colonocytes-expressed inflammatory markers	[155]
Rats	Improved gut integrity; modulated immune response to LPS; improved intestinal secretion of IgA	[158]
Piglets	Lowered intestinal pH, in synergy with OA; modulated several gut microbial taxa, potentially preventing postweaning diarrhea	[151]

M. sympodialis: *Malassezia sympodialis*; *M. furfur*: *Malassezia furfur*; LPS: lipopolysaccharide; TNBS: 2,4,6-trinitrobenzene sulphonic acid; MPO: myeloperoxidase.

5. Synthesis and Conclusions

This review aimed to highlight several aspects underlying the condition of obese subjects, which can be either metabolically unhealthy obese (MUHO) or metabolically healthy obese (MHO). While a panel of criteria serves to define the MUHO state, those defining metabolically healthy obesity remain the subject of current discussions. We underline the necessity of better defining the potential role of gut microbiota in the establishment of MUHO or MHO states. Moreover, we believe that gut microbiota structure may not only serve as a biomarker of those metabolic states, but can also be subjected to a diet-induced remodelling, modifying in turn the metabolic status of patients (MUHO *vs.* MHO or lean state). Dietary MCT, taken alone or with other supplements (such as prebiotics, probiotics, organic acids, *etc.*) could be used as anti-obesity interventions, in regards to their capacity to prevent intestinal permeability/endotoxemia by remodeling gut microbiota, and to prevent unhealthy storage by improving the lipid catabolism/anabolism balance. Figure 1 illustrates this concept.

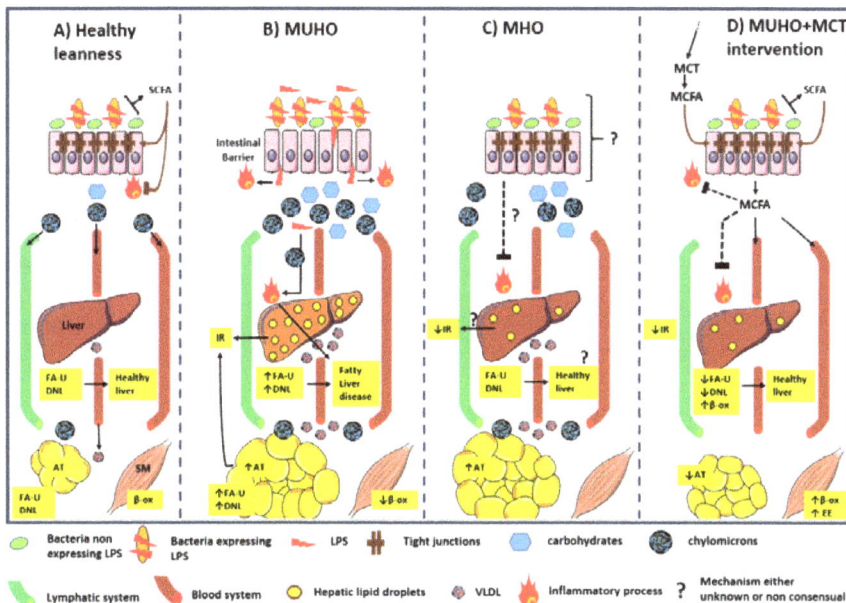

Figure 1. Crosstalk between gut, liver and peripheral metabolic tissues under 4 metabolic states. Under condition of healthy leanness (**A**) an optimal relative abundance of LPS-expressing *vs.* non-expressing bacteria contribute to gut impermeability, low intestinal and hepatic inflammation, and non-obesogenic/steatogenic nutrient supply. Under MUHO conditions (**B**), an elevation in the relative abundance of LPS-expressing bacteria (Gram-negative) induces LPS infiltration and leads to altered intestinal barrier integrity, local inflammation, liver injury and endotoxemia. At the same time, a high fat and carbohydrate supply contributes to adiposity, hepatic steatosis and peripheral insulin resistance. In MHO subjects (**C**), despite an adiposity sustained by a rich diet, a balanced gut microbiota would contribute to maintain intestinal and systemic metabolic health, prevent endotoxemia, and lower hepatic injury and peripheral insulin resistance. Our hypothetical model (**D**) suggests that diet MCT supplementation for MUHO subjects may facilitate a shift towards an MHO-like profile by improving lipid catabolism and lowering adiposity in part, but also by remodelling the gut microbiota into a metabolically beneficial structure. SCFA: short chain fatty acids; FA-U: Fatty acid uptake; AT: adipose tissue; DNL: *de novo* lipogenesis; SM: skeletal muscle; MUHO: metabolically unhealthy obese (or obesity); IR: Insulin resistance; β-ox: beta-oxidation; MHO: metabolically healthy obese (or obesity); MCT: medium chain triglycerides; MCFA: medium chain fatty acids; LPS: lipopolysaccharides; VLDL: very low density lipoproteins.

Acknowledgments: The authors are grateful to Rodolphe Soret and Quentin Escoula (UQAM, Canada) for suggestions, corrections and advice. Finally, authors are grateful to SERVIER Medical Art [159] creators for allowing free access to their images bank, which was used to construct Figure 1.

Author Contributions: S.A.R., A.D.K., K.F.B., and C.M. conceived, designed, revised and illustrated the ideas and the manuscript, and all approved its final version.

Conflicts of Interest: The authors declare no conflicts of interest.

References

1. Smith, K.B.; Smith, M.S. Obesity statistics. *Prim. Care* **2016**, *43*, 121–135. [CrossRef] [PubMed]
2. Ng, M.; Fleming, T.; Robinson, M.; Thomson, B.; Graetz, N.; Margono, C.; Mullany, E.C.; Biryukov, S.; Abbafati, C.; Abera, S.F.; *et al.* Global, regional, and national prevalence of overweight and obesity in children and adults during 1980–2013: A systematic analysis for the global burden of disease study 2013. *Lancet* **2014**, *384*, 766–781. [CrossRef]
3. Haslam, D.W.; James, W.P. Obesity. *Lancet* **2005**, *366*, 1197–1209. [CrossRef]
4. Graffy, P.M.; Pickhardt, P.J. Quantification of hepatic and visceral fat by ct and mr imaging: Relevance to the obesity epidemic, metabolic syndrome and nafld. *Br. J. Radiol.* **2016**, *89*, 20151024. [CrossRef] [PubMed]
5. Grundy, S.M. Metabolic syndrome update. *Trends Cardiovasc. Med.* **2016**, *26*, 364–373. [CrossRef] [PubMed]
6. Hryhorczuk, C.; Sharma, S.; Fulton, S.E. Metabolic disturbances connecting obesity and depression. *Front. Neurosci.* **2013**, *7*, 177. [CrossRef] [PubMed]
7. Reuter, C.P.; Silva, P.T.; Renner, J.D.; Mello, E.D.; Valim, A.R.; Pasa, L.; Silva, R.D.; Burgos, M.S. Dyslipidemia is associated with unfit and overweight-obese children and adolescents. *Arq. Brasil. Cardiol.* **2016**. [CrossRef] [PubMed]
8. Elmaogullari, S.; Tepe, D.; Ucakturk, S.A.; Karaca Kara, F.; Demirel, F. Prevalence of dyslipidemia and associated factors in obese children and adolescents. *J. Clin. Res. Pediatr. Endocrinol.* **2015**, *7*, 228–234. [CrossRef] [PubMed]
9. Cho, Y.; Shore, S.A. Obesity, asthma, and the microbiome. *Physiology* **2016**, *31*, 108–116. [CrossRef] [PubMed]
10. Payab, M.; Amoli, M.M.; Qorbani, M.; Hasani-Ranjbar, S. Adiponectin gene variants and abdominal obesity in an iranian population. *Eat. Weight Disord.* **2016**. [CrossRef] [PubMed]
11. Waleh, M.Q. Impacts of physical activity on the obese. *Prim. Care* **2016**, *43*, 97–107. [CrossRef] [PubMed]
12. Scott, E.M. Circadian clocks, obesity and cardiometabolic function. *Diabetes Obes. Metab.* **2015**, *17*, 84–89. [CrossRef] [PubMed]
13. Klingenberg, L.; Sjodin, A.; Holmback, U.; Astrup, A.; Chaput, J.P. Short sleep duration and its association with energy metabolism. *Obes. Rev. Off. J. Int. Assoc. Stud. Obes.* **2012**, *13*, 565–577. [CrossRef] [PubMed]
14. Choudhury, S.M.; Tan, T.M.; Bloom, S.R. Gastrointestinal hormones and their role in obesity. *Curr. Opin. Endocrinol. Diabetes Obes.* **2016**, *23*, 18–22. [CrossRef] [PubMed]
15. Lee, D.H.; Porta, M.; Jacobs, D.R., Jr.; Vandenberg, L.N. Chlorinated persistent organic pollutants, obesity, and type 2 diabetes. *Endocr. Rev.* **2014**, *35*, 557–601. [CrossRef] [PubMed]
16. Nova, E.; Perez de Heredia, F.; Gomez-Martinez, S.; Marcos, A. The role of probiotics on the microbiota: Effect on obesity. *Nutr. Clin. Pract.* **2016**. [CrossRef] [PubMed]
17. Patterson, E.; Ryan, P.M.; Cryan, J.F.; Dinan, T.G.; Ross, R.P.; Fitzgerald, G.F.; Stanton, C. Gut microbiota, obesity and diabetes. *Postgrad. Med. J.* **2016**. [CrossRef] [PubMed]
18. Drewnowski, A.; Almiron-Roig, E. Frontiers in neuroscience human perceptions and preferences for fat-rich foods. In *Fat Detection: Taste, Texture, and Post Ingestive Effects*; Montmayeur, J.P., Le Coutre, J., Eds.; CRC Press/Taylor & Francis Group, LLC.: Boca Raton, FL, USA, 2010.
19. Strable, M.S.; Ntambi, J.M. Genetic control of *de novo* lipogenesis: Role in diet-induced obesity. *Crit. Rev. Biochem. Mol. Biol.* **2010**, *45*, 199–214. [CrossRef] [PubMed]
20. Ameer, F.; Scandiuzzi, L.; Hasnain, S.; Kalbacher, H.; Zaidi, N. *De novo* lipogenesis in health and disease. *Metabol. Clin. Exp.* **2014**, *63*, 895–902. [CrossRef] [PubMed]
21. Povero, D.; Feldstein, A.E. Novel molecular mechanisms in the development of non-alcoholic steatohepatitis. *Diabetes Metabol. J.* **2016**, *40*, 1–11. [CrossRef] [PubMed]
22. Kaila, B.; Raman, M. Obesity: A review of pathogenesis and management strategies. *Can. J. Gastroenterol.* **2008**, *22*, 61–68. [CrossRef] [PubMed]
23. Rankinen, T.; Zuberi, A.; Chagnon, Y.C.; Weisnagel, S.J.; Argyropoulos, G.; Walts, B.; Perusse, L.; Bouchard, C. The human obesity gene map: The 2005 update. *Obesity* **2006**, *14*, 529–644. [CrossRef] [PubMed]
24. Waterland, R.A.; Travisano, M.; Tahiliani, K.G.; Rached, M.T.; Mirza, S. Methyl donor supplementation prevents transgenerational amplification of obesity. *Int. J. Obes.* **2008**, *32*, 1373–1379. [CrossRef] [PubMed]
25. McAllister, E.J.; Dhurandhar, N.V.; Keith, S.W.; Aronne, L.J.; Barger, J.; Baskin, M.; Benca, R.M.; Biggio, J.; Boggiano, M.M.; Eisenmann, J.C.; *et al.* Ten putative contributors to the obesity epidemic. *Crit. Rev. Food Sci. Nutr.* **2009**, *49*, 868–913. [CrossRef] [PubMed]

26. Kanayama, T.; Kobayashi, N.; Mamiya, S.; Nakanishi, T.; Nishikawa, J. Organotin compounds promote adipocyte differentiation as agonists of the peroxisome proliferator-activated receptor gamma/retinoid X receptor pathway. *Mol. Pharmacol.* **2005**, *67*, 766–774. [CrossRef] [PubMed]

27. Trayhurn, P.; Beattie, J.H. Physiological role of adipose tissue: White adipose tissue as an endocrine and secretory organ. *Proc. Nutr. Soc.* **2001**, *60*, 329–339. [CrossRef] [PubMed]

28. Maachi, M.; Pieroni, L.; Bruckert, E.; Jardel, C.; Fellahi, S.; Hainque, B.; Capeau, J.; Bastard, J.P. Systemic low-grade inflammation is related to both circulating and adipose tissue tnfalpha, leptin and il-6 levels in obese women. *Int. J. Obes. Relat. Metab. Disord.* **2004**, *28*, 993–997. [CrossRef] [PubMed]

29. Grover, S.A.; Kaouache, M.; Rempel, P.; Joseph, L.; Dawes, M.; Lau, D.C.; Lowensteyn, I. Years of life lost and healthy life-years lost from diabetes and cardiovascular disease in overweight and obese people: A modelling study. *Lancet Diabetes Endocrinol.* **2015**, *3*, 114–122. [CrossRef]

30. Roberts, C.K.; Hevener, A.L.; Barnard, R.J. Metabolic syndrome and insulin resistance: Underlying causes and modification by exercise training. *Compr. Physiol.* **2013**, *3*, 1–58. [PubMed]

31. Kyrou, I.; Randeva, H.S.; Weickert, M.O. Clinical problems caused by obesity. In *Endotext*; De Groot, L.J., Beck-Peccoz, P., Chrousos, G., Dungan, K., Grossman, A., Hershman, J.M., Koch, C., McLachlan, R., New, M., Rebar, R., *et al.*, Eds.; MDText.com, Inc.: South Dartmouth, MA, USA, 2000.

32. Poirier, P.; Giles, T.D.; Bray, G.A.; Hong, Y.; Stern, J.S.; Pi-Sunyer, F.X.; Eckel, R.H. Obesity and cardiovascular disease: Pathophysiology, evaluation, and effect of weight loss: An update of the 1997 american heart association scientific statement on obesity and heart disease from the obesity committee of the council on nutrition, physical activity, and metabolism. *Circulation* **2006**, *113*, 898–918. [PubMed]

33. Fabbrini, E.; Sullivan, S.; Klein, S. Obesity and nonalcoholic fatty liver disease: Biochemical, metabolic, and clinical implications. *Hepatology* **2010**, *51*, 679–689. [CrossRef] [PubMed]

34. Samocha-Bonet, D.; Dixit, V.D.; Kahn, C.R.; Leibel, R.L.; Lin, X.; Nieuwdorp, M.; Pietilainen, K.H.; Rabasa-Lhoret, R.; Roden, M.; Scherer, P.E.; *et al.* Metabolically healthy and unhealthy obese—The 2013 stock conference report. *Obes. Rev.* **2014**, *15*, 697–708. [CrossRef] [PubMed]

35. Karelis, A.D. Metabolically healthy but obese individuals. *Lancet* **2008**, *372*, 1281–1283. [CrossRef]

36. Primeau, V.; Coderre, L.; Karelis, A.D.; Brochu, M.; Lavoie, M.E.; Messier, V.; Sladek, R.; Rabasa-Lhoret, R. Characterizing the profile of obese patients who are metabolically healthy. *Int. J. Obes.* **2011**, *35*, 971–981. [CrossRef] [PubMed]

37. Velho, S.; Paccaud, F.; Waeber, G.; Vollenweider, P.; Marques-Vidal, P. Metabolically healthy obesity: Different prevalences using different criteria. *Eur. J. Clin. Nutr.* **2010**, *64*, 1043–1051. [CrossRef] [PubMed]

38. Wildman, R.P.; Muntner, P.; Reynolds, K.; McGinn, A.P.; Rajpathak, S.; Wylie-Rosett, J.; Sowers, M.R. The obese without cardiometabolic risk factor clustering and the normal weight with cardiometabolic risk factor clustering: Prevalence and correlates of 2 phenotypes among the US population (NHANES 1999–2004). *Arch. Intern. Med.* **2008**, *168*, 1617–1624. [CrossRef] [PubMed]

39. Plourde, G.; Karelis, A.D. Current issues in the identification and treatment of metabolically healthy but obese individuals. *Nutr. Metab. Cardiovasc. Dis.* **2014**, *24*, 455–459. [CrossRef] [PubMed]

40. Eckel, N.; Meidtner, K.; Kalle-Uhlmann, T.; Stefan, N.; Schulze, M.B. Metabolically healthy obesity and cardiovascular events: A systematic review and meta-analysis. *Eur. J. Prev. Cardiol.* **2015**. [CrossRef] [PubMed]

41. Loos, R.J. Integrating publicly available genome-wide association data to study the genetic basis of metabolically healthy obese and metabolically obese but normal-weight individuals. *Diabetes* **2014**, *63*, 4004–4007. [CrossRef] [PubMed]

42. Berezina, A.; Belyaeva, O.; Berkovich, O.; Baranova, E.; Karonova, T.; Bazhenova, E.; Brovin, D.; Grineva, E.; Shlyakhto, E. Prevalence, risk factors, and genetic traits in metabolically healthy and unhealthy obese individuals. *Biomed. Res. Int.* **2015**, *2015*, 548734. [CrossRef] [PubMed]

43. Kandasamy, A.D.; Sung, M.M.; Boisvenue, J.J.; Barr, A.J.; Dyck, J.R. Adiponectin gene therapy ameliorates high-fat, high-sucrose diet-induced metabolic perturbations in mice. *Nutr. Diabetes* **2012**, *2*, e45. [CrossRef] [PubMed]

44. Hur, K.Y.; Lee, M.S. Gut microbiota and metabolic disorders. *Diabetes Metab. J.* **2015**, *39*, 198–203. [CrossRef] [PubMed]

45. Guinane, C.M.; Cotter, P.D. Role of the gut microbiota in health and chronic gastrointestinal disease: Understanding a hidden metabolic organ. *Ther. Adv. Gastroenterol.* **2013**, *6*, 295–308. [CrossRef] [PubMed]

46. Chow, J.; Lee, S.M.; Shen, Y.; Khosravi, A.; Mazmanian, S.K. Host-bacterial symbiosis in health and disease. *Adv. Immunol.* **2010**, *107*, 243–274. [PubMed]

47. Kelly, C.J.; Zheng, L.; Campbell, E.L.; Saeedi, B.; Scholz, C.C.; Bayless, A.J.; Wilson, K.E.; Glover, L.E.; Kominsky, D.J.; Magnuson, A.; et al. Crosstalk between microbiota-derived short-chain fatty acids and intestinal epithelial hif augments tissue barrier function. *Cell Host Microb.* **2015**, *17*, 662–671. [CrossRef] [PubMed]

48. Den Besten, G.; Lange, K.; Havinga, R.; van Dijk, T.H.; Gerding, A.; van Eunen, K.; Muller, M.; Groen, A.K.; Hooiveld, G.J.; Bakker, B.M.; et al. Gut-derived short-chain fatty acids are vividly assimilated into host carbohydrates and lipids. *Am. J. Physiol. Gastrointest. Liver Physiol.* **2013**, *305*, G900–G910. [CrossRef] [PubMed]

49. Den Besten, G.; van Eunen, K.; Groen, A.K.; Venema, K.; Reijngoud, D.J.; Bakker, B.M. The role of short-chain fatty acids in the interplay between diet, gut microbiota, and host energy metabolism. *J. Lipid Res.* **2013**, *54*, 2325–2340. [CrossRef] [PubMed]

50. Singh, V.; Chassaing, B.; Zhang, L.; San Yeoh, B.; Xiao, X.; Kumar, M.; Baker, M.T.; Cai, J.; Walker, R.; Borkowski, K.; et al. Microbiota-dependent hepatic lipogenesis mediated by stearoyl coa desaturase 1 (scd1) promotes metabolic syndrome in tlr5-deficient mice. *Cell Metab.* **2015**, *22*, 983–996. [CrossRef] [PubMed]

51. LeBlanc, J.G.; Milani, C.; de Giori, G.S.; Sesma, F.; van Sinderen, D.; Ventura, M. Bacteria as vitamin suppliers to their host: A gut microbiota perspective. *Curr. Opin. Biotechnol.* **2013**, *24*, 160–168. [CrossRef] [PubMed]

52. Janssen, A.W.; Kersten, S. The role of the gut microbiota in metabolic health. *Fed. Am. Soc. Exp. Biol. J.* **2015**, *29*, 3111–3123. [CrossRef] [PubMed]

53. Everard, A.; Cani, P.D. Diabetes, obesity and gut microbiota. *Best Pract. Res. Clin. Gastroenterol.* **2013**, *27*, 73–83. [CrossRef] [PubMed]

54. Turnbaugh, P.J.; Ley, R.E.; Mahowald, M.A.; Magrini, V.; Mardis, E.R.; Gordon, J.I. An obesity-associated gut microbiome with increased capacity for energy harvest. *Nature* **2006**, *444*, 1027–1031. [CrossRef] [PubMed]

55. Cani, P.D.; Amar, J.; Iglesias, M.A.; Poggi, M.; Knauf, C.; Bastelica, D.; Neyrinck, A.M.; Fava, F.; Tuohy, K.M.; Chabo, C.; et al. Metabolic endotoxemia initiates obesity and insulin resistance. *Diabetes* **2007**, *56*, 1761–1772. [CrossRef] [PubMed]

56. Backhed, F.; Manchester, J.K.; Semenkovich, C.F.; Gordon, J.I. Mechanisms underlying the resistance to diet-induced obesity in germ-free mice. *Proc. Natl. Acad. Sci. USA* **2007**, *104*, 979–984. [CrossRef] [PubMed]

57. Cani, P.D.; Bibiloni, R.; Knauf, C.; Waget, A.; Neyrinck, A.M.; Delzenne, N.M.; Burcelin, R. Changes in gut microbiota control metabolic endotoxemia-induced inflammation in high-fat diet-induced obesity and diabetes in mice. *Diabetes* **2008**, *57*, 1470–1481. [CrossRef] [PubMed]

58. Amar, J.; Burcelin, R.; Ruidavets, J.B.; Cani, P.D.; Fauvel, J.; Alessi, M.C.; Chamontin, B.; Ferrieres, J. Energy intake is associated with endotoxemia in apparently healthy men. *Am. J. Clin. Nutr.* **2008**, *87*, 1219–1223. [PubMed]

59. Maron, D.F.; Smith, T.J.S.; Nachman, K.E. Restrictions on antimicrobial use in food animal production: An international regulatory and economic survey. *Glob. Health* **2013**, *9*, 48. [CrossRef] [PubMed]

60. Cazer, C.L.; Volkova, V.V.; Grohn, Y.T. Use of pharmacokinetic modeling to assess antimicrobial pressure on enteric bacteria of beef cattle fed chlortetracycline for growth promotion, disease control, or treatment. *Foodborne Pathog. Dis.* **2014**, *11*, 403–411. [CrossRef] [PubMed]

61. Van Boeckel, T.P.; Brower, C.; Gilbert, M.; Grenfell, B.T.; Levin, S.A.; Robinson, T.P.; Teillant, A.; Laxminarayan, R. Global trends in antimicrobial use in food animals. *Proc. Natl. Acad. Sci. USA* **2015**, *112*, 5649–5654. [CrossRef] [PubMed]

62. Johnson, T.A.; Stedtfeld, R.D.; Wang, Q.; Cole, J.R.; Hashsham, S.A.; Looft, T.; Zhu, Y.G.; Tiedje, J.M. Clusters of antibiotic resistance genes enriched together stay together in swine agriculture. *mBio* **2016**. [CrossRef] [PubMed]

63. Cani, P.D.; Possemiers, S.; Van de Wiele, T.; Guiot, Y.; Everard, A.; Rottier, O.; Geurts, L.; Naslain, D.; Neyrinck, A.; Lambert, D.M.; et al. Changes in gut microbiota control inflammation in obese mice through a mechanism involving glp-2-driven improvement of gut permeability. *Gut* **2009**, *58*, 1091–1103. [CrossRef] [PubMed]

64. Arslan, N. Obesity, fatty liver disease and intestinal microbiota. *World J. Gastroenterol.* **2014**, *20*, 16452–16463. [CrossRef] [PubMed]

65. Cani, P.D. Crosstalk between the gut microbiota and the endocannabinoid system: Impact on the gut barrier function and the adipose tissue. *Clin. Microbiol. Infect.* **2012**, *18*, 50–53. [CrossRef] [PubMed]

66. Membrez, M.; Blancher, F.; Jaquet, M.; Bibiloni, R.; Cani, P.D.; Burcelin, R.G.; Corthesy, I.; Mace, K.; Chou, C.J. Gut microbiota modulation with norfloxacin and ampicillin enhances glucose tolerance in mice. *Fed. Am. Soc. Exp. Biol. J.* **2008**, *22*, 2416–2426. [CrossRef] [PubMed]

67. Pereira, S.S.; Alvarez-Leite, J.I. Low-grade inflammation, obesity, and diabetes. *Curr. Obes. Rep.* **2014**, *3*, 422–431. [CrossRef] [PubMed]

68. Ley, R.E.; Backhed, F.; Turnbaugh, P.; Lozupone, C.A.; Knight, R.D.; Gordon, J.I. Obesity alters gut microbial ecology. *Proc. Natl. Acad. Sci. USA* **2005**, *102*, 11070–11075. [CrossRef] [PubMed]

69. Delzenne, N.M.; Cani, P.D. Interaction between obesity and the gut microbiota: Relevance in nutrition. *Annu. Rev. Nutr.* **2011**, *31*, 15–31. [CrossRef] [PubMed]

70. Abdallah Ismail, N.; Ragab, S.H.; Abd Elbaky, A.; Shoeib, A.R.; Alhosary, Y.; Fekry, D. Frequency of firmicutes and bacteroidetes in gut microbiota in obese and normal weight egyptian children and adults. *Arch. Med. Sci.* **2011**, *7*, 501–507. [CrossRef] [PubMed]

71. Clarke, S.F.; Murphy, E.F.; Nilaweera, K.; Ross, P.R.; Shanahan, F.; O'Toole, P.W.; Cotter, P.D. The gut microbiota and its relationship to diet and obesity: New insights. *Gut Microb.* **2012**, *3*, 186–202. [CrossRef] [PubMed]

72. Delzenne, N.M.; Neyrinck, A.M.; Backhed, F.; Cani, P.D. Targeting gut microbiota in obesity: Effects of prebiotics and probiotics. *Nat. Rev. Endocrinol.* **2011**, *7*, 639–646. [CrossRef] [PubMed]

73. Delzenne, N.M.; Neyrinck, A.M.; Cani, P.D. Modulation of the gut microbiota by nutrients with prebiotic properties: Consequences for host health in the context of obesity and metabolic syndrome. *Microb. Cell Fact.* **2011**, *10*, S10. [CrossRef] [PubMed]

74. Furet, J.P.; Kong, L.C.; Tap, J.; Poitou, C.; Basdevant, A.; Bouillot, J.L.; Mariat, D.; Corthier, G.; Dore, J.; Henegar, C.; *et al.* Differential adaptation of human gut microbiota to bariatric surgery-induced weight loss: Links with metabolic and low-grade inflammation markers. *Diabetes* **2010**, *59*, 3049–3057. [CrossRef] [PubMed]

75. Blaut, M. Gut microbiota and energy balance: Role in obesity. *Proc. Nutr. Soc.* **2015**, *74*, 227–234. [CrossRef] [PubMed]

76. Turnbaugh, P.J.; Ridaura, V.K.; Faith, J.J.; Rey, F.E.; Knight, R.; Gordon, J.I. The effect of diet on the human gut microbiome: A metagenomic analysis in humanized gnotobiotic mice. *Sci. Transl. Med.* **2009**, *1*, 6ra14. [CrossRef] [PubMed]

77. Ridaura, V.K.; Faith, J.J.; Rey, F.E.; Cheng, J.; Duncan, A.E.; Kau, A.L.; Griffin, N.W.; Lombard, V.; Henrissat, B.; Bain, J.R.; *et al.* Gut microbiota from twins discordant for obesity modulate metabolism in mice. *Science* **2013**, *341*, 1241214. [CrossRef] [PubMed]

78. Serino, M.; Luche, E.; Gres, S.; Baylac, A.; Berge, M.; Cenac, C.; Waget, A.; Klopp, P.; Iacovoni, J.; Klopp, C.; *et al.* Metabolic adaptation to a high-fat diet is associated with a change in the gut microbiota. *Gut* **2012**, *61*, 543–553. [CrossRef] [PubMed]

79. Neyrinck, A.M.; Van Hee, V.F.; Piront, N.; De Backer, F.; Toussaint, O.; Cani, P.D.; Delzenne, N.M. Wheat-derived arabinoxylan oligosaccharides with prebiotic effect increase satietogenic gut peptides and reduce metabolic endotoxemia in diet-induced obese mice. *Nutr. Diabetes* **2012**, *2*, e28. [CrossRef] [PubMed]

80. Sommer, F.; Stahlman, M.; Ilkayeva, O.; Arnemo, J.M.; Kindberg, J.; Josefsson, J.; Newgard, C.B.; Frobert, O.; Backhed, F. The gut microbiota modulates energy metabolism in the hibernating brown bear *Ursus arctos*. *Cell Rep.* **2016**, *14*, 1655–1661. [CrossRef] [PubMed]

81. Arinell, K.; Sahdo, B.; Evans, A.L.; Arnemo, J.M.; Baandrup, U.; Frobert, O. Brown bears (*Ursus arctos*) seem resistant to atherosclerosis despite highly elevated plasma lipids during hibernation and active state. *Clin. Transl. Sci.* **2012**, *5*, 269–272. [CrossRef] [PubMed]

82. Mar Rodriguez, M.; Perez, D.; Javier Chaves, F.; Esteve, E.; Marin-Garcia, P.; Xifra, G.; Vendrell, J.; Jove, M.; Pamplona, R.; Ricart, W.; *et al.* Obesity changes the human gut mycobiome. *Sci. Rep.* **2015**, *5*, 14600. [CrossRef] [PubMed]

83. McGuire, M.T.; Wing, R.R.; Hill, J.O. The prevalence of weight loss maintenance among american adults. *Int. J. Obes. Relat. Metab. Disord.* **1999**, *23*, 1314–1319. [CrossRef] [PubMed]

84. Field, A.E.; Malspeis, S.; Willett, W.C. Weight cycling and mortality among middle-aged or older women. *Arch. Intern. Med.* **2009**, *169*, 881–886. [CrossRef] [PubMed]

85. Hamm, P.; Shekelle, R.B.; Stamler, J. Large fluctuations in body weight during young adulthood and twenty-five-year risk of coronary death in men. *Am. J. Epidemiol.* **1989**, *129*, 312–318. [PubMed]

86. Chevrier, J.; Dewailly, E.; Ayotte, P.; Mauriege, P.; Despres, J.P.; Tremblay, A. Body weight loss increases plasma and adipose tissue concentrations of potentially toxic pollutants in obese individuals. *Int. J. Obes. Relat. Metab. Disord.* **2000**, *24*, 1272–1278. [CrossRef] [PubMed]

87. Hue, O.; Marcotte, J.; Berrigan, F.; Simoneau, M.; Dore, J.; Marceau, P.; Marceau, S.; Tremblay, A.; Teasdale, N. Increased plasma levels of toxic pollutants accompanying weight loss induced by hypocaloric diet or by bariatric surgery. *Obes. Surg.* **2006**, *16*, 1145–1154. [CrossRef] [PubMed]

88. Kim, M.J.; Marchand, P.; Henegar, C.; Antignac, J.P.; Alili, R.; Poitou, C.; Bouillot, J.L.; Basdevant, A.; Le Bizec, B.; Barouki, R.; *et al.* Fate and complex pathogenic effects of dioxins and polychlorinated biphenyls in obese subjects before and after drastic weight loss. *Environ. Health Perspect.* **2011**, *119*, 377–383. [CrossRef] [PubMed]

89. Kantartzis, K.; Machann, J.; Schick, F.; Rittig, K.; Machicao, F.; Fritsche, A.; Haring, H.U.; Stefan, N. Effects of a lifestyle intervention in metabolically benign and malign obesity. *Diabetologia* **2011**, *54*, 864–868. [CrossRef] [PubMed]

90. Shin, M.J.; Hyun, Y.J.; Kim, O.Y.; Kim, J.Y.; Jang, Y.; Lee, J.H. Weight loss effect on inflammation and ldl oxidation in metabolically healthy but obese (mho) individuals: Low inflammation and ldl oxidation in mho women. *Int. J. Obes.* **2006**, *30*, 1529–1534. [CrossRef] [PubMed]

91. McLaughlin, T.; Abbasi, F.; Lamendola, C.; Liang, L.; Reaven, G.; Schaaf, P.; Reaven, P. Differentiation between obesity and insulin resistance in the association with c-reactive protein. *Circulation* **2002**, *106*, 2908–2912. [CrossRef] [PubMed]

92. Janiszewski, P.M.; Ross, R. Effects of weight loss among metabolically healthy obese men and women. *Diabetes Care* **2010**, *33*, 1957–1959. [CrossRef] [PubMed]

93. Cui, Z.; Truesdale, K.P.; Bradshaw, P.T.; Cai, J.; Stevens, J. Three-year weight change and cardiometabolic risk factors in obese and normal weight adults who are metabolically healthy: The atherosclerosis risk in communities study. *Int. J. Obes.* **2015**, *39*, 1203–1208. [CrossRef] [PubMed]

94. Dalzill, C.; Nigam, A.; Juneau, M.; Guilbeault, V.; Latour, E.; Mauriege, P.; Gayda, M. Intensive lifestyle intervention improves cardiometabolic and exercise parameters in metabolically healthy obese and metabolically unhealthy obese individuals. *Can. J. Cardiol.* **2014**, *30*, 434–440. [CrossRef] [PubMed]

95. Liu, R.H.; Wharton, S.; Sharma, A.M.; Ardern, C.I.; Kuk, J.L. Influence of a clinical lifestyle-based weight loss program on the metabolic risk profile of metabolically normal and abnormal obese adults. *Obesity* **2013**, *21*, 1533–1539. [CrossRef] [PubMed]

96. Sesti, G.; Folli, F.; Perego, L.; Hribal, M.L.; Pontiroli, A.E. Effects of weight loss in metabolically healthy obese subjects after laparoscopic adjustable gastric banding and hypocaloric diet. *PLoS ONE* **2011**, *6*, e17737. [CrossRef] [PubMed]

97. Gilardini, L.; Vallone, L.; Cottafava, R.; Redaelli, G.; Croci, M.; Conti, A.; Pasqualinotto, L.; Invitti, C. Insulin sensitivity deteriorates after short-term lifestyle intervention in the insulin sensitive phenotype of obesity. *Obes. Facts* **2012**, *5*, 68–76. [CrossRef] [PubMed]

98. Karelis, A.D.; Messier, V.; Brochu, M.; Rabasa-Lhoret, R. Metabolically healthy but obese women: Effect of an energy-restricted diet. *Diabetologia* **2008**, *51*, 1752–1754. [CrossRef] [PubMed]

99. Evangelou, P.; Tzotzas, T.; Christou, G.; Elisaf, M.S.; Kiortsis, D.N. Does the presence of metabolic syndrome influence weight loss in obese and overweight women? *Metab. Syndr. Relat. Disord.* **2010**, *8*, 173–178. [CrossRef] [PubMed]

100. Nagao, K.; Yanagita, T. Bioactive lipids in metabolic syndrome. *Prog. Lipid Res.* **2008**, *47*, 127–146. [CrossRef] [PubMed]

101. Nagao, K.; Yanagita, T. Medium-chain fatty acids: Functional lipids for the prevention and treatment of the metabolic syndrome. *Pharmacol. Res.* **2010**, *61*, 208–212. [CrossRef] [PubMed]

102. Babayan, V.K. Medium chain triglycerides and structured lipids. *Lipids* **1987**, *22*, 417–420. [CrossRef] [PubMed]

103. Bach, A.C.; Babayan, V.K. Medium-chain triglycerides: An update. *Am. J. Clin. Nutr.* **1982**, *36*, 950–962. [PubMed]

104. Jensen, R.G. The composition of bovine milk lipids: January 1995 to december 2000. *J. Dairy Sci.* **2002**, *85*, 295–350. [CrossRef]

105. Papamandjaris, A.A.; MacDougall, D.E.; Jones, P.J. Medium chain fatty acid metabolism and energy expenditure: Obesity treatment implications. *Life Sci.* **1998**, *62*, 1203–1215. [CrossRef]

106. Marten, B.; Pfeuffer, M.; Schrezenmeir, J. Medium-chain triglycerides. *Int. Dairy J.* **2006**, *16*, 1374–1382. [CrossRef]

107. Noguchi, O.; Takeuchi, H.; Kubota, F.; Tsuji, H.; Aoyama, T. Larger diet-induced thermogenesis and less body fat accumulation in rats fed medium-chain triacylglycerols than in those fed long-chain triacylglycerols. *J. Nutr. Sci. Vitaminol.* **2002**, *48*, 524–529. [CrossRef] [PubMed]

108. Akpa, M.M.; Point, F.; Sawadogo, S.; Radenne, A.; Mounier, C. Inhibition of insulin and t3-induced fatty acid synthase by hexanoate. *Lipids* **2010**, *45*, 997–1009. [CrossRef] [PubMed]

109. Kersten, S. Mechanisms of nutritional and hormonal regulation of lipogenesis. *EMBO Rep.* **2001**, *2*, 282–286. [CrossRef] [PubMed]

110. Ambati, S.; Li, Q.; Rayalam, S.; Hartzell, D.L.; Della-Fera, M.A.; Hamrick, M.W.; Baile, C.A. Central leptin *versus* ghrelin: Effects on bone marrow adiposity and gene expression. *Endocrine* **2010**, *37*, 115–123. [CrossRef] [PubMed]

111. Berlanga, A.; Guiu-Jurado, E.; Porras, J.A.; Auguet, T. Molecular pathways in non-alcoholic fatty liver disease. *Clin. Exp. Gastroenterol.* **2014**, *7*, 221–239. [PubMed]

112. Goodridge, A.G.; Thurmond, D.C.; Baillie, R.A.; Hodnett, D.W.; Xu, G. Nutritional and hormonal regulation of the gene for malic enzyme. *Z. Ernahrungswissenschaft* **1998**, *37*, 8–13.

113. Roncero, C.; Goodridge, A.G. Hexanoate and octanoate inhibit transcription of the malic enzyme and fatty acid synthase genes in chick embryo hepatocytes in culture. *J. Biol. Chem.* **1992**, *267*, 14918–14927. [PubMed]

114. Thurmond, D.C.; Baillie, R.A.; Goodridge, A.G. Regulation of the action of steroid/thyroid hormone receptors by medium-chain fatty acids. *J. Biol. Chem.* **1998**, *273*, 15373–15381. [CrossRef] [PubMed]

115. Wang, B.; Fu, J.; Li, L.; Gong, D.; Wen, X.; Yu, P.; Zeng, Z. Medium-chain fatty acid reduces lipid accumulation by regulating expression of lipid-sensing genes in human liver cells with steatosis. *Int. J. Food Sci. Nutr.* **2016**, *67*, 288–297. [CrossRef] [PubMed]

116. Lieber, C.S.; Lefevre, A.; Spritz, N.; Feinman, L.; DeCarli, L.M. Difference in hepatic metabolism of long- and medium-chain fatty acids: The role of fatty acid chain length in the production of the alcoholic fatty liver. *J. Clin. Investig.* **1967**, *46*, 1451–1460. [CrossRef] [PubMed]

117. Ling, P.R.; Hamawy, K.J.; Moldawer, L.L.; Istfan, N.; Bistrian, B.R.; Blackburn, G.L. Evaluation of the protein quality of diets containing medium- and long-chain triglyceride in healthy rats. *J. Nutr.* **1986**, *116*, 343–349. [PubMed]

118. Traul, K.A.; Driedger, A.; Ingle, D.L.; Nakhasi, D. Review of the toxicologic properties of medium-chain triglycerides. *Food Chem. Toxicol.* **2000**, *38*, 79–98. [CrossRef]

119. Hill, J.O.; Peters, J.C.; Yang, D.; Sharp, T.; Kaler, M.; Abumrad, N.N.; Greene, H.L. Thermogenesis in humans during overfeeding with medium-chain triglycerides. *Metab. Clin. Exp.* **1989**, *38*, 641–648. [CrossRef]

120. Seaton, T.B.; Welle, S.L.; Warenko, M.K.; Campbell, R.G. Thermic effect of medium-chain and long-chain triglycerides in man. *Am. J. Clin. Nutr.* **1986**, *44*, 630–634. [PubMed]

121. Scalfi, L.; Coltorti, A.; Contaldo, F. Postprandial thermogenesis in lean and obese subjects after meals supplemented with medium-chain and long-chain triglycerides. *Am. J. Clin. Nutr.* **1991**, *53*, 1130–1133. [PubMed]

122. Dulloo, A.G.; Fathi, M.; Mensi, N.; Girardier, L. Twenty-four-hour energy expenditure and urinary catecholamines of humans consuming low-to-moderate amounts of medium-chain triglycerides: A dose-response study in a human respiratory chamber. *Eur. J. Clin. Nutr.* **1996**, *50*, 152–158. [PubMed]

123. Ishizawa, R.; Masuda, K.; Sakata, S.; Nakatani, A. Effects of different fatty acid chain lengths on fatty acid oxidation-related protein expression levels in rat skeletal muscles. *J. Oleo Sci.* **2015**, *64*, 415–421. [CrossRef] [PubMed]

124. Binnert, C.; Pachiaudi, C.; Beylot, M.; Hans, D.; Vandermander, J.; Chantre, P.; Riou, J.P.; Laville, M. Influence of human obesity on the metabolic fate of dietary long- and medium-chain triacylglycerols. *Am. J. Clin. Nutr.* **1998**, *67*, 595–601. [PubMed]

125. Nagata, J.; Kasai, M.; Watanabe, S.; Ikeda, I.; Saito, M. Effects of highly purified structured lipids containing medium-chain fatty acids and linoleic acid on lipid profiles in rats. *Biosci. Biotechnol. Biochem.* **2003**, *67*, 1937–1943. [CrossRef] [PubMed]

126. Nagata, J.; Kasai, M.; Negishi, S.; Saito, M. Effects of structured lipids containing eicosapentaenoic or docosahexaenoic acid and caprylic acid on serum and liver lipid profiles in rats. *BioFactors* **2004**, *22*, 157–160. [CrossRef] [PubMed]

127. Matsuo, T.; Matsuo, M.; Kasai, M.; Takeuchi, H. Effects of a liquid diet supplement containing structured medium- and long-chain triacylglycerols on bodyfat accumulation in healthy young subjects. *Asia Pac. J. Clin. Nutr.* **2001**, *10*, 46–50. [CrossRef] [PubMed]

128. Tsuji, H.; Kasai, M.; Takeuchi, H.; Nakamura, M.; Okazaki, M.; Kondo, K. Dietary medium-chain triacylglycerols suppress accumulation of body fat in a double-blind, controlled trial in healthy men and women. *J. Nutr.* **2001**, *131*, 2853–2859. [PubMed]

129. St-Onge, M.P.; Mayrsohn, B.; O'Keeffe, M.; Kissileff, H.R.; Choudhury, A.R.; Laferrere, B. Impact of medium and long chain triglycerides consumption on appetite and food intake in overweight men. *Eur. J. Clin. Nutr.* **2014**, *68*, 1134–1140. [CrossRef] [PubMed]

130. St-Onge, M.P.; Ross, R.; Parsons, W.D.; Jones, P.J. Medium-chain triglycerides increase energy expenditure and decrease adiposity in overweight men. *Obes. Res.* **2003**, *11*, 395–402. [CrossRef] [PubMed]

131. Lemarie, F.; Beauchamp, E.; Dayot, S.; Duby, C.; Legrand, P.; Rioux, V. Dietary caprylic acid (c8:0) does not increase plasma acylated ghrelin but decreases plasma unacylated ghrelin in the rat. *PLoS ONE* **2015**, *10*, e0133600. [CrossRef] [PubMed]

132. Lemarie, F.; Beauchamp, E.; Legrand, P.; Rioux, V. Revisiting the metabolism and physiological functions of caprylic acid (c8:0) with special focus on ghrelin octanoylation. *Biochimie* **2016**, *120*, 40–48. [CrossRef] [PubMed]

133. Li, Z.; Mulholland, M.; Zhang, W. Ghrelin o-acyltransferase (goat) and energy metabolism. *Sci. China Life Sci.* **2016**, *59*, 281–291. [CrossRef] [PubMed]

134. Kasai, M.; Nosaka, N.; Maki, H.; Negishi, S.; Aoyama, T.; Nakamura, M.; Suzuki, Y.; Tsuji, H.; Uto, H.; Okazaki, M.; *et al.* Effect of dietary medium- and long-chain triacylglycerols (mlct) on accumulation of body fat in healthy humans. *Asia Pac. J. Clin. Nutr.* **2003**, *12*, 151–160. [PubMed]

135. St-Onge, M.P.; Bourque, C.; Jones, P.J.; Ross, R.; Parsons, W.E. Medium- *versus* long-chain triglycerides for 27 days increases fat oxidation and energy expenditure without resulting in changes in body composition in overweight women. *Int. J. Obes. Relat. Metab. Disord.* **2003**, *27*, 95–102. [CrossRef] [PubMed]

136. St-Onge, M.P.; Jones, P.J. Greater rise in fat oxidation with medium-chain triglyceride consumption relative to long-chain triglyceride is associated with lower initial body weight and greater loss of subcutaneous adipose tissue. *Int. J. Obes. Relat. Metab. Disord.* **2003**, *27*, 1565–1571. [CrossRef] [PubMed]

137. Airhart, S.; Cade, W.T.; Jiang, H.; Coggan, A.R.; Racette, S.B.; Korenblat, K.; Spearie, C.A.; Waller, S.; O'Connor, R.; Bashir, A.; *et al.* A diet rich in medium-chain fatty acids improves systolic function and alters the lipidomic profile in patients with type 2 diabetes: A pilot study. *J. Clin. Endocrinol. Metab.* **2016**, *101*, 504–512. [CrossRef] [PubMed]

138. Assuncao, M.L.; Ferreira, H.S.; dos Santos, A.F.; Cabral, C.R., Jr.; Florencio, T.M. Effects of dietary coconut oil on the biochemical and anthropometric profiles of women presenting abdominal obesity. *Lipids* **2009**, *44*, 593–601. [CrossRef] [PubMed]

139. Rimbach, G.; Melchin, M.; Moehring, J.; Wagner, A.E. Polyphenols from cocoa and vascular health—A critical review. *Int. J. Mol. Sci.* **2009**, *10*, 4290–4309. [CrossRef] [PubMed]

140. Bourque, C.; St-Onge, M.P.; Papamandjaris, A.A.; Cohn, J.S.; Jones, P.J. Consumption of an oil composed of medium chain triacyglycerols, phytosterols, and *n*-3 fatty acids improves cardiovascular risk profile in overweight women. *Metabol. Clin. Exp.* **2003**, *52*, 771–777. [CrossRef]

141. St-Onge, M.P.; Lamarche, B.; Mauger, J.F.; Jones, P.J. Consumption of a functional oil rich in phytosterols and medium-chain triglyceride oil improves plasma lipid profiles in men. *J. Nutr.* **2003**, *133*, 1815–1820. [PubMed]

142. St-Onge, M.P.; Bosarge, A.; Goree, L.L.; Darnell, B. Medium chain triglyceride oil consumption as part of a weight loss diet does not lead to an adverse metabolic profile when compared to olive oil. *J. Am. Coll. Nutr.* **2008**, *27*, 547–552. [CrossRef] [PubMed]

143. Mumme, K.; Stonehouse, W. Effects of medium-chain triglycerides on weight loss and body composition: A meta-analysis of randomized controlled trials. *J. Acad. Nutr. Diet.* **2015**, *115*, 249–263. [CrossRef] [PubMed]

144. Mori, N.; Nakanishi, S.; Shiomi, S.; Kiyokawa, S.; Kakimoto, S.; Nakagawa, K.; Hosoe, K.; Minami, K.; Nadamoto, T. Enhancement of fat oxidation by licorice flavonoid oil in healthy humans during light exercise. *J. Nutr. Sci. Vitaminol.* **2015**, *61*, 406–416. [CrossRef] [PubMed]

145. Isaacs, C.E. The antimicrobial function of milk lipids. *Adv. Nutr. Res.* **2001**, *10*, 271–285. [PubMed]

146. Rios-Covian, D.; Ruas-Madiedo, P.; Margolles, A.; Gueimonde, M.; de Los Reyes-Gavilan, C.G.; Salazar, N. Intestinal short chain fatty acids and their link with diet and human health. *Front. Microbiol.* **2016**, *7*, 185. [CrossRef] [PubMed]

147. Schanler, R.J.; Goldblum, R.M.; Garza, C.; Goldman, A.S. Enhanced fecal excretion of selected immune factors in very low birth weight infants fed fortified human milk. *Pediatr. Res.* **1986**, *20*, 711–715. [CrossRef] [PubMed]

148. Papavassilis, C.; Mach, K.K.; Mayser, P.A. Medium-chain triglycerides inhibit growth of malassezia: Implications for prevention of systemic infection. *Crit. Care Med.* **1999**, *27*, 1781–1786. [CrossRef] [PubMed]

149. Kono, H.; Fujii, H.; Asakawa, M.; Yamamoto, M.; Matsuda, M.; Maki, A.; Matsumoto, Y. Protective effects of medium-chain triglycerides on the liver and gut in rats administered endotoxin. *Ann. Surg.* **2003**, *237*, 246–255. [CrossRef] [PubMed]

150. Zentek, J.; Buchheit-Renko, S.; Ferrara, F.; Vahjen, W.; Van Kessel, A.G.; Pieper, R. Nutritional and physiological role of medium-chain triglycerides and medium-chain fatty acids in piglets. *Anim. Health Res. Rev.* **2011**, *12*, 83–93. [CrossRef] [PubMed]

151. Zentek, J.; Ferrara, F.; Pieper, R.; Tedin, L.; Meyer, W.; Vahjen, W. Effects of dietary combinations of organic acids and medium chain fatty acids on the gastrointestinal microbial ecology and bacterial metabolites in the digestive tract of weaning piglets. *J. Anim. Sci.* **2013**, *91*, 3200–3210. [CrossRef] [PubMed]

152. Dierick, N.; Michiels, J.; Van Nevel, C. Effect of medium chain fatty acids and benzoic acid, as alternatives for antibiotics, on growth and some gut parameters in piglets. *Commun. Agric. Appl. Biol. Sci.* **2004**, *69*, 187–190. [PubMed]

153. Jacobi, S.K.; Odle, J. Nutritional factors influencing intestinal health of the neonate. *Adv. Nutr.* **2012**, *3*, 687–696. [CrossRef] [PubMed]

154. Kono, H.; Fujii, H.; Ogiku, M.; Tsuchiya, M.; Ishii, K.; Hara, M. Enteral diets enriched with medium-chain triglycerides and *n*-3 fatty acids prevent chemically induced experimental colitis in rats. *Transl. Res. J. Lab. Clin. Med.* **2010**, *156*, 282–291. [CrossRef] [PubMed]

155. Kono, H.; Fujii, H.; Ishii, K.; Hosomura, N.; Ogiku, M. Dietary medium-chain triglycerides prevent chemically induced experimental colitis in rats. *Transl. Res. J. Lab. Clin. Med.* **2010**, *155*, 131–141. [CrossRef] [PubMed]

156. Decuypere, J.A.; Dierick, N.A. The combined use of triacylglycerols containing medium-chain fatty acids and exogenous lipolytic enzymes as an alternative to in-feed antibiotics in piglets: Concept, possibilities and limitations. An overview. *Nutr. Res. Rev.* **2003**, *16*, 193–210. [CrossRef] [PubMed]

157. Liu, Y. Fatty acids, inflammation and intestinal health in pigs. *J. Anim. Sci. Biotechnol.* **2015**, *6*, 41. [CrossRef] [PubMed]

158. Kono, H.; Fujii, H.; Asakawa, M.; Maki, A.; Amemiya, H.; Hirai, Y.; Matsuda, M.; Yamamoto, M. Medium-chain triglycerides enhance secretory iga expression in rat intestine after administration of endotoxin. *Am. J. Physiol. Gastrointest. Liver Physiol.* **2004**, *286*, G1081–G1089. [CrossRef] [PubMed]

159. Servier Medical Art (Servier). Available online: http://www.servier.fr/smart/banque-dimages-powerpoint/ (acessed on 21 March 2016).

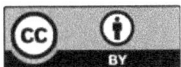

© 2016 by the authors. Licensee MDPI, Basel, Switzerland. This article is an open access article distributed under the terms and conditions of the Creative Commons Attribution (CC BY) license (http://creativecommons.org/licenses/by/4.0/).

nutrients

MDPI

Article

Elevation of Fasting Ghrelin in Healthy Human Subjects Consuming a High-Salt Diet: A Novel Mechanism of Obesity?

Yong Zhang [1,2], Fenxia Li [3], Fu-Qiang Liu [1,2,*], Chao Chu [2], Yang Wang [2], Dan Wang [2], Tong-Shuai Guo [2], Jun-Kui Wang [1], Gong-Chang Guan [1,2], Ke-Yu Ren [2] and Jian-Jun Mu [2,*]

[1]   Cardiovascular Department, Shaanxi Provincial People's Hospital, Xi'an 710068, China;
      zhangyong971292@163.com (Y.Z.); cardiowang@163.com (J.-K.W.); ntxhx2005@stu.xjtu.edu.cn (G.-C.G.)
[2]   Cardiovascular Department, First Affiliated Hospital of Medical College, Xi'an Jiaotong University,
      Xi'an 710061, China; iaacd@163.com (C.C.); wangyangxxk@126.com (Y.W.); m15991631129@163.com (D.W.);
      215guotongshuai@163.com (T.-S.G.); peizirong@yeah.net (K.-Y.R.)
[3]   Cardiovascular Department, Second Affiliated Hospital, Xi'an Medical University, Xi'an 710038, China;
      lfenxia@sina.com
*   Correspondence: liufuqiang0909@163.com (F.-Q.L.); mu_jjun@163.com (J.-J.M.);
     Tel.: +86-15029944259 (F.-Q.L.); +86-029-85323800 (J.-J.M.)

Received: 24 March 2016; Accepted: 19 May 2016; Published: 26 May 2016

Abstract: Overweight/obesity is a chronic disease that carries an increased risk of hypertension, diabetes mellitus, and premature death. Several epidemiological studies have demonstrated a clear relationship between salt intake and obesity, but the pathophysiologic mechanisms remain unknown. We hypothesized that ghrelin, which regulates appetite, food intake, and fat deposition, becomes elevated when one consumes a high-salt diet, contributing to the progression of obesity. We, therefore, investigated fasting ghrelin concentrations during a high-salt diet. Thirty-eight non-obese and normotensive subjects (aged 25 to 50 years) were selected from a rural community in Northern China. They were sequentially maintained on a normal diet for three days at baseline, a low-salt diet for seven days (3 g/day, NaCl), then a high-salt diet for seven days (18 g/day). The concentration of plasma ghrelin was measured using an immunoenzyme method (ELISA). High-salt intake significantly increased fasting ghrelin levels, which were higher during the high-salt diet (320.7 ± 30.6 pg/mL) than during the low-salt diet (172.9 ± 8.9 pg/mL). The comparison of ghrelin levels between the different salt diets was statistically-significantly different ($p < 0.01$). A positive correlation between 24-h urinary sodium excretion and fasting ghrelin levels was demonstrated. Our data indicate that a high-salt diet elevates fasting ghrelin in healthy human subjects, which may be a novel underlying mechanism of obesity.

Keywords: ghrelin; high salt; obesity; diet intervention

---

1. Introduction

Obesity has serious health consequences and is, therefore, a public health concern worldwide, according to the World Health Organization. By 2014 obesity was more than double what it had been in 1980. Of the 1.9 billion overweight adults in 2014, 600 million were classified as obese. Obesity at one time was a problem only in wealthy countries, but today it is common in low- and middle-income countries as well, particularly in the cities [1]. Health dangers caused by obesity include cardiovascular disease, the leading cause of death worldwide in 2012, diabetes mellitus, osteoarthritis, other degenerative joint diseases, and some forms of cancer, in particular endometrial, breast, and colon cancer. Increasing evidence shows that in both humans and experimental animals, obesity, like hypertension, is related to high salt consumption [2–11]. The belief that elevated sodium intake is a cause of obesity appears to have its origins in the idea that salt intake may increase the desire to eat certain types of foods and beverages, thus contributing to weight gain [2,3,8]. However, the pathophysiologic mechanisms remain unresolved.

Ghrelin is a 28-amino-acid peptide with an *N*-octanoyl alteration at serine-3, produced mainly in the stomach, which has been identified as the endogenous ligand of the growth hormone (GH) secretagogue receptor (GHS-R) [12]. Ghrelin has various physiological functions, such as stimulating the release of growth hormone and of appetite, as well as fat accumulation. Administration of exogenous ghrelin reportedly enhances appetite and increases food intake through the activation of hypothalamic neuropeptide Y/agouti-related peptide neurons, expressing GHS-R type 1a. In addition, ghrelin controls glucose homeostasis by regulating insulin secretion and sensitivity in pancreatic beta cells. Elimination of ghrelin in obese diabetic *ob/ob* mice increases basal insulin concentrations, enhances glucose-stimulated insulin secretion, and improves peripheral insulin sensitivity [12–15].

Data are still scarce in the literature with regard to the link between salt intake and ghrelin. We hypothesized that ghrelin contributes to the progression of obesity during high-salt loading. In the present study, which included non-obese and normotensive subjects, we investigated whether salt intake influences fasting ghrelin levels.

2. Materials and Methods

2.1. Subjects

From a total of 50 screened, normotensive subjects with similar dietary customs from a rural community in Northern China, 38 were enrolled in this study, and 12 were excluded because of hypertension or obesity. A brief medical questionnaire was administered. Subjects with a previous history of hypertension, obesity, liver, or renal disease or with diabetes mellitus were excluded. Hypertension was defined as mean systolic blood pressure $\geqslant$140 mmHg and/or mean diastolic blood pressure $\geqslant$90 mmHg. Obesity was defined as BMI $\geqslant$ 28 kg/m^2. All subjects were non-smokers. The institutional ethics committee of Xi'an Jiaotong University Medical School (Code: XJTU1AF2013LSL-056) approved the study protocol, and each subject gave written informed consent. All of the procedures were performed in accordance with institutional guidelines.

2.2. Protocol

The protocol consisted of a series of investigations, including a three-day baseline period in which a clinical history and physical examination (height, weight, and blood pressure (BP)) were obtained and subjects consumed a normal-salt diet, followed by seven days of a low-salt diet (51.3 mmol or 3 g of NaCl per day), then 7 days of a high-salt diet (307.7 mmol or 18 g of NaCl per day) [16]. During the baseline investigational period, each subject was given detailed dietary instructions to avoid table salt, cooking salt, high-sodium foods, and food rich in nitrite/nitrate for the subsequent 14 days. All meals were prepared in research kitchens and consumed onsite. Dietary total energy intake was supplied according to their baseline energy intake assessed by a brief food frequency questionnaire. Food consumption of study participants was carefully recorded at each meal by study staff members.

2.3. Biochemical Analyses

Blood glucose was measured using the glucose oxidase method. Serum lipids (total cholesterol, triglycerides, HDL-C) were measured. Blood samples for measurement of fasting plasma ghrelin concentrations were drawn with EDTA-aprotinin tubes and immediately placed on ice. All tubes were centrifuged at 4 °C for collection of plasma and stored at −80 °C until the time of analysis. Ghrelin was determined using a validated sandwich ELISA using a ghrelin-specific antibody (Wuhan USCN Science and Technology Co., Ltd., Wuhan, China). Five plasma samples were used to evaluate intra- and interassay coefficients of variation, which, for ghrelin, ranged from 2.1%–4.3% (mean, 3.2) to 6.4%–9.2% (mean, 7.8), respectively.

2.4. 24-h Urinary Sodium and Potassium Determination

Twenty-four-hour urine samples were collected at baseline and on day seven of each intervention period. Twenty-four hour urine collection was obtained with the first voided urine upon waking on the day of collection being discarded and participants then collecting all voided urine up to, and including, the first void the following morning. Participants were instructed to keep collected samples inside cooler bags provided and stored in a cool, dark place until completion when a research assistant was contacted to collect the sample. The times at the beginning and the end of urine collection were recorded. The samples were kept frozen at $-40\,^{\circ}\text{C}$ until analysis. Urinary concentrations of sodium were determined using ion-selective electrodes (Hitachi, Ltd., Tokyo, Japan). The 24-h urinary excretion of sodium and potassium was calculated by multiplying the concentration of sodium and potassium, respectively, by the 24-h total urine volume.

2.5. Statistical Analysis

The data are shown as mean $\pm$ SD. Differences between biochemical markers obtained at low- and high-salt intakes were calculated by analysis of variance with the repeated measures design. Age, sex, and body mass index (BMI) were adjusted using multivariable analysis. All calculations were performed with SPSS for Windows 16.0 software (SPSS, Inc., Chicago, IL, USA). Probability was assessed using a two-tailed p value of < 0.05 to describe statistical significance.

3. Result

3.1. Profiles of Study Subjects

All enrolled subjects completed this interventional study. Their average age was 50.9 ± 1.3 years and systolic BP and diastolic BP were 110.7 ± 2.2 and 72.6 ± 1.3 mmHg, respectively (Table 1). The 24-h urinary sodium excretion averaged 173.8 mmol/day (median: 131.5), which approximates an intake of 8 g of salt/day. Daily urinary potassium excretion averaged 48 ± 0.9 mmol/day (median: 44 mmol/day).

Table 1. Baseline demographic and clinical characteristics.

Parameter	Values
Mean age (year)	50.6 ± 2.1
Sex (male/female)	21/17
BMI (kg/m^2)	22.8 ± 0.4
Systolic BP (mmHg)	110.6 ± 5.8
Diastolic BP (mmHg)	72.1 ± 2.7
Glucose, mmol/L	3.91 ± 0.11
Total cholesterol, mmol/L	4.18 ± 0.14
Triglycerides, mmol/L	1.32 ± 0.11
LDL-cholesterol, mmol/L	2.35 ± 0.11
HDL-cholesterol, mmol/L	1.21 ± 0.04

3.2. Effects of Salt Intake on BP and 24-h Urinary Sodium Excretion

Table 2 shows BP responses to the low-salt and high-salt dietary interventions. BP significantly increased with the change from the low-salt to high-salt intervention ($p < 0.05$). The 24-h sodium excretions in the urine were calculated at the end of the intervention period to ensure compliance with the study protocol. As shown in Table 2, urinary sodium excretion significantly decreased with the change from baseline to the low-salt diet, but increased with the change from the low-salt to the high-salt diet (all $p < 0.05$). These results confirmed the subjects' compliance with the dietary intervention protocol.

Table 2. BP Levels (mmHg) and 24-h Urinary Sodium (mmol/day) at Baseline and During Dietary Interventions.

	SBP	DBP	24 h Urinary Na$^+$ (mmol/Day)
Baseline	110.6 ± 5.8	72.1 ± 2.7	175.8 ± 11.1
Low-salt diet	108.7 ± 2.8	73.5 ± 2.0	98.8 ± 9.3
High-salt diet	116.4 ± 5.8 *	77.3 ± 4.2 *	268 ± 10.2 *

$* p < 0.05$ *versus* low-salt diet.

3.3. The Effect of High-Salt Intake on Fasting Ghrelin Levels

As shown in Figure 1, the statistical difference was slight in the fasting ghrelin levels between the baseline and the low-salt dietary intervention (192.4 ± 12.6 pg/mL *vs.* 172.9 ± 8.9 pg/mL, $p = 0.037$). Moreover, high-salt intake clearly enhanced plasma ghrelin levels (320.7 ± 30.6 pg/mL *vs.* 172.9 ± 8.9 pg/mL, $p < 0.01$). Further analyses (Figure 2) showed that the fasting ghrelin concentration correlated with the 24-h urinary sodium excretion during among baseline, low-salt, and high-salt dietary intervention periods ($r = 0.637$, $p < 0.001$).

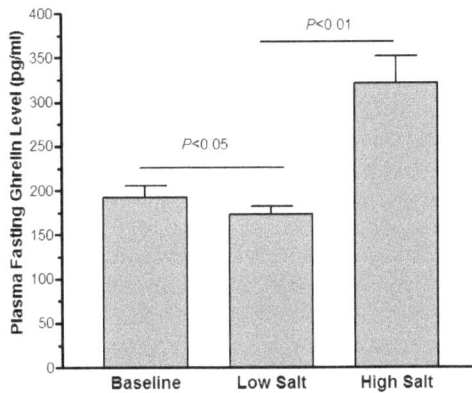

Figure 1. The effect of low-salt and high-salt intake on fasting ghrelin in all subjects.

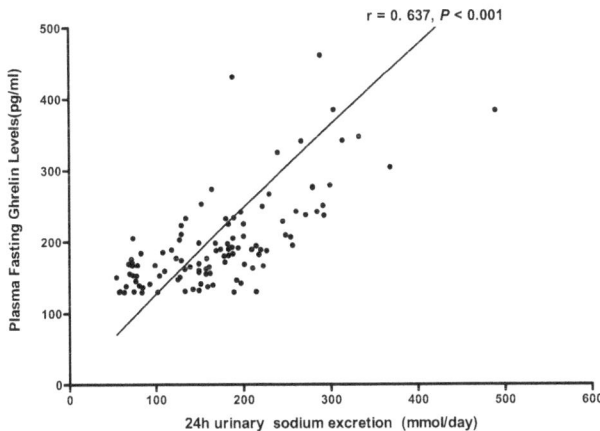

Figure 2. The correlation between plasma ghrelin levels and 24 h urinary sodium excretions in all subjects on baseline, a low-salt diet and on a high-salt diet.

4. Discussion

The initial finding of the present study is that high-salt intake is associated with fasting ghrelin elevation in non-obese and normotensive subjects. In addition, a positive correlation between 24-h urinary sodium excretion and fasting ghrelin levels was demonstrated in these Chinese subjects.

The well-established role of ghrelin as an important regulator of appetite and fat accumulation may be attributed to the pathogenesis of obesity. Chronic ghrelin administration increases body weight via diverse, concerted actions on food intake, energy expenditure, and fuel utilization [17–23]. On the contrary, congenital ablation of the ghrelin or ghrelin-receptor gene causes resistance to diet-induced obesity [24–26], and pharmacologic ghrelin blockade reduces food intake and body weight [21,27–30]. There may be a relationship between the genomic variation in the ghrelin gene and obesity [21–33]. In particular, the Leu72Met polymorphism in ghrelin was found to be associated with the early onset of obesity [31]. Ghrelin is produced primarily in the stomach, circulates in the blood, and serves as a peripheral signal, informing the arcuate nucleus of the central nervous system (via the vagus nerve) to stimulate hunger. Moreover, ghrelin also could be involved glucose metabolism through suppressing insulin secretion, which insulin plays a crucial role in obesity. It has been well documented that systemic administration of ghrelin or endogenous ghrelin could restrict glucose-induced insulin release and deteriorate glucose tolerance *in vivo* and *in vivo* [34–36], which leads to insulin resistance, indirectly take part in obesity. Therefore, ghrelin may possibly be a useful target against obesity.

Ghrelin may be the key to revealing the mechanisms of salt-induced obesity. Several epidemiological studies have demonstrated a clear relationship between salt intake and obesity [2,6,7], and interventional studies also show that a high-salt diet might induce subcutaneous and visceral adipose tissue [4,11]. A hypothesis has been proposed to explain the relationship between sodium intake and obesity: salty foods might be considered addictive substances that stimulate opioid receptors in the brain and the pleasure center, so that the consumption of salty foods every day produces an addiction to these foods, producing an increase in food consumption (tolerance to opiates), increased caloric intake, overweight, sedentary lifestyle, obesity, and related diseases [37,38]. In our study, we found that the high-salt diet elevated fasting ghrelin. Recently, Cai *et al.* reported that ghrelin is co-expressed with ENaC subunits in taste-receptor cells in fungiform papillae on the tongue and that Ghrelin/GHS-R/mice possess a significantly reduced salty taste sensitivity compared to wild-type mice [39]. Therefore, we conclude the salt-induced ghrelin increase may be a novel mechanism of obesity via informing the arcuate nucleus of the central nervous system to stimulate hunger.

Our study has several important strengths. First of all, the subjects were recruited from a rural community and were similar with respect to lifestyle and environmental risk factors, including diet and physical activity. Thus, confounding due to these exposures should be minimized. Moreover, participants with body mass index (BMI) more than 28 kg/m^2 was excluded, and adjustment for BMI was conducted; therefore, confounding effects of BMI probably had no influence on salt intake and ghrelin. Participation in the dietary interventions was high, and compliance with the study interventions, as assessed by urinary excretion of sodium during each intervention period, was excellent.

The present study has some limitations that should be addressed. Because all of the subjects were recruited from the Chinese population, whether or not our observation could be generalized to other racial populations is unknown. Further studies are required to validate our findings in a larger and more diverse sample and to elucidate the mechanisms by which salt loading affects plasma ghrelin. Meanwhile, insulin resistance could be involved in salt-induced obesity, and further studies will be needed to reveal the relationship between ghrelin and insulin during high-salt diet.

5. Conclusions

In conclusion, our human intervention study found that salt loading could increase circulating ghrelin production in normotensive Asian subjects. Our findings indicate that the elevation of ghrelin might be the underlying mechanism of salt-induced obesity, which sheds some new light on prevention and a possible therapeutic target for obesity in the future.

Acknowledgments: This study was supported by grant 81200512 (to Liu) from the Natural Science Foundation of China.

Author Contributions: F.-Q.L. and J.-J.M. conceived and designed the experiments; J.-J.M. was responsible for subject recruitment; F.-Q.L., K.-Y.R., T.-S.G., Y.W., C.C., D.W., Y.Z. and F.-X.L. performed the experiments; Y.Z. J.-K.W., G.-C.G. and F.-X.L. analyzed the data; Y.Z. wrote the paper. All authors read, critically revised and approved the final manuscript.

Conflicts of Interest: The authors declare no conflict of interest.

References

1. World Health Organization. Obesity and Overweight. Fact sheet N°311. Updated January 2015. Available online: http://www.who.int/mediacentre/factsheets/fs311/en/ (accessed on 27 July 2015).
2. Navia, B.; Aparicio, A.; Perea, J.M.; Pérez-Farinós, N.; Villar-Villalba, C.; Labrado, E.; Ortega, R.M. Sodium intake may promote weight gain: Results of the FANPE study in a representative sample of the adult Spanish population. *Nutr. Hosp.* **2014**, *29*, 1283–1289. [PubMed]
3. Fowler, S.P.; Williams, K.; Resendez, R.G.; Hunt, K.J.; Hazuda, H.P.; Stern, M.P. Fueling the obesity epidemic? Artificially sweetened beverage use and long-term weight gain. *Obesity* **2008**, *16*, 1894–1900. [CrossRef] [PubMed]
4. Zhou, X.; Yuan, F.; Ji, W.J.; Guo, Z.Z.; Zhang, L.; Lu, R.Y.; Liu, X.; Liu, H.M.; Zhang, W.C.; Jiang, T.M.; *et al.* High-salt intake induced visceral adipose tissue hypoxia and its association with circulating monocyte subsets in humans. *Obesity* **2014**, *22*, 1470–1476. [CrossRef] [PubMed]
5. Baudrand, R.; Campino, C.; Carvajal, C.A.; Olivieri, O.; Guidi, G.; Faccini, G.; Völhringer, P.A.; Cerda, J.; Owen, G.; Kalergis, A.M.; *et al.* High sodium intake is associated with increased glucocorticoid production, insulin resistance and metabolic syndrome. *Clin. Endocrinol.* **2014**, *80*, 677–684. [CrossRef] [PubMed]
6. Yoon, Y.S.; Oh, S.W. Sodium density and obesity; The Korea National Health and Nutrition Examination Survey 2007–2010. *Eur. J. Clin. Nutr.* **2013**, *67*, 141–146. [PubMed]
7. Hoffmann, I.S.; Cubeddu, L.X. Salt and the metabolic syndrome. *Nutr. Metab. Cardiovasc. Dis.* **2009**, *19*, 123–128. [CrossRef] [PubMed]
8. Cocores, J.A.; Gold, M.S. The Salted Food Addiction Hypothesis may explain overeating and the obesity epidemic. *Med. Hypotheses* **2009**, *73*, 892–899. [CrossRef] [PubMed]
9. Yuan, F.; Guo, Z.Z.; Ji, W.J.; Ji, W.J.; Ma, Y.Q.; Zhang, Z.L.; Zhou, X.; Li, Y.M. BOLD-MRI evaluation of subcutaneous and visceral adipose tissue oxygenation status: effect of dietary salt intake. *Am. J. Transl. Res.* **2015**, *7*, 598–606. [PubMed]
10. Ma, Y.; He, F.J.; MacGregor, G.A. High salt intake: Independent risk factor for obesity? *Hypertension* **2015**, *66*, 843–849. [CrossRef] [PubMed]
11. Lee, M.; Kim, M.K.; Kim, S.M.; Park, H.; Park, C.G.; Park, H.K. Gender-based differences on the association between salt-sensitive genes and obesity in Korean children aged between 8 and 9 years. *PLoS ONE* **2015**, *10*, e0120111. [CrossRef] [PubMed]
12. Kojima, M.; Hosoda, H.; Date, Y.; Nakazato, M.; Matsui, H.; Kangawa, K. Ghrelin is a growth-hormone-releasing acylated peptide from stomach. *Nature* **1999**, *402*, 656–660. [CrossRef] [PubMed]
13. Sato, T.; Ida, T.; Nakamura, Y.; Shiimura, Y.; Kangawqa, K.; Kojima, M. Physiological roles of ghrelin on obesity. *Obes. Res. Clin. Pract.* **2014**, *8*, e405–e413. [CrossRef] [PubMed]
14. Sato, T.; Nakamura, Y.; Shiimura, Y.; Ohgusu, H.; Kangawa, K.; Kojima, M. Structure, regulation and function of ghrelin. *J. Biochem.* **2012**, *151*, 119–128. [CrossRef] [PubMed]
15. Wiedmer, P.; Nogueiras, R.; Broglio, F.; D'Alessio, D.; Tschöp, M.H. Ghrelin, obesity and diabetes. *Nat. Clin. Pract. Endocrinol. Metab.* **2007**, *3*, 705–712. [CrossRef] [PubMed]

16. Wang, Y.; Liu, F.Q.; Wang, D.; Chu, C.; Mu, J.J.; Ren, K.Y.; Guo, T.S.; Chu, C.; Wang, L.; Geng, L.K.; *et al.* Effect of salt intake and potassium supplementation on serum renalase levels in Chinese adults: A randomized trial. *Medicine* **2014**, *93*, e44. [CrossRef] [PubMed]

17. Cummings, D.E. Ghrelin and the short-and long-term regulation of appetite and body weight. *Physiol. Behav.* **2006**, *89*, 71–84. [CrossRef] [PubMed]

18. Qi, Y.; Inoue, K.; Fu, M.; Inui, A.; Herzog, H. Chronic overproduction of ghrelin in the hypothalamus leads to temporal increase in food intake and body weight. *Neuropeptides* **2015**, *50*, 23–28. [CrossRef] [PubMed]

19. Nass, R.; Pezzoli, S.S.; Oliver, M.C.; Patrie, J.T.; Harrell, F.E.; Clasey, J.L.; Heymsfield, S.B.; Bach, M.A.; Vance, M.L.; Thorner, M.O. Effects of an oral ghrelin mimetic on body composition and clinical outcomes in healthy older adults: A randomized trial. *Ann. Intern. Med.* **2008**, *149*, 601–611. [CrossRef] [PubMed]

20. Tschop, M.; Smiley, D.L.; Heiman, M.L. Ghrelin induces adiposity in rodents. *Nature* **2000**, *407*, 908–913. [CrossRef] [PubMed]

21. Nakazato, M.; Murakami, N.; Date, Y.; Kojima, M.; Matsuo, H.; Kangawa, K.; Matsukura, S. A role for ghrelin in the central regulation of feeding. *Nature* **2001**, *409*, 194–198. [CrossRef] [PubMed]

22. Wren, A.M.; Small, C.J.; Abbott, C.R.; Dhillo, W.S.; Seal, L.J.; Cohen, M.A.; Batterham, R.L.; Taheri, S.; Stanley, S.A.; Ghatei, M.A.; *et al.* Ghrelin causes hyperphagia and obesity in rats. *Diabetes* **2001**, *50*, 2540–2547. [CrossRef] [PubMed]

23. Keen-Rhinehart, E.; Bartness, T.J. Peripheral ghrelin injections stimulate food intake, foraging and food hoarding in Siberian hamsters. *Am. J. Physiol.* **2005**, *288*, R716–R722. [CrossRef] [PubMed]

24. Sun, Y.; Wang, P.; Zheng, H.; Smith, R.G. Ghrelin stimulation of growth hormone release and appetite is mediated through the growth hormone secretagogue receptor. *Proc. Natl. Acad. Sci. USA* **2004**, *101*, 4679–4684. [CrossRef] [PubMed]

25. Wortley, K.E.; Anderson, K.D.; Garcia, K.; Murray, J.D.; Malinova, L.; Liu, R.; Moncrieffe, M.; Thabet, K.; Cox, H.J.; Yancopoulos, G.D.; *et al.* Genetic deletion of ghrelin does not decrease food intake but influences metabolic fuel preference. *Proc. Natl. Acad. Sci. USA* **2004**, *101*, 8227–8232. [CrossRef] [PubMed]

26. Sun, Y.; Ahmed, S.; Smith, R.G. Deletion of ghrelin impairs neither growth nor appetite. *Mol. Cell. Biol.* **2003**, *23*, 7973–7981. [CrossRef] [PubMed]

27. Asakawa, A.; Inui, A.; Kaga, T.; Katsuura, G.; Fujimiya, M.; Fujino, M.A.; Kasuga, M. Antagonism of ghrelin receptor reduces food intake and body weight gain in mice. *Gut* **2003**, *52*, 947–952. [CrossRef] [PubMed]

28. Shuto, Y.; Shibasaki, T.; Otagiri, A.; Kuriyama, H.; Ohata, H.; Tamura, H.; Kamegai, J.; Sugihara, H.; Oikawa, S.; Wakabayashi, I. Hypothalamic growth hormone secretagogue receptor regulates growth hormone secretion, feeding, and adiposity. *J. Clin. Investig.* **2002**, *109*, 1429–1436. [CrossRef] [PubMed]

29. Bagnasco, M.; Tulipano, G.; Melis, M.R.; Argiolas, A.; Cocchi, D.; Muller, E.E. Endogenous ghrelin is an orexigenic peptide acting in the arcuate nucleus in response to fasting. *Regul. Pept.* **2003**, *111*, 161–167. [CrossRef]

30. Murakami, N.; Hayashida, T.; Kuroiwa, T.; Nakahara, K.; Ida, T.; Mondal, M.S.; Nakazato, M.; Kojima, M.; Kangawa, K. Role for central ghrelin in food intake and secretion profile of stomach ghrelin in rats. *J. Endocrinol.* **2002**, *174*, 283–288. [CrossRef] [PubMed]

31. Del Giudice, M.; Santoro, N.; Cirillo, G.; Raimondo, P.; Grandone, A.; D'Aniello, A.; Di Nardo, M.; Perrone, L. Molecular screening of the ghrelin gene in Italian obese children: The Leu72Met variant is associated with an earlier onset of obesity. *Int. J. Obes.* **2004**, *28*, 447–450. [CrossRef] [PubMed]

32. Pöykkö, S.; Ukkola, O.; Kauma, H.; Savolainen, M.J.; Kesäniemi, Y.A. Ghrelin Arg51Gln mutation is a risk factor for Type 2 diabetes and hypertension in a random sample of middle-aged subjects. *Diabetologia* **2003**, *46*, 455–458. [PubMed]

33. Ukkola, O.; Ravussin, E.; Jacobson, P.; Pérusse, L.; Rankinen, T.; Tschöp, M.; Heiman, M.L.; Leon, A.S.; Rao, D.C.; Skinner, J.S.; *et al.* Role of ghrelin polymorphisms in obesity based on three different studies. *Obes. Res.* **2002**, *10*, 782–791. [CrossRef] [PubMed]

34. Reimer, M.K.; Pacini, G.; Ahrén, B. Dose-dependent inhibition by ghrelin of insulin secretion in the mouse. *Endocrinology* **2003**, *44*, 916–921. [CrossRef] [PubMed]

35. Dezaki, K.; Hosoda, H.; Kakei, M.; Hashiguchi, S.; Watanabe, M.; Kangawa, K.; Yada, T. Endogenous ghrelin in pancreatic islets restricts insulin release by attenuating Ca^{2+} signaling in beta-cells: Implication in the glycemic control in rodents. *Diabetes* **2004**, *53*, 3142–3151. [CrossRef] [PubMed]

36. Tong, J.; Prigeon, R.L.; Davis, H.W.; Bidlingmaier, M.; Kahn, S.E.; Cummings, D.E.; Tschöp, M.H.; D'Alessio, D. Ghrelin suppresses glucose-stimulated insulin secretion and deteriorates glucose tolerance in healthy humans. *Diabetes* **2010**, *59*, 2145–2151. [CrossRef] [PubMed]
37. Na, E.S.; Morris, M.J.; Johnson, A.K. Opioid mechanisms that mediate the palatability of and appetite for salt in sodium replete and deficient states. *Physiol. Behav.* **2012**, *106*, 164–170. [CrossRef] [PubMed]
38. Bolhuis, D.P.; Costanzo, A.; Newman, L.P.; Keast, R.S. Salt Promotes Passive Overconsumption of Dietary Fat in Humans. *J. Nutr.* **2016**, *146*, 838–845. [CrossRef] [PubMed]
39. Cai, H.; Cong, W.N.; Daimon, C.M.; Wang, R.; Tschöp, M.H.; Sévigny, J.; Martin, B.; Maudsley, S. Altered lipid and salt taste responsivity in ghrelin and GOAT null mice. *PLoS ONE* **2013**, *8*, e76553. [CrossRef] [PubMed]

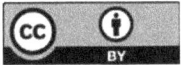

© 2016 by the authors. Licensee MDPI, Basel, Switzerland. This article is an open access article distributed under the terms and conditions of the Creative Commons Attribution (CC BY) license (http://creativecommons.org/licenses/by/4.0/).

nutrients

MDPI

Article

Association between Metabolite Profiles, Metabolic Syndrome and Obesity Status

Bénédicte Allam-Ndoul [1,2], Frédéric Guénard [1,2], Véronique Garneau [1,2], Hubert Cormier [1,2], Olivier Barbier [3], Louis Pérusse [1,4] and Marie-Claude Vohl [1,2,*]

[1]   Institute of Nutrition and Functional Foods (INAF), Laval University, Quebec City, QC G1V0A6, Canada; allamndoulbenedicte@gmail.com (B.A.-N.); Frederic.Guenard@fsaa.ulaval.ca (F.G.); Veronique.Garneau@fsaa.ulaval.ca (V.G.); cormier.hubert@yahoo.com (H.C.); louis.perusse@kin.ulaval.ca (L.P.)
[2]   School of Nutrition, Laval University, Quebec City, QC G1V0A6, Canada
[3]   Laboratory of Molecular Pharmacology, CHU-Quebec Research Center, and Faculty of Pharmacy, Laval University, Quebec City, QC G1V4G2, Canada; Olivier.barbier@crchul.ulaval.ca
[4]   Department of Kinesiology, Laval University, Quebec City, QC G1V0A6, Canada
*   Correspondence: marie-claude.vohl@fsaa.ulaval.ca; Tel.: +1-418-656-2131 (ext. 4676); Fax: +1-418-656-5877

Received: 13 April 2016; Accepted: 20 May 2016; Published: 27 May 2016

Abstract: Underlying mechanisms associated with the development of abnormal metabolic phenotypes among obese individuals are not yet clear. Our aim is to investigate differences in plasma metabolomics profiles between normal weight (NW) and overweight/obese (Ov/Ob) individuals, with or without metabolic syndrome (MetS). Mass spectrometry-based metabolite profiling was used to compare metabolite levels between each group. Three main principal components factors explaining a maximum of variance were retained. Factor 1's (long chain glycerophospholipids) metabolite profile score was higher among Ov/Ob with MetS than among Ov/Ob and NW participants without MetS. This factor was positively correlated to plasma total cholesterol (total-C) and triglyceride levels in the three groups, to high density lipoprotein -cholesterol (HDL-C) among participants without MetS. Factor 2 (amino acids and short to long chain acylcarnitine) was positively correlated to HDL-C and negatively correlated with insulin levels among NW participants. Factor 3's (medium chain acylcarnitines) metabolite profile scores were higher among NW participants than among Ov/Ob with or without MetS. Factor 3 was negatively associated with glucose levels among the Ov/Ob with MetS. Factor 1 seems to be associated with a deteriorated metabolic profile that corresponds to obesity, whereas Factors 2 and 3 seem to be rather associated with a healthy metabolic profile.

Keywords: metabolic syndrome; obesity; metabolites

1. Introduction

Metabolic syndrome (MetS) is defined as the association of obesity, insulin resistance (IR), hypertension and dyslipidemia [1]. MetS predisposes an individual to several metabolic diseases such as type 2 diabetes and cardiovascular diseases (CVD) [2]. Obesity is mainly considered to be responsible for the rising prevalence of MetS [2], associated with higher plasma triglyceride (TG) levels, lower high density lipoprotein-cholesterol (HDL-C) levels, hyperglycemia and increased CVD risk [1]. The prevalence of obesity has been increasing dramatically worldwide over the past three decades [3].

Obesity results from a complex interaction between predisposing genetic factors and changes in environmental factors such as diet. It is recommended that obesity be the primary target of intervention for MetS [4]. Nevertheless, it is important to point out the fact that 10%–30% of obese individuals are insulin sensitive and have normal plasma lipid profile and blood pressure, thus being considered as obese but metabolically healthy [5–7].

Metabolites are intermediate products of different metabolic pathways. Their levels can be modulated by genetic factors, environmental factors or gene–environment interactions. In recent years, advanced laboratory techniques, such as metabolomics have been developed. It has allowed the investigation of a large number of metabolites in human biological fluids or tissues [8]. Metabolomics is a powerful tool which provides the possibility to study metabolite differences between several groups at any given time and thus allows capturing the dynamic physiological conditions corresponding to disease outcomes or metabolic alterations.

Several studies used metabolomics to investigate metabolite profiles associated with obesity. For instance, Lee *et al.* observed a shift in metabolite composition in obese individuals compared to normal-weight individuals [9]. In a study examining the influence of fat free mass on metabolite profile, Jourdan *et al.* showed that the serum metabolite composition was strongly associated with obesity stages [10]. Therefore, investigation of serum metabolite concentrations provides an ideal way to uncover the underlying mechanisms associated with the development of abnormal metabolic status in obese individuals. We hypothesize that metabolite profiles differ between lean and obese subjects with or without MetS. The aim of the present study was to apply comprehensive metabolic profiling tools to gain broader understanding of metabolic differences between lean and obese subjects with or without MetS.

2. Materials and Methods

2.1. Subjects

Two hundred subjects aged between 18 and 55 years were randomly selected from the INFOGENE study [11]. The recruitment took place between May 2004 and March 2007 in the Quebec City metropolitan area. The final study sample consisted of 664 individuals. Participants were recruited using advertisements in local newspapers and radio stations, in addition to electronic group messages sent to university and hospital employees. During their visit at the clinical investigation unit, participants completed a questionnaire on socio-demographic characteristics and lifestyle habits. All participants signed a written consent to participate in this study that has been approved by the ethics committee of Laval University.

2.2. Anthropometric Measurements

A trained research assistant measured height, weight, waist (WC) and hip circumferences. Systolic (SBP) and diastolic (DBP) blood pressure were measured after a 5 min rest while participants were lying on their backs, with arms and legs uncrossed. Fat and lean masses were assessed using a bioelectrical impedance meter (101-RJL Systems, Detroit, MI, USA). Body mass index (BMI) was calculated by dividing weight in kilograms by height in meters squared. The obesity status of the participants was assessed using BMI and the body fat mass percentage. Subjects were classified in the overweight and obese (Ov/Ob) group if they had a BMI $\geqslant$ 25 kg/m^2. Body fat $\geqslant$25% of total body fat mass in men and $\geqslant$30% in women were considered to classify an individual as being obese [12].

2.3. Biochemical Parameters

Fasting blood samples were obtained from an antecubital vein into vacutainer tubes containing Ethylenediaminetetraacetic acid (EDTA) after a 12 h overnight fast. Total cholesterol (total-C) and TG levels were determined from plasma and lipoprotein fractions using the Olympus AU400e system (Plympus America Inc., Melville, NY, USA). A precipitation of low-density lipoprotein cholesterol (LDL-C) fraction in the infranatant with heparin-manganese chloride [13] was used to obtain the HDL-C fraction. LDL-C concentrations were estimated using the Friedewald's equation [14,15]. Radioimmunoassay with polyethylene glycol separation was used to measure fasting insulin [16].

Fasting glucose concentrations were enzymatically measured [17]. Homeostasis model assessment of insulin resistance (HOMA-IR) was obtained using: (fasting glucose × fasting insulin)/22.5 [18].

2.4. Metabolite Profiling

To assess the metabolite profiling, the Absolute ID p180 Kit (Biocrates Life Sciences AG, Innsbruck, Australia) for mass spectrometry was used. The quantification of 95 metabolites was done for 200 participants. Metabolites were composed of 67 Glycerophospholipids (GPs), 12 Acylcarnitines (ACs), 10 Sphingolipids (SGs) and 6 amino acids (AA). For GPs, ACs and SGs x:y notation was used, x denotes the number of carbons in the side chain and y the number of double bonds. The lipids were subdivided into different classes: 28 Phosphatidylcholines diacyl (PCaa); 36 Phosphatidylcholines acyl-alkyl (PCae); 3 LysoPhosphatidylcholines acyl (LysoPC); 4 Hydroxyshingomyelins; and 6 Shingomyelins (SM). GPs are differentiated with respect to the presence of ester (a) and ether (e) bonds in the glycerol moiety. Two letters indicate that the first and second positions of glycerol unit are bound to a fatty acid residue, while a single letter (a or e) indicates a bond with only one fatty acid residue. The concentration of all metabolites was reported in µM. Metabolites for which more than half of the values were below the limit of detection and or with standard out of range were excluded.

2.5. Statistical Analyses

Transformations were applied to the variables that were not normally distributed. Logarithmic transformations were performed for fasting insulin, total-C and HDL-C, and an inverse transformation for TG and fasting glucose. All analyses were conducted on age- and sex-adjusted data; analysis of variance was used to underline the differences in metabolic characteristics between obese/overweight with or without MetS and normal-weight participants with or without MetS. Individuals with MetS had at least 3 of the following five criteria: waist circumference (WC) >88 cm for women and 102 cm for men, fasting plasma triglycerides (TG) ⩾1.7 mmol/L, high-density lipoprotein cholesterol (HDL-C) levels ⩽1.03 mmol/L for men and 1.29 mmol/L for women, glucose levels ⩾ 5.6 mmol/L and resting blood pressure ⩾130/85 mmHg.

The significance level of all analyses was set at $p \leqslant 0.05$. Differences between groups were assessed using the least square means. Principal component analysis (PCA) was used to reduce the large number of correlated metabolites into clusters of fewer uncorrelated factors. Factors derived from PCA that had eigenvalues greater than or equal to 1 were identified and considered for further analyses. Metabolites with a factor loading ⩾0.50 or −0.50 were reported as composing a given PCA-derived factor. Then, scoring coefficients were used to calculate baseline metabolite factor scores for each individual. These scores corresponded to the sum of metabolic signature groups multiplied by their respective factor loading. These scores represented the degree of each participant's metabolic signature conforming to each factor. To detect association between factors and MetS criteria, Pearson correlations were used. All statistical analyses were performed using SAS statistical software version 9.2 (SAS Institute, Inc., Cary, NC, USA).

3. Results

3.1. Descriptive Characteristics

Descriptive characteristics of study participants are presented in Table 1. Groups were defined according to BMI and MetS status. Ov/Ob individuals with or without MetS were older than normal weight (NW) subjects. Among obese individuals, subjects with MetS were older than those without MetS. As expected, WC and fat mass increased progressively with the deterioration of metabolic state (*i.e.*, obesity and MetS status). The same trend was observed for fasting insulin levels and SBP. The Ov/Ob subjects with the MetS had a more deteriorated plasma lipid profile including increased plasma TG levels and decreased plasma HDL-C levels compared to Ov/Ob without MetS or NW individuals. There was no significant difference between groups for plasma LDL-C levels. NW individuals had lower HOMA-IR index values than Ov/Ob with or without MetS.

Table 1. Baseline characteristics.

	MetS−		MetS+	*p*-Value
	Ov/Ob (*n* = 83)	NW (*n* = 65)	Ov/Ob (*n* = 46)	
Age (years)	35.7 ± 10.4 [2]	28.9 ± 7.4 [1]	37.9 ± 10.0 [3]	<0.0001
BMI (kg/m^2)	31.4 ± 4.2 [2]	22.2 ± 1.8 [1]	34.3 ± 4.9 [3]	<0.0001
Waist circumference (cm) [a]	97.8 ± 10.8 [2]	74.7 ± 5.7 [1]	109.0 ± 11.9 [3]	<0.0001
Fat mass (kg)	31.3 ± 9.0 [2]	14.5 ± 4.3 [1]	36.5 ± 10.5 [3]	<0.0001
Lean mass (kg)	57.5 ± 11.1 [2]	48.9 ± 8.9 [1]	65.3 ± 12.1 [3]	<0.0001
Systolic blood pressure (mmHg)	119.9 ± 9.0 [2]	115.9 ± 9.8 [1]	130.1 ± 10.6 [3]	<0.0001
Diastolic blood pressure (mmHg)	77.7 ± 7.7 [1]	74.0 ± 9.9 [1]	83.5 ± 9.5 [2]	<0.0001
Fasting glucose (mmol/L)	5.4 ± 0.5 [2]	5.8 ± 1.3 [1]	6.1 ± 1.1 [3]	0.002
Fasting insulin (pmol/L)	86.1 ± 56.3 [2]	48.7 ± 17.1 [1]	133.1 ± 72.3 [3]	<0.0001
HOMA-IR	2.98 ± 1.77 [2]	1.84 ± 0.94 [1]	5.33 ± 3.70 [3]	<0.0001
Total-C (mmol/L)	4.57 ± 1.00 [2]	4.13 ± 0.67 [1]	4.84 ± 1.14 [2]	0.02
LDL-C (mmol/L)	2.81 ± 0.91	2.52 ± 0.70	2.99 ± 1.23	0.29
HDL-C (mmol/L)	1.32 ± 0.30 [2]	1.60 ± 0.45 [1]	0.99 ± 0.24 [3]	<0.0001
TG (mmol/L)	1.15 ± 0.56 [2]	0.77 ± 0.31 [1]	2.16 ± 1.21 [3]	<0.0001

Values are means ± SD. [a] *p* values are adjusted for age, sex and BMI. *p* values in bold were considered significantly different. [1,2,3] Represents the differences between groups using generalized linear models (GLM). Abbreviations: Ov/Ob, overweight/obese; NW, Normal weight; MetS+, with the metabolic syndrome; MetS−, without the metabolic syndrome.

3.2. Serum Metabolite Score

Using PCA, we retained three main factors that explained a maximum of variance in the data (Figure 1). Factor 1 was composed of 81 metabolites, including long chain PCaa and PCae, and few medium to long chain SGs. Factor 2 was composed of short and long chain ACs and several AA (C0, C16, C18, C3, C4, glutamic acid, isoleucine, leucine, methionine, phenylalanine, tyrosine and valine), whereas factor 3 was composed of few medium chain ACs (C12, C14:1-OH, C14:2, C18:2). Lists of metabolites composing each factor are available in Tables S1–S3.

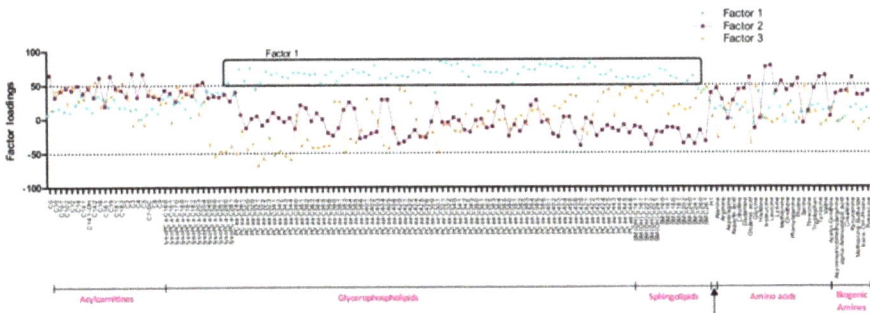

Figure 1. Metabolites patterns of the INFOGENE study. Metabolites with absolute factor loadings ⩾0.5 or −0.5 were regarded as significant contributors to the pattern. The blue line represents factor 1, the purple factor 2 and the orange factor 3.

In Table 2, factor scores are presented according to BMI and MetS status (Table 2A), and according to bioelectrical impedance analysis (BIA) measurement and MetS status (Table 2B). In fact, since body composition is difficult to predict based on a single indicator such as BMI, we also classified the subjects as being obese or not according to their percentage of body fat mass assessed by BIA. Briefly, when the BMI status was used, factor 1 score was higher among Ov/Ob participants with

MetS (0.36 ± 1.01) than among Ov/Ob participants without MetS (0.01 ± 1.01) or NW participants (-0.31 ± 0.84). Factor 2 score was higher among NW subjects (0.14 ± 1.03) than among Ov/Ob subjects with (-0.22 ± 0.73) or without (-0.05 ± 1.04) MetS. NW subjects had higher factor 3 scores (0.34 ± 0.95) than Ov/Ob subjects with (-0.36 ± 0.95) or without MetS (-0.01 ± 0.99). When the fat percentage was used, factor 1 score was higher among Ov/Ob participants with MetS (0.30 ± 0.16) than among Ov/Ob participants without MetS (0.03 ± 0.11) or NW participants (-0.35 ± 0.14). Factor 2 score was higher among NW subjects (0.29 ± 0.14) than among Ov/Ob subjects with (0.03 ± 0.17) or without (-0.08 ± 0.12) MetS. However, associations with factor 3 were lost. The association of obesity, metabolic syndrome and metabolite profile remained similar in the present study sample even though BMI or BIA measurements are used to define obesity. Thus, for the rest of the study, the obesity will be defined using BMI criteria.

Table 2A. Metabolite factor scores (obesity classification of subjects according to BMI criteria).

	MetS−		MetS+	*p*-Value
	Ov/Ob (*n* = 83)	NW (*n* = 65)	Ov/Ob (*n* = 46)	
Factor 1	0.01 ± 1.01 [2]	-0.31 ± 0.84 [3]	0.36 ± 1.01 [1]	0.003
Factor 2	-0.05 ± 1.04 [2]	0.14 ± 1.03 [3]	-0.22 ± 0.73 [1]	0.02
Factor 3	-0.01 ± 0.99 [2]	0.34 ± 0.95 [3]	-0.36 ± 0.95 [1]	0.03

Table 2B. Metabolite factor scores (obesity classification of subjects according to BIA criteria).

	MetS−		MetS+	*p*-Value
	Ob (*n* = 84)	NW (*n* = 65)	Ob (*n* = 36)	
Factor 1	0.03 ± 0.11 [3]	-0.35 ± 0.14 [2]	0.30 ± 0.16 [1]	0.005
Factor 2	-0.20 ± 0.11 [1]	0.29 ± 0.14 [2]	-0.17 ± 0.16 [1]	0.03
Factor 3	-0.08 ± 0.12 [1]	0.12 ± 0.15 [1]	0.03 ± 0.17 [1]	0.59

3.3. Relation between Cardiometabolic Risk Factors and PCA Factors

Table 3 shows that factor 1 was positively correlated with total-C and TG levels in all three groups. HDL-C was also positively correlated with factor 1 but only in subjects without MetS (Ov/Ob: $r = 0.27$; $p = 0.01$ and NW: $r = 0.26$; $p = 0.04$) while LDL-C was correlated with factor 1 only in Ov/Ob people with MetS ($r = 0.31$; $p = 0.04$). In Table 4, we observe that factor 2 was negatively correlated to WC among Ov/Ob with MetS ($r = -0.36$; $p = 0.02$). Factor 2 was also associated with HDL-C ($r = 0.34$; $p = 0.008$) and insulin levels ($r = -0.25$; $p = 0.05$) in NW individuals without MetS. In addition, factor 2 was associated with LDL-C ($r = 0.30$; $p = 0.007$) and total-C ($r = 0.34$; $p = 0.002$) among Ov/Ob subjects without MetS. Finally, Table 5 shows that factor 3 is negatively associated with glucose among Ov/Ob with MetS ($r = -0.30$; $p = 0.05$) and with insulin ($r = -0.27$; $p = 0.02$) and HOMA-IR ($r = -0.24$; $p = 0.03$) among Ov/Ob without MetS.

Table 3. Correlations between cardiometabolic risk factors and factor 1.

		MetS−		MetS+
		Ov/Ob (*n* = 83)	NW (*n* = 65)	Ov/Ob (*n* = 46)
WC	*r*	0.14	0.23	0.01
	p	0.23	0.07	0.95
Total-C	*r*	0.32	0.38	0.63
	p	0.003	0.003	<0.0001
TG	*r*	0.61	0.45	0.44
	p	<0.0001	0.0002	0.003
HDL-C	*r*	0.27	0.26	0.19
	p	0.01	0.04	0.22

Table 3. *Cont.*

		MetS−		MetS+
		Ov/Ob (*n* = 83)	NW (*n* = 65)	Ov/Ob (*n* = 46)
LDL-C	*r*	0.11	0.22	0.31
	p	0.33	0.09	**0.04**
Glucose	*r*	−0.03	0.03	0.16
	p	0.81	0.81	0.32
Insulin	*r*	0.12	−0.05	−0.03
	p	0.39	0.69	0.86
SBP	*r*	0.03	−0.07	0.23
	p	0.81	0.64	0.19
DBP	*r*	−0.1	−0.04	0.16
	p	0.39	0.74	0.29
HOMA-IR	*r*	0.08	−0.03	0.002
	p	0.47	0.82	0.91

Pearson correlation coefficients (*r*) and associated *p* values are provided. Abbreviations: Ov/Ob, overweight/obese; NW, Normal weight; MetS+, with the metabolic syndrome; MetS−, without the metabolic syndrome.

Table 4. Correlations between cardiometabolic risk factors and factor 2.

		MetS−		MetS+
		Ov/Ob (*n* = 83)	NW (*n* = 65)	Ov/Ob (*n* = 46)
WC	*r*	−0.10	0.09	−0.36
	p	0.35	0.47	**0.02**
Total-C	*r*	0.34	0.18	0.17
	p	**0.002**	0.17	0.28
TG	*r*	0.01	−0.09	0.05
	p	0.91	0.46	0.75
HDL-C	*r*	0.09	0.34	0.12
	p	0.42	**0.008**	0.53
LDL-C	*r*	0.30	−0.02	0.16
	p	**0.007**	0.91	0.31
Glucose	*r*	−0.02	0.002	0.14
	p	0.83	0.99	0.36
Insulin	*r*	0.08	−0.25	0.15
	p	0.49	**0.05**	0.32
SBP	*r*	0.05	−0.04	0.09
	p	0.67	0.79	0.58
DBP	*r*	0.09	0.08	0.06
	p	0.44	0.56	0.71
HOMA-IR	*r*	0.07	−0.14	0.16
	p	0.54	0.30	0.30

Pearson correlation coefficients (*r*) and associated *p* values are provided. Abbreviations: Ov/Ob, overweight/obese; NW, Normal weight; MetS+, with the metabolic syndrome; MetS−, without the metabolic syndrome.

Table 5. Correlations between cardiometabolic risk factors and factor 3.

		MetS−		MetS+
		Ov/Ob (*n* = 83)	NW (*n* = 65)	Ov/Ob (*n* = 46)
WC	*r*	−0.07	0.02	0.17
	p	0.55	0.89	0.28
Total-C	*r*	−0.06	0.14	0.13
	p	0.62	0.29	0.41

Table 5. *Cont.*

		MetS−		MetS+
		Ov/Ob (*n* = 83)	NW (*n* = 65)	Ov/Ob (*n* = 46)
TG	*r*	−0.16	0.04	−0.22
	p	0.16	0.75	0.15
HDL-C	*r*	0.16	0.22	0.14
	p	0.16	0.09	0.36
LDL-C	*r*	−0.08	0.01	0.11
	p	0.46	0.93	0.48
Glucose	*r*	0.0009	−0.10	−0.32
	p	0.99	0.42	**0.05**
Insulin	*r*	−0.27	−0.21	−0.1
	p	**0.02**	0.09	0.52
SBP	*r*	0.07	0.06	−0.06
	p	0.51	0.67	0.71
DBP	*r*	−0.04	0.01	0.25
	p	0.71	0.92	0.11
HOMA-IR	*r*	−0.24	−0.23	−0.17
	p	**0.03**	0.08	0.26

Pearson correlation coefficients (*r*) and associated *p* values are provided. Abbreviations: Ov/Ob, overweight/obese; NW, Normal weight; MetS+, with the metabolic syndrome; MetS−, without the metabolic syndrome.

4. Discussion

Abdominal obesity is a feature of MetS. The risk of developing metabolic disorders is proportional to the degree of obesity [19]. However, all obese individuals do not have MetS [4,20]. Mechanisms explaining the development of MetS are poorly understood and must be intensely investigated since their understanding may favor the design of prevention and therapeutic strategies. Metabolites are the intermediate products of different metabolic pathways. In the present study, employing metabolomics, we investigated differences in plasma composition between lean and Ov/Ob people, with or without MetS.

Obesity is defined as an excess of body fat. Unfortunately, body fat is tricky to measure. Several methods can be used to determine whether a human being is obese or not [21]. Depending on the method used, the definition of obesity can be surprisingly different. In the present study, obesity status was assessed using BMI and fat mass quantification by BIA. Metabolite score remained similar when either BMI or percent body fat were used. Thus, the rest of the analyses were done using BMI criteria to classify study subjects as being obese or not.

Using PCAs, we identified three metabolite clusters: factor 1, 2 and 3. Factor 1 is composed of long chain phosphatidylcholines and SMs. It regroups metabolites that seem to be linked with MetS but also with obesity itself. In fact, factor 1 score was higher and positive among Ov/Ob participants with and without MetS and negative among NW people. PCaa and SMs composing factor 1 are involved in lipid metabolism and are important for lipid transport. Their concentrations have been related to fat accumulation in liver of obese subjects [22], possibly explaining higher plasma levels of these metabolites in this population. In a study realised by Eisingerand *et al.*, an increase of total PCs and SMs was observed in mice fed a high fat diet in comparison with mice fed with a standard chow diet [23].

Plasmalogens (PLs) are a subclass of GPs characterized by the presence of a vinyl-ether bond and an ester bond at the sn-1 and sn-2 positions, respectively, of the glycerol backbone [24]. They have several cell functions; in fact, they act as reservoirs for second messengers or as structural attributes in the plasma membrane. They are also anti-oxidants preventing lipoprotein peroxidation; the hydrogen atoms adjacent to the vinyl-ether bond have relatively low disassociation energies and are preferentially oxidized over diacyl GP when exposed to various free radicals and singlet oxygen. PLs are consumed in this reaction. This was proposed to spare the oxidation of polyunsaturated fatty acids and other vulnerable membrane lipids, suggesting a role for PLs as sacrificial oxidants [25]. Sinder and collaborators showed that the oxidative products of PLs are unable to further propagate lipid peroxidation; thus PLs may terminate lipid oxidation. In the present study, a global reduction of PL concentrations was seen among Ov/Ob subjects (Table S1) in line with increased oxidative state observed in obesity [26]. To investigate environmental factors related to obesity, Pietilainen *et al.* led a study in monozygotic twins discordant for obesity. A change in the general metabolites serum composition was seen between obese and non-obese twins [27]. A decrease of ether phospholipids was observed among obese twins compared to lean twins [27,28]. Jordan *et al.* also reported a diminution of PCae with an increase of subject's fat mass. Studies among children have shown a decrease of PCae between lean and obese children [9,29]. As far as PCaa are concerned, Oberbach *et al.* showed an increase of several PCaa including C32:0, C32:1 and C40:5 levels among obese as compared to lean individuals [30,31], a trend that was also observed for PCaa C32:1 and C40:5 in the present study. Globally, our current study adds to others arguing that development of obesity comes along with a global decrease of PCae and with an increase of several PCaa by demonstrating that these changes are more important in the group of subjects with MetS.

Factor 2 is composed of AA including branch chained AA (BCAAs) (isoleucine, leucine and valine) and few ACs. BCAAs are essential AA that must be supplied by the diet [32]. BCAAs play a variety of physiological roles. They are regulatory molecules that have several cellular functions. They are nutrient signals that regulate protein synthesis, degradation and insulin secretion [33–35]. Although BCAAs are essential to the human body, studies have shown a dysregulation of their plasma concentrations with diseases [15]. For instance, in obese and insulin resistant subjects, an increase of BCAA levels is often observed when compared to lean individuals [30,36,37]. Factor 2 was comprised of a few ACs including free and odd short-chain ACs (C3 and C5). These two ACs are by-products of BCAA catabolism, thus their presence may be related to the degradation of BCAAs.

Factor 2 and factor 3 scores are higher among NW than among Ov/Ob individuals. It seems that the clusters of metabolites belonging to factors 2 and 3 are more tightly linked to a healthy metabolic state than factor 1. Several authors reported that increased plasma BCAA and AC levels were linked to several metabolic diseases [32,38]. In the present study, factor 2 and 3 scores were higher among NW subjects with a more favorable metabolic state. Factor 2 and 3 metabolite scores were lower among Ov/Ob participants with MetS and intermediate for Ov/Ob without MetS. This suggests a relation between metabolites composing these factors, MetS and obesity status. In the present study, an increase of the BCAA levels can be seen from NW participants to Ov/Ob ones, this increase being more important among Ov/Ob subjects with MetS. The same situation was observed for short chain ACs such as C0, C3 and C5.

Correlations between factor 1 and cardiometabolic risk factors were investigated. A positive correlation of factor 1 with plasma total-C and TG levels was observed in each group. This suggests that the association between factor 1, total-C and TG is independent of the metabolic state of study participants. A positive correlation was also seen between factor 1 and LDL-C levels but only among Ov/Ob participants with MetS. LDL-C is an established risk factor for CVDs but is not included as one of the five components of the MetS [39]. In literature, evidence regarding the association between LDL-C levels and MetS is not abundant, thus the contribution of LDL-C levels to the altered plasma lipid profile in MetS is unclear. HDL-C levels are known to be negatively associated with a deteriorated metabolic health. Here, we observed a positive association between factor 1 and HDL-C levels but only in groups without MetS irrespective of their obesity status. Factor 1 discriminates participants according to their MetS status rather than on obesity status. Factor 1 is mostly composed of GPs and SGs. Since these lipids are present in membranes and are involved in lipoprotein metabolism and transport, the association between blood lipids and these metabolites was expected. In a study led by Graessen *et al.*, bariatric surgery was associated with an improvement of the plasma lipid profile. In fact, they reported an improvement of the LDL-C levels along with a decrease of PC concentrations in obese subjects with MetS [15,40].

Factor 2 is composed of AA including BCAAs and few ACs. BCAAs have several physiological functions [41,42]. However, despite these beneficial effects on metabolic health, studies have shown that increased levels of circulating BCAAs were associated with poor metabolic health. In the present study, factor 2 was positively correlated with HDL-C and negatively correlated with insulin levels among NW participants without MetS. A negative correlation was also noted between WC and factor 2 but only among Ov/Ob with MetS. These results are concordant with what was observed with the metabolite scores; in fact, NW participants had higher metabolite scores and lower concentrations of BCAAs and short chain ACs. The association of factor 2 with a better health profile seems to be positively linked to HDL-C and negatively to insulin levels. Factor 3 is composed of medium ACs and is negatively correlated with glucose levels among Ov/Ob subjects with MetS and also negatively correlated to insulin levels and HOMA-IR among Ov/Ob individuals without MetS. In a study led by our group, a cluster of metabolites composed of medium to long chain ACs was negatively associated to a Western dietary pattern [43]. These results strengthen the hypothesis that the medium to long chain AC parts of factor 3 are positively associated with metabolic health.

5. Conclusions

Using metabolomic profiling, we identified a handful of relevant metabolites distinguishing obesity and MetS. For instance, long chain PCaa, PCae and medium chain SMs composing factor 1 were distributed differently between Ov/Ob and the other groups. They seem to be rather associated with a deteriorated metabolic profile. In contrast, factors 2 and 3 are associated with a healthy metabolic profile. So far, mechanisms explaining the shift of metabolite levels from normal to abnormal metabolic phenotypes are not clear. More validation studies are needed to better understand the underlying mechanisms triggering the dysregulation of metabolic traits in obesity.

Supplementary Materials: The following are available online at http://www.mdpi.com/2072-6643/8/6/324/s1, Table S1: Factor 1 metabolites composition categorized by obesity and MetS status, Table S2: Factor 2 metabolites composition categorized by obesity and MetS status, Table S3: Factor 3 metabolites composition categorized by obesity and MetS status.

Acknowledgments: This research would not have been possible without the excellent collaboration of all the participants. We would like to thank Marie-Eve Bouchard, Steve Amireault, Diane Drolet, and Dominique Beaulieu for their involvement in the study coordination, recruitment of the subjects, and data collection. We would also like to thank Chenomx Inc. (Edmonton, AB, Canada) who performed the mass spectrometry analyses to measure plasma metabolite levels. Marie-Claude Vohl is Canada Research Chair in Genomics Applied to Nutrition and Health.

Author Contributions: P.L. and M.-C.V. conceived and designed the experiments; V.G., B.A.-N., F.G. and H.C. analyzed the data; B.A.-N. and O.B. interpreted data; B.A.-N. wrote the paper.

Conflicts of Interest: The authors declare no conflict of interest.

References

1. Expert Panel on Detection, Evaluation. Executive summary of the third report of the national cholesterol education program (NCEP) expert panel on detection, evaluation, and treatment of high blood cholesterol in adults (Adult Treatment Panel III). *JAMA* **2001**, *285*, 2486–2497.
2. Sowers, J.R. Obesity as a cardiovascular risk factor. *Am. J. Med.* **2003**, *115*, S37–S41. [CrossRef]
3. James, P.T. Obesity: The worldwide epidemic. *Clin. Dermatol.* **2004**, *22*, 276–280. [CrossRef] [PubMed]
4. Karelis, A.D.; St-Pierre, D.H.; Conus, F.; Rabasa-Lhoret, R.; Poehlman, E.T. Metabolic and body composition factors in subgroups of obesity: What do we know? *J. Clin. Endocrinol. Metab.* **2004**, *89*, 2569–2575. [CrossRef] [PubMed]
5. Aguilar-Salinas, C.A.; Garcia, E.G.; Robles, L.; Riano, D.; Ruiz-Gomez, D.G.; Garcia-Ulloa, A.C.; Melgarejo, M.A.; Zamora, M.; Guillen-Pineda, L.E.; Mehta, R.S.; *et al.* High adiponectin concentrations are associated with the metabolically healthy obese phenotype. *J. Clin. Endocrinol. Metab.* **2008**, *93*, 4075–4079. [CrossRef] [PubMed]

6. Hamer, M.; Stamatakis, E. Metabolically healthy obesity and risk of all-cause and cardiovascular disease mortality. *J. Clin. Endocrinol. Metab.* **2012**, *97*, 2482–2488. [CrossRef] [PubMed]
7. Wildman, R.P.; Muntner, P.; Reynolds, K.; McGinn, A.P.; Rajpathak, S.; Wylie-Rosett, J.; Sowers, M.R. The obese without cardiometabolic risk factor clustering and the normal weight with cardiometabolic risk factor clustering: Prevalence and correlates of 2 phenotypes among the US population (NHANES 1999–2004). *Arch. Intern. Med.* **2008**, *168*, 1617–1624. [CrossRef] [PubMed]
8. Bain, J.R.; Stevens, R.D.; Wenner, B.R.; Ilkayeva, O.; Muoio, D.M.; Newgard, C.B. Metabolomics applied to diabetes research: Moving from information to knowledge. *Diabetes* **2009**, *58*, 2429–2443. [CrossRef] [PubMed]
9. Lee, A.; Jang, H.B.; Ra, M.; Choi, Y.; Lee, H.J.; Park, J.Y.; Kang, J.H.; Park, K.H.; Park, S.I.; Song, J. Prediction of future risk of insulin resistance and metabolic syndrome based on Korean boy's metabolite profiling. *Obes. Res. Clin. Pract.* **2014**, *9*, 336–345. [CrossRef] [PubMed]
10. Jourdan, C.; Petersen, A.K.; Gieger, C.; Doring, A.; Illig, T.; Wang-Sattler, R.; Meisinger, C.; Peters, A.; Adamski, J.; Prehn, C.; *et al.* Body fat free mass is associated with the serum metabolite profile in a population-based study. *PLoS ONE* **2012**, *7*, e40009. [CrossRef] [PubMed]
11. Paradis, A.M.; Perusse, L.; Godin, G.; Vohl, M.C. Validity of a self-reported measure of familial history of obesity. *Nutr. J.* **2008**, *7*, 27. [CrossRef] [PubMed]
12. Frankenfield, D.C.; Rowe, W.A.; Cooney, R.N.; Smith, J.S.; Becker, D. Limits of body mass index to detect obesity and predict body composition. *Nutrition* **2001**, *17*, 26–30. [CrossRef]
13. Albers, J.J.; Warnick, G.R.; Wiebe, D.; King, P.; Steiner, P.; Smith, L.; Breckenridge, C.; Chow, A.; Kuba, K.; Weidman, S.; *et al.* Multi-laboratory comparison of three heparin-Mn2+ precipitation procedures for estimating cholesterol in high-density lipoprotein. *Clin. Chem.* **1978**, *24*, 853–856. [PubMed]
14. Kubo, N. Evaluation of LDL-cholesterol measurement. *Rinsho Byori* **2002**, *50*, 242–247. [PubMed]
15. Newgard, C.B.; An, J.; Bain, J.R.; Muehlbauer, M.J.; Stevens, R.D.; Lien, L.F.; Haqq, A.M.; Shah, S.H.; Arlotto, M.; Slentz, C.A.; *et al.* A branched-chain amino acid-related metabolic signature that differentiates obese and lean humans and contributes to insulin resistance. *Cell Metab.* **2009**, *9*, 311–326. [CrossRef] [PubMed]
16. Desbuquois, B.; Aurbach, G.D. Use of polyethylene glycol to separate free and antibody-bound peptide hormones in radioimmunoassays. *J. Clin. Endocrinol. Metab.* **1971**, *33*, 732–738. [CrossRef] [PubMed]
17. Richterich, R.; Kuffer, H.; Lorenz, E.; Colombo, J.P. The determination of glucose in plasma and serum (hexokinase-glucose-6-phosphate dehydrogenase method) with the Greiner electronic selective analyzer GSA II (author's transl). *Z. Klin. Chem. Klin. Biochem.* **1974**, *12*, 5–13. [PubMed]
18. Matthews, D.R.; Hosker, J.P.; Rudenski, A.S.; Naylor, B.A.; Treacher, D.F.; Turner, R.C. Homeostasis model assessment: Insulin resistance and beta-cell function from fasting plasma glucose and insulin concentrations in man. *Diabetologia* **1985**, *28*, 412–419. [CrossRef] [PubMed]
19. Despres, J.P.; Lemieux, I.; Bergeron, J.; Pibarot, P.; Mathieu, P.; Larose, E.; Rodes-Cabau, J.; Bertrand, O.F.; Poirier, P. Abdominal obesity and the metabolic syndrome: Contribution to global cardiometabolic risk. *Arterioscler. Thromb. Vasc. Biol.* **2008**, *28*, 1039–1049. [CrossRef] [PubMed]
20. Fernandez-Real, J.M.; Menendez, J.A.; Moreno-Navarrete, J.M.; Bluher, M.; Vazquez-Martin, A.; Vazquez, M.J.; Ortega, F.; Dieguez, C.; Fruhbeck, G.; Ricart, W.; *et al.* Extracellular fatty acid synthase: A possible surrogate biomarker of insulin resistance. *Diabetes* **2010**, *59*, 1506–1511. [CrossRef] [PubMed]
21. Andreoli, A.; Garaci, F.; Cafarelli, F.P.; Guglielmi, G. Body composition in clinical practice. *Eur. J. Radiol.* **2016**. [CrossRef] [PubMed]
22. Heilbronn, L.K.; Coster, A.C.; Campbell, L.V.; Greenfield, J.R.; Lange, K.; Christopher, M.J.; Meikle, P.J.; Samocha-Bonet, D. The effect of short-term overfeeding on serum lipids in healthy humans. *Obesity* **2013**, *21*, E649–E659. [CrossRef] [PubMed]
23. Eisinger, K.; Krautbauer, S.; Hebel, T.; Schmitz, G.; Aslanidis, C.; Liebisch, G.; Buechler, C. Lipidomic analysis of the liver from high-fat diet induced obese mice identifies changes in multiple lipid classes. *Exp. Mol. Pathol.* **2014**, *97*, 37–43. [CrossRef] [PubMed]
24. Engelmann, B. Plasmalogens: Targets for oxidants and major lipophilic antioxidants. *Biochem. Soc. Trans.* **2004**, *32*, 147–150. [CrossRef] [PubMed]
25. Braverman, N.E.; Moser, A.B. Functions of plasmalogen lipids in health and disease. *Biochim. Biophys. Acta* **2012**, *1822*, 1442–1452. [CrossRef] [PubMed]

26. Kelly, A.S.; Jacobs, D.R.; Sinaiko, A.R., Jr.; Moran, A.; Steffen, L.M.; Steinberger, J. Relation of circulating oxidized LDL to obesity and insulin resistance in children. *Pediatr. Diabetes* **2010**, *11*, 552–555. [CrossRef] [PubMed]

27. Pietilainen, K.H.; Sysi-Aho, M.; Rissanen, A.; Seppanen-Laakso, T.; Yki-Jarvinen, H.; Kaprio, J.; Oresic, M. Acquired obesity is associated with changes in the serum lipidomic profile independent of genetic effects—A monozygotic twin study. *PLoS ONE* **2007**, *2*, e218. [CrossRef] [PubMed]

28. Chen, H.H.; Tseng, Y.J.; Wang, S.Y.; Tsai, Y.S.; Chang, C.S.; Kuo, T.C.; Yao, W.J.; Shieh, C.C.; Wu, C.H.; Kuo, P.H. The metabolome profiling and pathway analysis in metabolic healthy and abnormal obesity. *Int. J. Obes.* **2015**, *39*, 1241–1248. [CrossRef] [PubMed]

29. Wahl, S.; Yu, Z.; Kleber, M.; Singmann, P.; Holzapfel, C.; He, Y.; Mittelstrass, K.; Polonikov, A.; Prehn, C.; Romisch-Margl, W.; *et al.* Childhood obesity is associated with changes in the serum metabolite profile. *Obes. Facts* **2012**, *5*, 660–670. [CrossRef] [PubMed]

30. Huffman, K.M.; Shah, S.H.; Stevens, R.D.; Bain, J.R.; Muehlbauer, M.; Slentz, C.A.; Tanner, C.J.; Kuchibhatla, M.; Houmard, J.A.; Newgard, C.B.; *et al.* Relationships between circulating metabolic intermediates and insulin action in overweight to obese, inactive men and women. *Diabetes Care* **2009**, *32*, 1678–1683. [CrossRef] [PubMed]

31. Oberbach, A.; Bluher, M.; Wirth, H.; Till, H.; Kovacs, P.; Kullnick, Y.; Schlichting, N.; Tomm, J.M.; Rolle-Kampczyk, U.; Murugaiyan, J.; *et al.* Combined proteomic and metabolomic profiling of serum reveals association of the complement system with obesity and identifies novel markers of body fat mass changes. *J. Proteom. Res.* **2011**, *10*, 4769–4788. [CrossRef] [PubMed]

32. Layman, D.K. The role of leucine in weight loss diets and glucose homeostasis. *J. Nutr.* **2003**, *133*, S261–S267.

33. Cota, D.; Proulx, K.; Smith, K.A.; Kozma, S.C.; Thomas, G.; Woods, S.C.; Seeley, R.J. Hypothalamic mTOR signaling regulates food intake. *Science* **2006**, *312*, 927–930. [CrossRef] [PubMed]

34. Fajans, S.S. Leucine-Induced hypoglycemia. *N. Engl. J. Med.* **1965**, *272*, 1224–1227. [CrossRef] [PubMed]

35. Hay, N.; Sonenberg, N. Upstream and downstream of mTOR. *Genes Dev.* **2004**, *18*, 1926–1945. [CrossRef] [PubMed]

36. Shah, S.H.; Crosslin, D.R.; Haynes, C.S.; Nelson, S.; Turer, C.B.; Stevens, R.D.; Muehlbauer, M.J.; Wenner, B.R.; Bain, J.R.; Laferrere, B.; *et al.* Branched-chain amino acid levels are associated with improvement in insulin resistance with weight loss. *Diabetologia* **2012**, *55*, 321–330. [CrossRef] [PubMed]

37. Wilson, P.W.; Meigs, J.B.; Sullivan, L.; Fox, C.S.; Nathan, D.M.; D'Agostino, R.B., Sr. Prediction of incident diabetes mellitus in middle-aged adults: The Framingham Offspring Study. *Arch. Intern. Med.* **2007**, *167*, 1068–1074. [CrossRef] [PubMed]

38. Wang, T.J.; Larson, M.G.; Vasan, R.S.; Cheng, S.; Rhee, E.P.; McCabe, E.; Lewis, G.D.; Fox, C.S.; Jacques, P.F.; Fernandez, C.; *et al.* Metabolite profiles and the risk of developing diabetes. *Nat. Med.* **2011**, *17*, 448–453. [CrossRef] [PubMed]

39. Superko, H.R.; Krauss, R.M. Coronary artery disease regression. Convincing evidence for the benefit of aggressive lipoprotein management. *Circulation* **1994**, *90*, 1056–1069. [CrossRef] [PubMed]

40. Graessler, J.; Bornstein, T.D.; Goel, D.; Bhalla, V.P.; Lohmann, T.; Wolf, T.; Koch, M.; Qin, Y.; Licinio, J.; Wong, M.L.; *et al.* Lipidomic profiling before and after Roux-en-Y gastric bypass in obese patients with diabetes. *Pharmacogenom. J.* **2014**, *14*, 201–207. [CrossRef] [PubMed]

41. Doi, M.; Yamaoka, I.; Nakayama, M.; Mochizuki, S.; Sugahara, K.; Yoshizawa, F. Isoleucine, a blood glucose-lowering amino acid, increases glucose uptake in rat skeletal muscle in the absence of increases in AMP-activated protein kinase activity. *J. Nutr.* **2005**, *135*, 2103–2108. [PubMed]

42. Doi, M.; Yamaoka, I.; Nakayama, M.; Sugahara, K.; Yoshizawa, F. Hypoglycemic effect of isoleucine involves increased muscle glucose uptake and whole body glucose oxidation and decreased hepatic gluconeogenesis. *Am. J. Physiol. Endocrinol. Metab.* **2007**, *292*, E1683–E1693. [CrossRef] [PubMed]

43. Bouchard-Mercier, A.; Rudkowska, I.; Lemieux, S.; Couture, P.; Vohl, M.C. The metabolic signature associated with the Western dietary pattern: A cross-sectional study. *Nutr. J.* **2013**, *12*, 158. [CrossRef] [PubMed]

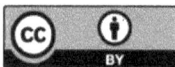

© 2016 by the authors. Licensee MDPI, Basel, Switzerland. This article is an open access article distributed under the terms and conditions of the Creative Commons Attribution (CC BY) license (http://creativecommons.org/licenses/by/4.0/).

nutrients

MDPI

Article

Complementary Effects of Genetic Variations in *LEPR* on Body Composition and Soluble Leptin Receptor Concentration after 3-Month Lifestyle Intervention in Prepubertal Obese Children

Joanna Gajewska [1,*], Alina Kuryłowicz [2], Ewa Mierzejewska [3], Jadwiga Ambroszkiewicz [1], Magdalena Chełchowska [1], Halina Weker [4] and Monika Puzianowska-Kuźnicka [2,5]

[1] Screening Department, Institute of Mother and Child, Kasprzaka 17a, Warsaw 01-211, Poland; jagoda.ambroszkiewicz@imid.med.pl (J.A.); magdalena.chelchowska@imid.med.pl (M.C.)
[2] Department of Human Epigenetics, Mossakowski Medical Research Center, Polish Academy of Sciences, Warsaw 02-106, Poland; kurylowiczala@gazeta.pl (A.K.); mpuzianowska@wum.edu.pl (M.P.-K.)
[3] Department of Epidemiology and Biostatistics, Institute of Mother and Child, Warsaw 01-211, Poland; ewa.mierzejewska@imid.med.pl
[4] Department of Nutrition, Institute of Mother and Child, Warsaw 01-211, Poland; halina.weker@imid.med.pl
[5] Department of Geriatrics and Gerontology, Medical Center of Postgraduate Education, Warsaw 01-826, Poland
* Correspondence: joanna.gajewska@imid.med.pl; Tel.: +48-22-327-7260; Fax: +48-22-327-7161

Received: 30 March 2016; Accepted: 24 May 2016; Published: 27 May 2016

Abstract: In obese individuals, weight loss might be affected by variants of the adipokine-encoding genes. We verified whether selected functional single nucleotide polymorphisms in *LEP*, *LEPR* and *ADIPOQ* are associated with changes in serum levels of the respective adipokines and weight loss in 100 prepubertal obese (SDS-BMI > 2) Caucasian children undergoing lifestyle intervention. Frequencies of the -2548G > A *LEP*, Q223R *LEPR*, K656N *LEPR*, -11377C > G and -11426A > G *ADIPOQ* polymorphisms were analyzed by restriction fragment length polymorphism. Serum adipokine and soluble leptin receptor (sOB-R) concentrations were measured using the ELISA method. Among the analyzed polymorphisms, only *LEPR* polymorphisms were associated with changes of SDS-BMI or sOB-R concentrations in children after therapy. Carriers of the wild-type K665N and at least one minor Q223R allele had the greatest likelihood of losing weight (OR = 5.09, p = 0.006), an increase in sOB-R (p_{trend} = 0.022) and decrease in SDS-BMI correlated with the decrease of fat mass (p < 0.001). In contrast, carrying of the wild-type Q223R and at least one minor K665N allele were associated with a decrease in sOB-R concentrations and a decrease in SDS-BMI correlated with a decrease in fat-free mass (p = 0.002). We suggest that the combination of different LEPR variants, not a single variant, might determine predisposition to weight loss in the prepubertal period.

Keywords: leptin receptor; polymorphisms; weight loss; adipokines; prepubertal period

1. Introduction

It is widely recognized that the response to lifestyle interventions, such as changes in dietary habits and physical activity, can be heterogeneous and largely genetically determined [1]. Functional variants of genes involved in appetite regulation, energy metabolism and fat storage are considered candidates to confer susceptibility to weight loss, and their identification may be helpful in the prevention of future health problems.

Among several genetic variants investigated in relation to the effectiveness of weight loss therapy in obese subjects are Q223R (or Gln223Arg, rs1137101) and K656N (or Lys656Asn, rs8129183)

polymorphisms in the leptin receptor gene (*LEPR*) [2–4]. Leptin receptor, which is a member of the cytokine receptor family, has several isoforms of different locations and functions [5]. For example, the weight-regulating effects of leptin are mediated by binding to and activation of the specific receptor (long isoform, OB-R$_L$) in the brain, while a soluble form of this receptor (one of its short isoforms, sOB-R) modulates leptin levels by binding free leptin in the circulation and preventing the hormone from degradation and clearance [6].

The Q223R A > G (A668G) and K656N G > C (G1968C) polymorphisms in *LEPR* result in nonconservative changes: glutamine to arginine at codon 223 and lysine to asparagine at codon 656, respectively [7,8]. These amino acid substitutions result in changes of the electric charge from neutral to positive for Q223→R and from positive to neutral for K656→N and, therefore, are likely to have functional consequences resulting in changed leptin signaling and, in the broader perspective, an affected response to energy restriction [7]. However, there are only a few studies that have evaluated the impact of these polymorphisms on changes in metabolic parameters during weight loss.

The diverse response of leptin levels and body mass changes depending on polymorphic variants of *LEP* and *LEPR* has been investigated mainly in obese adults [2,3,9–13]. There are also studies suggesting a gene-gene interaction between the *LEP* and *LEPR* variants in a genetic susceptibility to the development of obesity [14]. A cumulative effect of *LEPR* polymorphisms with other obesity susceptibility loci, including variants in the adiponectin locus (*ADIPOQ*), on weight loss was also observed in Spanish obese adolescents after a multidisciplinary intervention [15]. Case-control studies on the association between polymorphisms in genes encoding adipokines with childhood obesity have been conducted [16–20], but to our knowledge, there is no data concerning the influence of these polymorphisms on weight loss and adipokine concentrations after multidisciplinary intervention. Therefore, the aim of our study was to investigate the effect of selected functional single nucleotide polymorphisms (SNPs) in *LEPR*, *LEP*, and *ADIPOQ* loci on metabolic response and weight loss after a 3-month lifestyle intervention in prepubertal obese children.

2. Methods

2.1. Subjects

One hundred obese prepubertal Caucasian children aged 5–10 years were recruited between 2010 and 2012 from a group of consecutive patients seeking dietary counseling in the Department of Nutrition at the Institute of Mother and Child in Warsaw. Obesity was classified as standard deviation score-body mass index (SDS-BMI) >2. Exclusion criteria were: (a) presence of endocrine disorders or genetic syndromes, including syndromic obesity; (b) other chronic medical conditions; (c) intake of medications that could affect growth, pubertal development, nutritional or dietary status. Pubertal stage was determined according to the Tanner scale and subjects who showed pubertal development were excluded. Written informed consent was obtained from the parents of all the examined children. The study was performed in accordance with the Helsinki Declaration for Human Research and the study protocol was approved (No. 25/2006) by the Ethics Committee of the Institute of Mother and Child in Warsaw, Poland.

2.2. Dietary Intervention

To evaluate changes in clinical, anthropometric and biochemical parameters in response to lifestyle changes, the obese prepubertal patients underwent a 3-month intervention program consisting of dietary and physical activity modifications and behavioral therapy, including individual psychological care for the child and his/her family. The dietary guidelines, recommending a low-energy diet based on a balanced distribution of carbohydrates, proteins and lipids, for children and their parents, were described in a previous study [21]. The recommended daily energy intake was 1200–1400 kcal/day. The diet was composed of 20% protein, 30% fat and of 50% carbohydrates. Patients had 3–5 meals every day. Study participants did not receive vitamins or mineral supplements. Patients received instructions concerning physical activity, details of which were also previously described [22]. Children were advised to reduce sedentary activities, including watching television and playing computer games to less than two hours a day. Two weeks before the visit in the Department of Nutrition, study participants completed a 10–14 days food diary using a standard questionnaire. Next, randomly selected 3-day records: two consecutive weekdays and one weekend day, before (visit T0) and after 3 months of therapy (visit T3) were analyzed. The subjects and their parents were asked to record the type and amount of food and beverages consumed for the selected days. We evaluated the average daily energy intake and the percentage of energy intake from protein, fat and carbohydrates in the children's diets. Average daily food rations and their nutritional value were calculated using nutritional analysis software (Dietetyk®, National Food and Nutrition Institute, version 2.0, Warsaw, Poland) [23]. The age- and sex-specific dietary reference intake (DRI) percentage was calculated using reference values of daily energy intake for children and adolescents according to Jarosz *et al.* [24].

2.3. Anthropometric Parameters

Physical examinations, including body height and weight measurements, were performed before (visit T0) and after 3 months of therapy (visit T3). Body height was measured using a standing stadiometer and recorded with a precision of 1 mm. Body weight was assessed unclothed, to the nearest 0.1 kg, with a calibrated balance scale. BMI was calculated as body weight divided by height squared (kg/m^2). The BMI of each individual was converted to a standard SDS-BMI for the child's age and sex using Polish reference tables [25]. The data of this reference population were derived from a study concerning the physical development of Warsaw children and adolescents aged 1–18 years, which was conducted in the years 1996–1999 by the Department of Development of Children and Adolescents at the Institute of Mother and Child. Skinfolds were measured with a Holtain skinfold caliper (Holtain Ltd., Wales, UK). Fat mass percentage was calculated according to Lohman's formula [26].

2.4. Biochemical Measurements

Biochemical parameters were determined twice: before (visit T0) and after 3 months of therapy (visit T3). Venous blood samples were collected between 8:00 and 10:00 a.m. after an overnight fast, and centrifuged at $1000\times g$ for 10 min at 4 °C. Serum specimens were stored at -70 °C prior to assay. Commercially available ELISA kits (DRG Diagnostics, Marburg, Germany) were used to determine leptin and sOB-R concentrations. Inter-assay variations (CV%) were 5.3% and 3.3% for total leptin and sOB-R, respectively. Serum levels of total adiponectin and high molecular weight (HMW) adiponectin were determined using ELISA kit (ALPCO Diagnostics, Salem, NH, USA). Adiponectin multimers were selectively measured after sample pretreatment with two proteases that specifically digested the trimeric forms or both the hexameric and trimeric forms. In this assay, total adiponectin and HMW adiponectin levels were determined directly. Inter-assay variations were 5.0% and 5.7% for total adiponectin and HMW adiponectin, respectively. Glucose, total cholesterol, LDL and HDL-cholesterol and triglycerides were measured by standard methods (Roche Diagnostics, Basel, Switzerland). To reduce interassay variance, samples obtained before and after therapy were analyzed in one assay.

2.5. DNA Isolation and Genetic Analysis

DNA was isolated from 4 mL of venous blood samples by a salting-out procedure [27]. Genotyping of the -2548G > A *LEP* (rs7799039), Q223R (*A668G*, rs1137101) and K656N (*G1968C*, rs8129183) *LEPR*, as well as -11377C > G (rs266729) and -11426A > G (rs16861194) *ADIPOQ* polymorphisms was performed by PCR amplification followed by digestion with an appropriate restriction enzyme [20]. The obtained restriction fragments were visualized on 2%–3% agarose gels. For quality control of genetic testing: (i) amplification blank controls consisting of only amplification reagents without DNA were performed during each PCR reaction; (ii) randomly selected DNA samples were analyzed by sequencing; (iii) control samples with genotypes identified by sequencing were included into each PCR-RFLP reaction.

2.6. Statistical Analysis

The results are presented as means ± standard deviation (SD) for normally distributed data or medians and interquartile range (25th–75th percentiles) for non-normally distributed variables. The Kolmogorov-Smirnov test and graphical inspections of data were used to evaluate the distribution for normality.

Due to the fact that an increase in height between visit T0 and T3 could be partially responsible for a decrease in SDS-BMI in that time period, weight loss during intervention was defined as SDS-BMI change (Δ) $\leqslant$ −0.5. Differences in anthropometric characteristics and biochemical parameters between children who lost weight and those who have not were assessed using the Student t test for normally distributed data and the nonparametric Mann-Whitney test for non-normally distributed data. Paired Student *t* test or nonparametric Wilcoxon test were used to compare the parameters mentioned above before and after intervention in the whole group and in subgroups of children who lost weight and those that did not.

The Hardy-Weinberg equilibrium analysis was performed using a chi-square test with one degree of freedom. Additive, dominant, recessive and allelic models were tested for every polymorphism for associations with weight loss. Under each model, the odds ratios (ORs) with their 95% confidence intervals (CI) were calculated, and the chi-square test, Fisher exact test and Cochran-Armitage test for trend were used, as appropriate. The procedure described by Benjamini and Hochberg was used to correct *p*-values for multiple testing [28]. Linkage disequilibrium (LD) was analyzed using the pairwise LD measure D', and haplotype blocks were constructed from population genotype data using Haploview software [29], with the default algorithm for generating haplotype blocks based on methods established by Gabriel *et al.* [30]. A D' value of 1 indicates complete LD between the two markers; a D' value greater than 0.8—strong LD; 0.2–0.8—incomplete LD; whereas a D' of less than 0.2—negligible LD. Multiple logistic regression analysis was conducted to assess the combined impact of two *LEPR* polymorphisms on weight loss during therapy.

Changes in SDS-BMI, body composition and biochemical parameters were expressed as delta variables, calculated by subtracting values at baseline (T0) from values measured after 3 months of therapy (T3). Differences in anthropometric characteristics and biochemical parameters between different genotypes were assessed using the Student *t* test for normally distributed data and the nonparametric Mann-Whitney test for non-normally distributed data. To study associations of the combined genotypes of the *LEPR* polymorphisms Q223R and K656N with changes in soluble leptin receptor concentration, the multivariate linear regression model adjusted for age and sex was used. Genetic variants of the studied polymorphisms were treated as a continuous variable and put in order from the exclusive presence of at least one copy of Q223R minor allele to the exclusive presence of at least one copy of K656N minor allele. Test for linear trend was applied.

The correlation coefficients between changes in body composition and changes in SDS-BMI due to the intervention in children with combined genotypes of the *LEPR* Q223R and K656N polymorphisms were calculated using Pearson correlation.

Statistical significance was set at 0.05. Statistical analysis was performed using SPSS v.18.0 software (SPSS Inc., Chicago, IL, USA) and StatXact-3 software, version 3.1 (Cytel Software Corporation, Cambridge, MA, USA).

3. Results

3.1. Distribution of Polymorphisms in LEPR, LEP and ADIPOQ in Obese Children

One hundred obese children aged 4–10 years (47% male) were included in the analysis. After 3 months of therapy, mean height and SDS-height in the whole group increased (from 136 cm to 138 cm and from 0.98 to 1.29, respectively, both $p < 0.001$), while median weight, BMI and SDS-BMI decreased (from 47.2 kg to 45.2 kg, 25.1 kg/m^2 to 23.1 kg/m^2, and 3.46 to 2.82, respectively, all $p < 0.001$).

We categorized the children into two subgroups according to the level of SDS-BMI change during the intervention: with weight loss (ΔSDS-BMI ⩽ −0.5, n = 71) and without weight loss (ΔSDS-BMI > −0.5, n = 29).

Genotype and allele frequencies of the studied polymorphisms are shown in Table 1. All analyzed genotypes fulfilled the criteria of the Hardy-Weinberg equilibrium. Genotype frequencies of the *LEPR* Q223R (*A* > *G*) polymorphism were significantly different in obese children with and without weight loss. Analysis revealed the strongest association in the dominant genetic model when the presence of the *AG* or the *GG* genotype was associated with more than a three-fold higher likelihood of weight loss (OR = 3.45 (95% CI: 1.38–8.78), *p* = 0.007, adjusted FDR (False Discovery Rate) *p* = 0.035) compared with the *AA* genotype. The frequency of the *G* allele was also higher in obese patients with weight loss than without weight loss (52.1% *vs.* 32.8%; OR = 2.23 (95% CI: 1.18–4.23), *p* = 0.013, adjusted FDR *p* = 0.065).

We found no differences between the studied groups in genotype and allele distribution for K656N (G > C) *LEPR*, -2548G > A *LEP*, -11377C > G *ADIPOQ* and -11426A > G *ADIPOQ* SNPs.

Table 1. Distribution of *LEP*, *LEPR*, and *ADIPOQ* genotypes and alleles in prepubertal obese children with or without weight loss.

Gene/SNP	Obese Children with Weight Loss (ΔSDS-BMI ⩽ −0.5) n (%)	Obese Children without Weight Loss (ΔSDS-BMI > −0.5) n (%)	Inheritance Model	OR (95% CI)	Unadjusted *p*-Value	FDR Adjusted *p*-Value
LEP -2548G > A						
Genotypes						
GG	23 (32.4)	10 (34.5)	additive	–	0.767	0.767
GA	31 (43.7)	10 (34.5)	dominant	1.10 (0.44, 2.74)	0.840	0.840
AA	17 (23.9)	9 (31.0)	recessive	0.70 (0.27, 1.82)	0.463	0.926
Alleles						
G	77 (54.2)	30 (51.7)				
A	65 (45.8)	28 (48.3)	allelic	0.90 (0.49, 1.67)	0.748	0.748
LEPR Q223R A > G						
Genotypes						
AA	15 (21.1)	14 (48.3)	additive	–	0.014	0.056
AG	38 (53.5)	11 (37.9)	dominant	3.48 (1.38, 8.78)	0.007	**0.035**
GG	18 (25.4)	4 (13.8)	recessive	2.12 (0.65, 6.93)	0.205	0.820
Alleles						
A	68 (47.9)	39 (67.2)				
G	74 (52.1)	19 (32.8)	allelic	2.23 (1.18, 4.23)	0.013	0.065
LEPR K656N G > C						
Genotypes						
GG	58 (81.7)	19 (65.5)	additive	–	0.206	0.412
GC	11 (15.5)	10 (34.5)	dominant	0.43 (0.16, 1.13)	0.081	0.203
CC	2 (2.8)	0 (0.0)	recessive	–	1.000	1.000
Alleles						
G	127 (89.4)	48 (82.8)				
C	15 (10.6)	10 (17.2)	allelic	0.57 (0.24, 1.35)	0.195	0.488
ADIPOQ -11426A > G						
Genotypes						
AA	59 (83.1)	23 (79.3)	additive	–	–	–
AG	12 (16.9)	6 (20.7)	dominant	0.78 (0.26, 2.32)	0.655	1.092
GG	0 (0.0)	0 (0.0)	recessive	–	–	
Alleles						
A	130 (91.5)	52 (89.7)				
G	12 (8.5)	6 (10.3)	allelic	0.80 (0.28, 2.24)	0.671	0.839
ADIPOQ -11377C > G						
Genotypes						
CC	31 (43.7)	12 (41.4)	additive	–	0.657	0.876
CG	31 (43.7)	12 (41.4)	dominant	0.91 (0.38, 2.18)	0.834	1.043
GG	9 (12.6)	5 (17.2)	recessive	0.70 (0.21, 2.29)	0.540	0.720
Alleles						
C	93 (65.5)	36 (62.1)				
G	49 (34.5)	22 (37.9)	allelic	0.86 (0.46, 1.62)	0.646	1.077

FDR, false discovery rate; OR, odds ratio; BMI, body mass index; SDS, standard deviation score; SNP, single nucleotide polymorphism; CI, confidence interval.

3.2. Associations of Combination of Q223R and K656N LEPR Polymorphisms with Weight Loss in Obese Children after a 3-Month Intervention

Combined genotype frequencies of the *LEPR* Q223R/K656N polymorphisms are shown in Table 2. A complete LD between the two polymorphisms was observed (D' = 1). The *LEPR* genotype combinations Q223R/K656N: AG/CC, GG/GC and GG/CC were not observed. All children homozygous for one *LEPR* minor allele were wild-type homozygotes for the other.

Table 2. Distribution of Q223R and K656N *LEPR* genotypes in prepubertal obese children.

		LEPR K656N n (%)			Total
		GG	*GC*	*CC*	
	AA	18 (18.0%)	9 (9.0%)	2 (2.0%)	29.0%
LEPR Q223R	*AG*	37 (37.0%)	12 (12.0%)	–	49.0%
	GG	22 (22.0%)	–	–	22.0%
	Total	77.0%	21.0%	2.0%	100.0%

Based on the finding that the presence of only one minor allele in *LEPR* Q223R was sufficient for a higher likelihood of weight loss, we divided the children into four categories (Table 3): (1) the reference group: wild-type homozygotes for both polymorphisms; (2) subjects with at least one minor allele in Q223R only (genotypes *AG* or *GG*) and wild-type homozygotes for K656N; (3) wild-type homozygotes for Q223R with at least one minor allele in K656N only (genotypes *GC* or *CC*); (4) combined heterozygotes for both loci (Q223R *AG* and K656N *GC*). In the logistic regression model, we confirmed that obese children with at least one minor allele in Q223R and wild-type homozygotes for K656N had a 5-fold higher likelihood of losing weight (ΔSDS-BMI ≤ −0.5) (OR = 5.09 (95% CI: 1.60–16.24), p = 0.006) when compared with wild-type homozygotes for both loci. We did not find significant effects of other combinations of *LEPR* polymorphisms on weight loss.

Table 3. Logistic regression model of the combined influence of Q223R and K656N *LEPR* polymorphisms on weight loss (ΔSDS-BMI ≤ −0.5) in prepubertal obese children.

Variable	Children with Weight Loss (ΔSDS-BMI ≤ −0.5) n (%)	Children without Weight Loss (ΔSDS-BMI > −0.5) n (%)	OR	95% CI	p
Q223R/K656N genotypes					
Wild-type/Wild-type	9 (12.7%)	9 (31%)	Ref	-	-
AG or GG/Wild-type	49 (69.0%)	10 (34.5%)	5.09	(1.60, 16.24)	0.006
Wild-type/GC or CC	6 (8.5%)	5 (17.2%)	1.19	(0.25, 5.60)	0.828
AG/GC	7 (9.9%)	5 (17.2%)	1.53	(0.34, 6.85)	0.580
Sex					
Male	35 (49.3%)	12 (41.4%)	Ref	-	-
Female	36 (50.7%)	17 (58.6%)	0.95	(0.36, 2.51)	0.912
Age (year)	–		0.85	(0.62, 1.16)	0.301

OR, odds ratio; CI, confidence interval; Ref, reference.

3.3. Body Composition, Biochemical Parameters and Energy Intake before and after Intervention

Of the 100 children enrolled in the study, the full set of biochemical and anthropometric parameters as well as data on nutrition intake before and after intervention were available from 76 (aged 5–10 years, 42.1% male). Genotype and allele frequencies of the *LEPR* Q223R polymorphism in these 76 children were similar to those observed in the whole group. As in the whole group (n = 100), it was shown that the subjects carrying at least one minor allele in Q223R polymorphism (the *AG* or *GG* genotype) had a higher likelihood of weight loss (OR = 3.67 (95% CI: 1.24–10.84), p = 0.016) than wild-type homozygotes. Moreover, the presence of the G allele (in the allelic model) was associated with a higher probability of ΔSDS-BMI ⩽ −0.5 (OR = 2.23 (95% CI: 1.05–4.76), p = 0.036) when compared with A allele.

Both groups of children, who lost weight and those who did not, reduced their energy intake during the therapy (p < 0.001) (Table 4). In addition, the proportions of protein, fat and carbohydrates in daily energy intake and percentage of DRI were similar in both groups. Children with and without weight loss at visit T3, at the beginning of the intervention (T0) did not differ significantly in terms of anthropometric parameters, whereas at visit T3 the two groups had a similar height, SDS-height, and SDS-BMI, but significantly different body weight (p = 0.037) and BMI (p = 0.013). In the obese children with a change in SDS-BMI ⩽ −0.5 after the intervention, the median weight decrease was 5% (p < 0.001), the median fat mass decrease was 15% (p < 0.001), and the mean fat-free mass decrease was 3% (p < 0.001), while children with a change in SDS-BMI > −0.5 had similar values of these parameters before and after therapy.

Leptin levels after a 3-month intervention were significantly reduced in both groups, but at visit T3 this parameter was more than 2-fold lower (p < 0.001) in patients with weight loss compared with those with a change in SDS-BMI > −0.5 (Table 4). Soluble leptin receptor concentration increased only in children with weight loss (p < 0.001) and after the therapy its median concentration was about 30% higher than in those without weight loss (p < 0.001). Total adiponectin and HMW-adiponectin levels increased (both p < 0.05), while LDL-cholesterol and triglycerides decreased (p < 0.05 and p = 0.001, respectively) after the therapy only in children who lost weight (Table 4).

3.4. Associations of the LEPR Q223R and K656N Polymorphisms with the Level of Adipokines and Body Composition after 3-Month Intervention

We observed significant differences in the mean decrease in SDS-BMI and percentage of fat mass between individuals carrying different genotypes of the *LEPR* Q223R polymorphism (Table 5). The carriers of at least one minor allele (*AG* heterozygotes and *GG* homozygotes) had significantly greater mean changes of these parameters than the wild-type homozygotes (−0.97 *vs.* −0.63, p = 0.01 and −3.3% *vs.* −0.8%, p = 0.003, respectively). However, therapy-induced decrease in leptin, sOB-R level, leptin/sOB-R and leptin/adiponectin ratios were similar in the AG + GG and AA groups.

In contrast, we found significant differences in the mean, therapy-induced, decrease of sOB-R level between individuals carrying different genotypes of the *LEPR* K656N polymorphism. The wild-type homozygotes had significantly greater changes of sOB-R than carriers of at least one minor allele (*GC* heterozygotes and *CC* homozygotes), (4.0 ng/mL *vs.* 0.0 ng/mL, p = 0.032), despite the fact that therapy-induced changes in body composition were similar in the wild-type homozygotes and carriers of the K656N minor allele (Table 5).

In the linear regression model, after adjustment for age and sex, the differences in change of sOB-R concentrations among the four groups with different combinations of *LEPR* Q223R and K656N genotypes remained significant (p_{trend} = 0.022) with the trend from the highest values in the carriers of at least one minor allele in Q223R only towards lowest values in the carriers of at least one minor allele in K656N only (Figure 1).

Table 4. Clinical and biochemical characteristics and dietary intake in prepubertal obese children with and without weight loss.

	Obese Children with Weight Loss (ΔSDS-BMI ≤ −0.5) n = 56			Obese Children without Weight Loss (ΔSDS-BMI > −0.5) n = 20			p (T0 vs. T0)	p (T3 vs. T3)
	T0	T3	p (T3 vs. T0)	T0	T3	p (T3 vs. T0)		
Age (years)	8.1 (6.8–9.2)			8.8 (7.3–9.6)			0.110	
Male (%)	44.6			35.0			0.453	
Anthropometric parameters								
Height (cm)	135 ± 10	137 ± 10	<0.001	139 ± 10	141 ± 10	<0.001	0.137	0.152
SDS–height	0.99 ± 1.01	1.31 ± 1.00	<0.001	1.14 ± 1.08	1.42 ± 1.12	<0.001	0.572	0.700
Weight (kg)	45.2 (39.6–56.5)	42.9 (35.7–51.8)	<0.001	50.7 (39.7–56.6)	50.8 (39.8–56.3)	0.779	0.501	0.037
BMI	24.7 (23.1–28.1)	22.6 (20.4–25.5)	<0.001	25.8 (23.5–27.0)	25.2 (22.8–26.8)	0.002	0.929	0.013
SDS–BMI	3.52 (2.71–4.81)	2.41 (1.73–3.89)	<0.001	3.40 (2.88–4.02)	3.10 (2.50–3.87)	0.002	0.596	0.081
Body composition								
Fat mass (%)	41.1 (39.3–44.5)	38.4 (33.9–41.5)	<0.001	39.6 (36.7–43.4)	40.3 (37.2–43.5)	0.911	0.183	0.253
Fat mass (kg)	19.9 (15.7–23.7)	16.8 (13.5–20.9)	<0.001	20.8 (16.9–22.9)	20.3 (16.1–24.3)	0.881	0.832	0.031
Fat-free mass (kg)	27.5 ± 6.9	26.8 ± 6.5	<0.001	30.3 ± 6.8	30.3 ± 6.7	0.876	0.130	0.048
Biochemical measurements								
Leptin (ng/mL)	37.0 (23.5–54.7)	11.8 (5.9–26.6)	<0.001	42.9 (29.3–66.2)	26.5 (15.1–45.0)	0.004	0.288	0.001
Soluble leptin receptor (ng/mL)	23.0 (18.2–26.8)	28.4 (23.2–31.7)	<0.001	22.8 (18.7–26.2)	21.5 (19.3–24.1)	0.444	0.911	0.000
Leptin/soluble leptin receptor	1.51 (0.88–2.92)	0.46 (0.19–0.98)	<0.001	1.85 (1.18–2.67)	1.33 (0.65–2.24)	0.030	0.509	0.000
Total adiponectin (μg/mL)	6.6 (5.0–7.4)	7.0 (5.8–8.3)	0.046	5.7 (4.4–6.5)	6.9 (4.5–7.7)	0.332	0.135	0.233
HMW adiponectin (μg/mL)	3.3 (2.1–4.5)	3.9 (3.0–4.7)	0.001	2.9 (2.1–4.1)	3.1 (2.0–4.9)	0.687	0.615	0.166
HMW/total adiponectin (%)	49.0 ± 14.4	53.5 ± 12.3	0.010	53.1 ± 14.8	49.9 ± 17.1	0.394	0.319	0.353
Leptin/adiponectin	6.26 (3.23–9.69)	1.87 (0.91–4.09)	<0.001	8.79 (5.34–12.02)	4.22 (3.49–7.87)	0.003	0.104	0.001
Glucose (mg/dL)	84 ± 6	82 ± 6	0.087	83 ± 4	84 ± 5	0.255	0.475	0.190
Total cholesterol (mg/dL)	154 (144–165)	152 (140–165)	0.117	156 (145–163)	158 (139–176)	0.478	0.591	0.224
HDL–cholesterol (mg/dL)	49 (42–60)	50 (41–57)	0.763	48 (39–54)	53 (43–61)	0.190	0.425	0.439
LDL–cholesterol (mg/dL)	95 (85–99)	89 (76–101)	0.028	91 (83–103)	95 (79–113)	0.260	0.671	0.278
Triglycerides (mg/dL)	91 (69–115)	75 (49–96)	0.001	93 (58–135)	82 (58–117)	0.601	0.962	0.330
Dietary intake								
Energy (kcal/24 h)	1727 (1431–2136)	1215 (962–1369)	<0.001	1822 (1493–2080)	1278 (1018–1546)	<0.001	0.972	0.305
Energy (% of DRI)	93.9 (78.5–112.5)	63.4 (49.0–73.3)	<0.001	82.1 (72.1–113.8)	55.4 (41.3–78.1)	<0.001	0.288	0.716
Proteins (% of energy intake)	13.5 (12.3–15.7)	16.8 (15.1–18.6)	<0.001	13.3 (12.7–15.3)	16.1 (14.0–19.1)	0.009	0.732	0.508
Carbohydrates (% of energy intake)	53.4 (47.7–55.9)	51.2 (48.2–55.5)	0.956	52.3 (47.8–56.1)	51.3 (49.4–55.5)	0.936	0.906	0.928
Fat (% of energy intake)	33.5 (31.0–38.0)	30.9 (28.7–34.0)	0.008	35.1 (31.2–37.3)	33.3 (27.5–38.2)	0.376	0.813	0.406
Proteins (% of DRI)	219 (170–266)	172 (142–210)	<0.001	201 (160–270)	169 (123–195)	0.006	0.436	0.516
Carbohydrates (% of DRI)	337 (285–428)	231 (189–287)	<0.001	312 (277–414)	257 (199–300)	<0.001	0.870	0.716
Fat (% of DRI)	104 (90–136)	71 (53–82)	<0.001	111 (83–144)	70 (53–102)	0.001	0.870	0.428

Results are presented as means ± standard deviations for normally distributed data, or medians and interquartile ranges (25th–75th percentiles) for non-normally distributed variables; SDS: standard deviation score, BMI: body mass index, HMW: high molecular weight, DRI: dietary reference intake.

Table 5. Associations of *LEPR* Q223R and K656N polymorphisms with level of adipokines and body composition before and after 3-month intervention.

	LEPR Q223R A > G			LEPR K656N G > C		
	Q223 (AA) (n = 22)	223R (AG + GG) (n = 54)	p AA vs. AG + GG	K656 (GG) (n = 60)	656N (GC + CC) (n = 16)	p GG vs. GC + CC
Baseline SDS-BMI	3.52 (3.11–4.12)	3.32 (2.60–5.05)	0.630	3.48 (2.65–4.75)	3.40 (2.96–5.74)	0.495
Delta SDS-BMI	−0.63 ± 0.53	−0.97 ± 0.50	0.010	−0.89 ± 0.53	−0.79 ± 0.55	0.494
Baseline fat mass (%)	40.2 (37.3–44.0)	41.1 (38.9–44.3)	0.464	40.7 (37.5–43.8)	42.2 (37.9–44.2)	0.499
Delta fat mass (%)	−0.8 ± 2.9	−3.3 ± 3.2	0.003	−2.9 ± 3.4	−1.2 ± 2.7	0.068
Baseline fat-free mass (kg)	29.7 ± 5.8	27.7 ± 7.4	0.114	28.2 ± 6.9	28.4 ± 7.3	0.819
Delta fat-free mass (kg)	−0.7 ± 1.1	−0.4 ± 1.2	0.402	−0.4 ± 1.2	−0.8 ± 1.0	0.342
Baseline Leptin (ng/mL)	44.0 (28.3–65.9)	37.0 (22.8–54.6)	0.166	37.0 (21.5–55.1)	46.0 (32.4–61.4)	0.125
Delta Leptin (ng/mL)	−26.6 ± 24.4	−21.2 ± 20.5	0.334	−22.2 ± 21.4	−24.9 ± 23.2	0.670
Baseline sOB-R (ng/mL)	22.0 (17.6–27.6)	23.1 (19.6–26.6)	0.639	23.1 (18.2–26.5)	22.3 (19.3–28.3)	0.828
Delta sOB-R (ng/mL)	1.2 ± 6.3	3.9 ± 6.7	0.108	4.0 ± 6.4	0.0 ± 6.9	0.032
Baseline Leptin/sOB-R	2.24 (1.09–3.29)	1.50 (0.89–2.50)	0.204	1.42 (.86–2.69)	2.27 (1.43–3.02)	0.198
Delta Leptin/sOB-R	−0.82 (−2.52—−0.15)	−0.85 (−1.68—−0.36)	0.891	−0.82 (−1.94—−0.34)	−1.02 (−2.07—−0.09)	0.674
Baseline Leptin/adiponectin	7.79 (5.37–11.86)	6.05 (3.32–9.98)	0.248	6.63 (3.34–10.63)	7.06 (5.13–10.98)	0.333
Delta Leptin/adiponectin	−4.5 ± 3.7	−4.0 ± 3.8	0.628	−4.22 ± 3.62	−3.72 ± 4.36	0.678

Results are presented as means ± standard deviations for normally distributed data, or medians and interquartile ranges (25th–75th percentiles) for non-normally distributed variables; SDS: standard deviation score, BMI: body mass index, sOB-R: soluble leptin receptor.

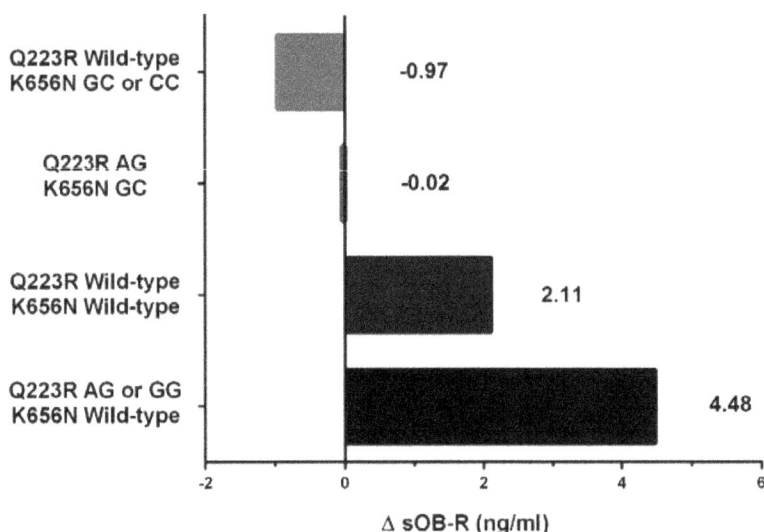

Figure 1. Changes in soluble leptin receptor concentrations in obese children with different genotypes of *LEPR* Q223R and K656N polymorphisms after 3 months of dietary intervention; results of linear regression model adjusted for age and sex.

In addition, we found a positive correlation between therapy-induced change in SDS-BMI and change in percentage of fat mass in the carriers of at least one minor allele in Q223R only as well as in the wild-type homozygotes for both polymorphisms (both $p < 0.001$), while we did not observe a significant correlation between changes in SDS-BMI and fat-free mass in these two groups (Table 6). In contrast, in carriers of at least one minor allele in K656N only, a positive correlation between change in SDS-BMI and change in fat-free mass was observed ($p = 0.002$), while no association between change in SDS-BMI and change in percentage of fat mass was found. No correlation between change in SDS-BMI and changes in body composition was found in the combined heterozygotes for both *LEPR* polymorphisms.

Table 6. Correlations of changes in fat mass and fat-free mass with change in SDS-BMI in children with different genotypes of Q223R and K656N *LEPR* polymorphisms after 3 months of dietary intervention.

Q223R/K656N Genotype	Change in Fat Mass (%)		Change in Fat-Free Mass (kg)	
	Pearson r	p	Pearson r	p
Wild-type/Wild-type	0.858	<0.001	0.334	0.244
AG or GG/Wild-type	0.519	<0.001	0.194	0.197
Wild-type/GC or CC	0.372	0.364	0.904	0.002
AG/GC	0.566	0.144	0.683	0.062

We found no differences in baseline levels and changes during intervention in BMI-SDS, body composition, and adipokine concentrations between carriers of different genotypes of -2548G > A *LEP*, -11377C > G *ADIPOQ* and -11426A > G *ADIPOQ* SNPs.

4. Discussion

Our study shows that both Q223R and K656N polymorphisms in the leptin receptor gene may modulate the effect of lifestyle intervention in obese individuals during the prepubertal period, whereas other investigated SNPs in genes encoding leptin and adiponectin were not related to a reduction in body mass. We also demonstrated that combinations of genotypes of the investigated polymorphisms in *LEPR* may determine predisposition to therapy-induced changes in body composition and soluble leptin receptor concentration in prepubertal children.

Based on the finding that obese subjects have higher serum levels of leptin and lower levels of its soluble receptor, it has been suggested that human obesity is associated with leptin resistance [31]. Since both the Q223R and the K656N polymorphisms are located within the region encoding the extracellular domain of the leptin receptor, the substitution of one amino acid by another can affect the functional characteristics of the receptor leading to its modified signaling capacity and resulting in various levels of leptin in circulation [1].

In our previous work, consistently with the results of other authors, we did not observe an association between these two *LEPR* SNPs and obesity in children and adolescents [20,32,33]. However, none of these studies took into account the combined effect of the Q223R and K656N variants on susceptibility to obesity and the level of serum adipokines. Such an interaction was described by Lu *et al.* [14] who found that a combination of a polymorphism in the *LEP* 3' flanking region with two polymorphisms in *LEPR* (K109R and K656N) was associated with obesity in a Chinese population, even though none of them individually were associated with body weight or BMI.

Lifestyle interventions, including modification of dietary habits and increased physical activity, are recommended as an effective therapy for weight reduction as well as for an improvement of biochemical parameters in obese children and adolescents [34]. Like other authors and in accordance with our previous findings, after therapy-induced weight loss we observed a significant decrease in leptin concentration with a parallel increase in soluble leptin receptor and adiponectin levels [35–37]. However, about 30% of the studied group did not have a change in body mass or body composition despite having energy intake and percentage of DRI before and after therapy similar to the children with weight loss. This finding implies that response to lifestyle interventions may be genetically determined.

Given the important role of leptin in the regulation of energy metabolism, we suggest that genetic variants of *LEPR* may modulate physiological responses to lifestyle interventions and its influence on health in prepubertal obese children. When analyzed separately, the Q223R and K656N polymorphisms were related to different parameters in children after weight loss therapy: the Q223R *LEPR* SNP was associated with changes in BMI and fat mass percentage, while the K656N with changes in soluble leptin receptor serum concentrations. In contrast, we did not find any differences in serum leptin levels in relation to the studied *LEPR* polymorphisms in obese children before and after intervention. The results of previous studies on the relationship between *LEPR* variants and leptin concentrations in the circulation are ambiguous. Mars *et al.* [10] also demonstrated no effect of the K109R, Q223R and K656N SNPs on an acute decline in leptin levels after only 4 days of energy restriction in men. However, Luis *et al.* [38] observed in Spanish adults a significant decrease in weight, fat mass as well as leptin concentrations in wild-type homozygotes of K656N after a 3months lifestyle intervention, whereas carriers of the minor allele had no decrease in fat mass or leptin levels after this period. In addition, carriers of the minor K656N allele did not respond with a decrease in insulin level or HOMA-IR after weight loss induced by a hypocaloric diet [3]. Similarly to other authors studying the K656N polymorphism in adults, we also suggest that children with the minor allele, which is associated with a lack of soluble leptin receptor changes after therapy, may be more resistant to multidisciplinary intervention than wild-type homozygotes [4].

Repasy *et al.* [19] when analyzing the relationship between the Q223R polymorphism and indicators of energy expenditure in obese children (aged 13 ± 2.7 years), also found no association between leptin concentrations and different genotypes of this SNP. However, the wild-type homozygotes compared with other genotypes showed a significantly lower post-absorptive and postprandial respiratory quotient, which could indicate a lower binding capacity of leptin to the soluble form of the receptor in plasma [19]. In our study, we also did not observe any differences in leptin levels between the carriers of the Q223R genotypes before and after therapy in contrast with an adult population in whom differences in leptin concentrations had been observed [39]. These differences could be explained by the younger age of Repasy *et al.*'s [19] study population and our patients, in whom the full effect of Q223R polymorphism has not yet been developed. Nevertheless, our study points at the association between this polymorphism and weight loss in children after lifestyle intervention. Carriers of the Q223R wild-type variant lost significantly less weight and less fat mass after therapy than carriers of the minor allele; therefore, we suggest that wild-type variant carriers may be more resistant to weight loss therapy than carriers of the minor variant. Other authors observed that in adults the wild-type variant of Q223R correlated not only with leptin concentrations but also with higher BMI and body fat, impaired glucose metabolism and dyslipidemia, as well as lower respiratory quotient during low-intensity exercise [40,41]. Therefore, it is suggested that this variant of *LEPR* polymorphism may carry a risk of insulin resistance and liver steatosis in later life. Other genetic variant at the *LEPR* locus (rs3790433) was also associated with increased risk of metabolic syndrome and insulin resistance in adults with metabolic syndrome [12]. In addition, authors found that low plasma level of (*n*-3) and high level of (*n*-6) polyunsaturated fatty acids exacerbated impact of this polymorphism on the risk of hiperinsulinemia and insulin resistance. Many studies have shown that fatty acids influence leptin expression and concentration, but the influence of genetic variations on this is still unknown [42,43]. However, the knowledge of gene-nutrient interactions might be useful in developing personalized dietary recommendations in obese adults as well as obese children.

To our knowledge, the combined influence of both *LEPR* polymorphisms on soluble leptin receptor levels and weight loss in obese subjects has not yet been analyzed. Our results indicate that the studied *LEPR* polymorphisms may have a complementary effect on the weight loss process in obese prepubertal children during lifestyle intervention. Among different combinations of both *LEPR* SNPs, we found that children with at least one minor allele in Q223R coupled with wild-type K665N had the greatest likelihood of losing weight (5-fold), the greatest increase in soluble leptin receptor concentrations and decrease in SDS-BMI correlated with a decrease in fat mass during intervention. In contrast, carriers of the wild-type Q223R together with at least one minor allele in K665N, presented no difference in likelihood of weight loss when compared with the reference genotype combination. Moreover, only this tested combination showed a tendency towards a decrease in soluble leptin receptor concentration and towards a decrease in SDS-BMI correlated with a decrease in fat-free mass after therapy. It is known that a change of amino acid physico-chemical properties is one of the mechanisms of SNPs affecting protein stability and function, as well as protein-protein interactions [44]. Amino acid substitutions in leptin receptor domain due to SNP in *LEPR* result in changes of the electric charge from neutral to positive for Q223→R and from positive to neutral for K656→N [7]. In our study, in the first combination of both *LEPR* SNPs, mentioned above, resulting in higher odds of weight loss, 223R and K565 were associated with positive electric charge, while in the latter combination, resulting in the lack of the higher likelihood to lose weight, both SNP variants, Q223 and 565N, were associated with neutral electric charge. Therefore, it seems that the consequence of a substitution of one amino acid by another can be a change in leptin-leptin receptor interactions caused by the differences in charge of amino acids, that may alter the efficiency of the weight loss process in children.

In some studies, functional SNPs in *ADIPOQ* were found to have a significant effect on human body composition, but other reports did not confirm an association between these polymorphisms and obesity [45,46]. In our previous study we found that the -11377C > G *ADIPOQ* polymorphism may modulate the risk of childhood obesity and this polymorphism had a significant impact on the adipokine profile in prepubertal obese children [20]. In the present study, we observed an increase in adiponectin concentrations in obese children with weight loss, while levels of this adipokine remained unchanged in children without weight loss. However, we did not observe any associations between the two analyzed *ADIPOQ* polymorphisms and reduction in body mass in prepubertal children after 3 months of therapy. Sorensen *et al.* [47], when analyzing the -11377C > G *ADIPOQ* SNP in a panel of obesity-related candidate genes in approximately 800 adults, suggested its minor role, if any, in modulating weight changes induced by a moderate hypo-energetic low-fat diet. However, other authors studying 2 SNPs in genes encoding adiponectin (-11377C > G *ADIPOQ*) and its receptor

1 suggested that these polymorphisms may play a role in the responsiveness to dietary fatty acid modification in adults with metabolic syndrome [13]. Several *ADIPOQ* polymorphisms were also studied in Spanish obese adolescents, but none of them were associated with SDS-BMI and fat mass changes after 3 months of multidisciplinary treatment [15], which is in concordance with our results.

This study has a few potential limitations. Firstly, adiposity was assessed by indirect estimations (BMI, BMI-SDS, skinfold thickness); nevertheless, the same methods were used before and after intervention, so analyzing differences in these parameters should obviate possible measurement errors. Secondly, our findings were obtained from a relatively small sample of subjects, though thoroughly characterized in terms of phenotypes. Therefore, ethnically matched studies should be performed to confirm our results in different populations of prepubertal obese children. Thirdly, the 3-day records provide only fragmentary information about dietary intake. However, these food records were reported to yield the strongest agreement with actual dietary intake compared with 24-h recall and 5-day food frequency records in children [48]. Finally, the lifestyle intervention period in this study was only 3 months and a study of a long-term intervention is needed to verify the relationship between the polymorphisms in adipokine genes and adipokine levels in relation to clinical outcomes.

5. Conclusions

We found that out of the 5 analyzed polymorphisms, only the Q223R and K656N in the leptin receptor gene may modulate the weight loss process after lifestyle intervention during the prepubertal period. We also demonstrated a complementary effect of these *LEPR* variants on the predisposition to weight loss, changes in body composition, and to leptin receptor concentrations in obese children. Children with at least one minor allele in Q223R and wild-type K665N had the best likelihood of losing weight which was associated with a decrease in fat mass and an increase in soluble leptin receptor concentrations. We suggest that even though the contribution of a single *LEPR* polymorphism may not be sufficient to influence the weight loss process, the combination of different *LEPR* variants might more precisely determine a child's predisposition to reduction of body mass in the prepubertal period.

Acknowledgments: This work was supported by grant No. NN 407173534 from the Polish Ministry of Science and Higher Education.

Author Contributions: J.G., J.A. and M.C. gathered the biochemical measurements and analyzed data. A.K. carried out the genetic experiments and analyzed data. E.M. undertook statistical analysis and interpretation of data. H.W. calculated the basic nutrients value in average daily food rations. J.G. and M.P.-K. participated in the project development. All authors were involved in writing the paper and had final approval of the submitted version.

Conflicts of Interest: The authors declare no conflicts of interest.

References

1. Ghalandari, H.; Hosseini-Esfahani, F.; Mirmiran, P. The association of polymorphisms in leptin/leptin receptor genes and ghrelin/ghrelin receptor genes with overweight/obesity and the related metabolic disturbances: A review. *Int. J. Endocrinol. Metab.* **2015**, *13*. [CrossRef] [PubMed]
2. De Luis Roman, D.; Aller, R.; Izaola, O.; Sagrado, M.G.; Conde, R. Influence of Lys656Asn polymorphism of leptin receptor gene on leptin response secondary to two hypocaloric diets: A randomized clinical trial. *Ann. Nutr. Metab.* **2008**, *52*, 209–214. [CrossRef] [PubMed]
3. De Luis Roman, D.; Aller, R.; Izaola, O.; Gonzalez Sagrado, M.; Conde, R.; de la Fuente, B.; Primo, D. Effect of Lys656Asn polymorphism of leptin receptor gene on cardiovascular risk factors and serum adipokine levels after a high polyunsaturated fat diet in obese patients. *J. Clin. Lab. Anal.* **2015**, *29*, 432–436. [CrossRef] [PubMed]
4. Rudkowska, I.; Pérusse, L. Individualized weight management: What can be learned from nutrigenomics and nutrigenetics? *Prog. Mol. Biol. Transl. Sci.* **2012**, *108*, 347–382. [PubMed]
5. Farooqi, I.S.; Wangensteen, T.; Collins, S.; Kimber, W.; Matarese, G.; Keogh, J.M.; Lank, E.; Bottomley, B.; Lopez-Fernandez, J.; Ferraz-Amaro, I.; *et al.* Clinical and molecular genetic spectrum of congenital deficiency of the leptin receptor. *N. Engl. J. Med.* **2007**, *356*, 237–247. [CrossRef] [PubMed]

6. Zastrow, O.; Seidel, B.; Kiess, W.; Thiery, J.; Keller, E.; Bottuer, A.; Kratzsch, J. The soluble leptin receptor is crucial for leptin action: Evidence from clinical and experimental data. *Int. J. Obes. Relat. Metab. Disord.* **2003**, *27*, 1472–1478. [CrossRef] [PubMed]

7. Chung, W.K.; Power-Kehoe, L.; Chua, M.; Chu, F.; Aronne, L.; Huma, Z.; Sothern, M.; Udall, J.N.; Kahle, B.; Leibel, R.L. Exonic and intronic sequence variation in the human leptin receptor gene (LEPR). *Diabetes* **1997**, *46*, 1509–1511. [CrossRef] [PubMed]

8. Richert, L.; Chevalley, T.; Manen, D.; Bonjour, J.P.; Rizzoli, R.; Ferrari, S. Bone mass in prepubertal boys is associated with a Gln223Arg amino acid substitution in the leptin receptor. *J. Clin. Endocrinol. Metab.* **2007**, *92*, 4380–4386. [CrossRef] [PubMed]

9. Lakka, T.A.; Rankinen, T.; Weisnagel, S.J.; Chagnon, Y.C.; Lakka, H.M.; Ukkola, O.; Boulé, N.; Rice, T.; Leon, A.S.; Skinner, J.S.; *et al.* Leptin and leptin receptor gene polymorphisms and changes in glucose homeostasis in response to regular exercise in nondiabetic individuals: The HERITAGE family study. *Diabetes* **2004**, *53*, 1603–1608. [CrossRef] [PubMed]

10. Mars, M.; van Rossum, C.T.; de Graaf, C.; Hoebee, B.; de Groot, L.C.; Kok, F.J. Leptin responsiveness to energy restriction: Genetic variation in the leptin receptor gene. *Obes. Res.* **2004**, *12*, 442–444. [CrossRef] [PubMed]

11. Bašić, M.; Butorac, A.; Landeka Jurčević, I.; Bačun-Družina, V. Obesity: Genome and environment interactions. *Arh. Hig. Rada Toksikol.* **2012**, *63*, 395–405. [CrossRef] [PubMed]

12. Phillips, C.M.; Goumidi, L.; Bertrais, S.; Field, M.R.; Ordovas, J.M.; Cupples, L.A.; Defoort, C.; Lovegrove, J.A.; Drevon, C.A.; Blaak, E.E.; *et al.* Leptin receptor polymorphisms interact with polyunsaturated fatty acids to augment risk of insulin resistance and metabolic syndrome in adults. *J. Nutr.* **2010**, *140*, 238–244. [CrossRef] [PubMed]

13. Ferguson, J.F.; Phillips, C.M.; Tierney, A.C.; Pérez-Martínez, P.; Defoort, C.; Helal, O.; Lairon, D.; Planells, R.; Shaw, D.I.; Lovegrove, J.A.; *et al.* Gene-nutrient interactions in the metabolic syndrome: Single nucleotide polymorphisms in ADIPOQ and ADIPOR1 interact with plasma saturated fatty acids to modulate insulin resistance. *Am. J. Clin. Nutr.* **2010**, *91*, 794–801. [CrossRef] [PubMed]

14. Lu, J.; Zou, D.; Zheng, L.; Chen, G.; Lu, J.; Feng, Z. Synergistic effect of LEP and LEPR gene polymorphism on body mass index in a Chinese population. *Obes. Res. Clin. Pract.* **2013**, *7*, 445–449. [CrossRef] [PubMed]

15. Moleres, A.; Rendo-Urteaga, T.; Zulet, M.A.; Marcos, A.; Campoy, C.; Garagorri, J.M.; Martínez, J.A.; Azcona-Sanjulián, M.C.; Marti, A. Obesity susceptibility loci on body mass index and weight loss in Spanish adolescents after a lifestyle intervention. *J. Pediatr.* **2012**, *161*, 466–470. [CrossRef] [PubMed]

16. Petrone, A.; Zavarella, S.; Caiazzo, A.; Leto, G.; Spoletini, M.; Potenziani, S.; Osborn, J.; Vania, A.; Buzzetti, R. The promoter region of the adiponectin gene is a determinant in modulating insulin sensitivity in childhood obesity. *Obesity* **2006**, *14*, 1498–1504. [CrossRef] [PubMed]

17. Tabassum, R.; Mahendran, Y.; Dwivedi, O.P.; Chauhan, G.; Ghosh, S.; Marwaha, R.K.; Tandon, N.; Bharadwaj, D. Common variants of IL6, LEPR, and PBEF1 are associated with obesity in Indian children. *Diabetes* **2012**, *61*, 626–631. [CrossRef] [PubMed]

18. León-Mimila, P.; Villamil-Ramírez, H.; Villalobos-Comparán, M.; Villarreal-Molina, T.; Romero-Hidalgo, S.; López-Contreras, B.; Gutiérrez-Vidal, R.; Vega-Badillo, J.; Jacobo-Albavera, L.; Posadas-Romeros, C.; *et al.* Contribution of common genetic variants to obesity and obesity-related traits in Mexican children and adults. *PLoS ONE* **2013**, *8*, e70640. [CrossRef]

19. Répásy, J.; Bokor, S.; Erhardt, É.; Molnár, D. Association of Gln223 Arg polymorphism of the leptin receptor gene with indicators of energy expenditure in obese children. *Nutrition* **2014**, *30*, 837–840. [CrossRef] [PubMed]

20. Gajewska, J.; Kuryłowicz, A.; Ambroszkiewicz, J.; Mierzejewska, E.; Chełchowska, M.; Szamotulska, K.; Weker, H.; Puzianowska-Kuźnicka, M. ADIPOQ -11377C > G polymorphism increases the risk of adipokine abnormalities and child obesity regardless of dietary intake. *J. Pediatr. Gastroenterol. Nutr.* **2016**, *62*, 122–129. [CrossRef] [PubMed]

21. Weker, H. Simple obesity in children. A study on the role of nutritional factors. *Med. Wieku Rozwoj.* **2006**, *10*, 3–191. [PubMed]

22. Oblacińska, A.; Weker, H. *Prevention of Obesity in Children and Adolescents*; HELP-MED: Kraków, Poland, 2008.

23. Dzieniszewski, J.; Szponar, L.; Szczygieł, B.; Socha, J. *Scientific Foundations of Nutrition in Hospitals in Poland*; National Food and Nutrition Institute: Warsaw, Poland, 2001.

24. Jarosz, M.; Traczyk, I.; Rychlik, E. Energia. In *Normy Żywienia dla Populacji Polskiej—Nowelizacja*; Jarosz, M., Ed.; National Food and Nutrition Institute: Warsaw, Poland, 2012; pp. 18–32.

25. Palczewska, I.; Niedzwiedzka, Z. Somatic development indices in children and youth of Warsaw. *Med. Wieku Rozwoj.* **2001**, *5*, 18–118. [PubMed]

26. Lohman, T.G. Skinfolds and body density and their relation to body fatness: A review. *Hum. Biol.* **1981**, *53*, 181–225. [PubMed]

27. Miller, S.A.; Dykes, D.D.; Polesky, H.F. A simple salting out procedure for extracting DNA from human nucleated cells. *Nucleic Acids Res.* **1988**, *16*, 1215. [CrossRef] [PubMed]

28. Benjamini, Y.; Hochberg, Y. Controlling the false discovery rate: A practical and powerful approach to multiple testing. *J. R. Stat. Soc. B* **1995**, *57*, 289–300.

29. Barrett, J.C.; Fry, B.; Maller, J.; Daly, M.J. Haploview: Analysis and visualization of LD and haplotype maps. *Bioinformatics* **2005**, *21*, 263–265. [CrossRef] [PubMed]

30. Gabriel, S.B.; Schaffner, S.F.; Nguyen, H.; Moore, J.M.; Roy, J.; Blumenstiel, B.; Higgins, J.; DeFelice, M.; Lochner, A.; Faggart, M.; *et al.* The structure of haplotype blocks in the human genome. *Science* **2002**, *296*, 2225–2229. [CrossRef] [PubMed]

31. Xu, S.; Xue, Y. Pediatric obesity: Causes, symptoms, prevention and treatment. *Exp. Ther. Med.* **2016**, *11*, 15–20. [CrossRef] [PubMed]

32. Zandoná, M.R.; Rodrigues, R.O.; Albiero, G.; Campagnolo, P.D.; Vitolo, M.R.; Almeida, S.; Mattevi, V.S. Polymorphisms in LEPR, PPARG and APM1 genes: Associations with energy intake and metabolic traits in young children. *Arq. Bras. Endocrinol. Metab.* **2013**, *57*, 603–611. [CrossRef]

33. Komşu-Ornek, Z.; Demirel, F.; Dursun, A.; Ermiş, B.; Pişkin, E.; Bideci, A. Leptin receptor gene Gln223Arg polymorphism is not associated with obesity and metabolic syndrome in Turkish children. *Turk. J. Pediatr.* **2012**, *54*, 20–24. [PubMed]

34. Ho, M.; Garnett, S.P.; Baur, L.; Burrows, T.; Stewart, L.; Neve, M.; Collins, C. Effectiveness of lifestyle interventions in child obesity: Systematic review with meta-analysis. *Pediatrics* **2012**, *130*, 1647–1671. [CrossRef] [PubMed]

35. Reinehr, T.; Roth, C.; Menke, T.; Andler, W. Adiponectin before and after weight loss in obese children. *J. Clin. Endocrinol. Metab.* **2004**, *89*, 3790–3794. [CrossRef] [PubMed]

36. Cambuli, V.M.; Musiu, M.C.; Incani, M.; Paderi, M.; Serpe, R.; Marras, V.; Cossu, E.; Cavallo, M.G.; Mariotti, S.; Loche, S.; *et al.* Assessment of adiponectin and leptin as biomarkers of positive metabolic outcome after lifestyle intervention in overweight and obese children. *J. Clin. Endocrinol. Metab.* **2008**, *93*, 3051–3057. [CrossRef] [PubMed]

37. Gajewska, J.; Weker, H.; Ambroszkiewicz, J.; Szamotulska, K.; Chełchowska, M.; Franek, E.; Laskowska-Klita, T. Alterations in markers of bone metabolism and adipokines following a 3-month lifestyle intervention induced weight loss in obese prepubertal children. *Exp. Clin. Endocrinol. Diabetes* **2013**, *121*, 498–504. [CrossRef] [PubMed]

38. De Luis Roman, D.; de la Fuente, R.A.; Sagrado, M.G.; Izaola, O.; Vicente, R.C. Leptin receptor Lys656Asn polymorphism is associated with decreased leptin response and weight loss secondary to a lifestyle modification in obese patients. *Arch. Med. Res.* **2006**, *37*, 854–859. [CrossRef] [PubMed]

39. Quinton, N.D.; Lee, A.J.; Ross, R.J.; Eastell, R.; Blakemore, A.I. A single nucleotide polymorphism (SNP) in the leptin receptor is associated with BMI, fat mass and leptin levels in postmenopausal Caucasian women. *Hum. Genet.* **2001**, *108*, 233–236. [CrossRef] [PubMed]

40. Furusawa, T.; Naka, I.; Yamauchi, T.; Natsuhara, K.; Kimura, R.; Nakazawa, M.; Ishida, T.; Inaoka, T.; Matsumura, Y.; Ataka, Y.; *et al.* The Q223R polymorphism in LEPR is associated with obesity in Pacific Islanders. *Hum. Genet.* **2010**, *127*, 287–294. [CrossRef] [PubMed]

41. Loos, R.J.; Rankinen, T.; Chagnon, Y.; Tremblay, A.; Pérusse, L.; Bouchard, C. Polymorphisms in the leptin and leptin receptor genes in relation to resting metabolic rate and respiratory quotient in the Québec Family Study. *Int. J. Obes.* **2006**, *30*, 183–190. [CrossRef] [PubMed]

42. Reseland, J.E.; Syversen, U.; Bakke, I.; Qvigstad, G.; Eide, L.G.; Hjertner, O.; Gordeladze, J.O.; Drevon, C.A. Leptin is expressed in and secreted from primary cultures of human osteoblasts and promotes bone mineralization. *J. Bone. Miner. Res.* **2001**, *16*, 1426–1433. [CrossRef] [PubMed]

43. Lombardo, Y.B.; Hein, G.; Chicco, A. Metabolic syndrome: Effects of *n*-3 PUFAs on a model of dyslipidemia, insulin resistance and adiposity. *Lipids* **2007**, *42*, 427–437. [CrossRef] [PubMed]

44. Kucukkal, T.G.; Petukh, M.; Li, L.; Alexov, E. Structural and physico-chemical effects of disease and non-disease nsSNPs on proteins. *Curr. Opin. Struct. Biol.* **2015**, *32*, 18–24. [CrossRef] [PubMed]
45. An, S.S.; Hanley, A.J.; Ziegler, J.T.; Brown, W.M.; Haffner, S.M.; Norris, J.M.; Rotter, J.I.; Guo, X.; Chen, Y.D.; Wagenknecht, L.E.; *et al.* Association between ADIPOQ SNPs with plasma adiponectin and glucose homeostasis and adiposity phenotypes in the IRAS Family Study. *Mol. Genet. Metab.* **2012**, *107*, 721–728. [CrossRef] [PubMed]
46. Karmelic, I.; Lovric, J.; Bozina, T.; Ljubić, H.; Vogrinc, Ž.; Božina, N.; Sertić, J. Adiponectin level and gene variability are obesity and metabolic syndrome markers in young population. *Arch. Med. Res.* **2012**, *43*, 145–153. [CrossRef] [PubMed]
47. Sørensen, T.I.; Boutin, P.; Taylor, M.A.; Larsen, L.H.; Verdich, C.; Petersen, L.; Holst, C.; Echwald, S.M.; Dina, C.; Toubro, S.; *et al.* Genetic polymorphisms and weight loss in obesity: A randomised trial of hypo-energetic high- *versus* low-fat diets. *PLoS Clin. Trials* **2006**, *1*, e12. [CrossRef]
48. Crawford, P.B.; Obarzanek, E.; Morrison, J.; Sabry, Z.I. Comparative advantage of 3-day food records over 24-h recall and 5-day food frequency validated by observation of 9- and 10-year-old girls. *J. Am. Diet. Assoc.* **1994**, *94*, 626–630. [CrossRef]

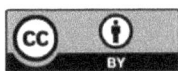

© 2016 by the authors. Licensee MDPI, Basel, Switzerland. This article is an open access article distributed under the terms and conditions of the Creative Commons Attribution (CC BY) license (http://creativecommons.org/licenses/by/4.0/).

nutrients

MDPI

Review

Does Metabolically Healthy Obesity Exist?

Araceli Muñoz-Garach [1,2,*], Isabel Cornejo-Pareja [1] and Francisco J. Tinahones [1,2]

[1] Department of Endocrinology and Nutrition, Virgen de la Victoria Hospital, Málaga University,
    Málaga 29010, Spain; isabelmaria_cornejo@hotmail.com (I.C.-P.); fjtinahones@hotmail.com (F.J.T.)
[2] CIBER Fisiopatologia Obesidad y Nutricion (CIBEROBN), Instituto de Salud Carlos III, Madrid 28029, Spain
* Correspondence: aracelimugar@gmail.com; Tel.: +34-64-603-2764

Received: 31 March 2016; Accepted: 17 May 2016; Published: 1 June 2016

Abstract: The relationship between obesity and other metabolic diseases have been deeply studied. However, there are clinical inconsistencies, exceptions to the paradigm of "more fat means more metabolic disease", and the subjects in this condition are referred to as metabolically healthy obese (MHO). They have long-standing obesity and morbid obesity but can be considered healthy despite their high degree of obesity. We describe the variable definitions of MHO, the underlying mechanisms that can explain the existence of this phenotype caused by greater adipose tissue inflammation or the different capacity for adipose tissue expansion and functionality apart from other unknown mechanisms. We analyze whether these subjects improve after an intervention (traditional lifestyle recommendations or bariatric surgery) or if they stay healthy as the years pass. MHO is common among the obese population and constitutes a unique subset of characteristics that reduce metabolic and cardiovascular risk factors despite the presence of excessive fat mass. The protective factors that grant a healthier profile to individuals with MHO are being elucidated.

Keywords: metabolically healthy obesity; metabolic syndrome; adipose tissue; inflammation

1. Introduction

Obesity is a major health problem and an important risk factor for the development of diseases such as diabetes mellitus. The mechanism by which obesity leads to the development of insulin resistance still needs to be elucidated. There is a large body of epidemiological evidence on the relationship between obesity and other metabolic diseases. However, there are clinical inconsistencies that are exceptions to the paradigm of "more fat, more metabolic disease". There are subjects with long-standing obesity and morbid obesity who can be considered healthy despite a high degree of obesity. This phenomenon was described 15 years ago [1], and these subjects were referred to as metabolically healthy obese (MHO).

There is great inconsistency in the definitions of MHO, with a high degree of variability surrounding the prevalence of this phenotype, which has been estimated to be between 10% and 34% depending on the criteria used [2–5]. MHO appears to be more prevalent in women than in men and its prevalence appears to decrease with age in both sexes [6]. At the same time, there are individuals who, despite having "normal" weight, have an increased risk of disease.

Historically, the primary concern regarding obesity was the concurrent metabolic and cardiovascular risk. In recent years, there has been increased awareness of those individuals who do not fit into this traditional phenotype. This suggests that fat storage is not the only determinant in the association between obesity and insulin resistance, and the term "adiposopathy" is beginning to be used.

Existing guidelines also fail to individualize the management of MHO or metabolically unhealthy/abnormal obese (MUO) patients. This is further complicated because of a gap in the recognition and appropriate management of those normal-weight individuals who demonstrate high metabolic risk profiles.

2. Definition of Metabolically Healthy Obesity

Most studies suggest the definition of MHO (body mass index (BMI) $\geqslant$ 30 kg/m^2) to be obesity without the presence of metabolic diseases such as type 2 diabetes (T2DM), dyslipidemia or hypertension [1,7,8]. To date there are no accepted criteria for identifying MHO [7] individuals. The identification of individuals with MHO is hampered by the absence of a standardized definition of the condition. Several approaches were used to identify or define the MHO phenotype. The most referenced are:

1. Hyperinsulinemic-euglycemic clamp [8–10].
2. The upper quartile of glucose disposal rate [10].
3. The upper quartile of an index of insulin sensitivity after an oral glucose tolerance test [11,12].
4. Less than two of the following cardiometabolic disorders (systolic blood pressure $\geqslant$130 mmHg, diastolic blood pressure $\geqslant$85 mmHg, triglycerides $\geqslant$1.7 mmol/L or $\geqslant$150 mg/dL, fasting glucose $\geqslant$5.6 mmol/L, homeostasis model assessment of insulin resistance (HOMA-IR) $\geqslant$5, ultrasensitive C-reactive protein (CRP) $\geqslant$0.1 mg/L, HDL cholesterol $\leqslant$1.03 mmol/L or 40 mg/dL in men and $\leqslant$1.3 mmol/L or 50 mg/dL in women [3,13].
5. Less than three metabolic syndrome criteria [14].
6. Subjects with BMI above 30 kg/m^2 and HDL cholesterol levels of at least 40 mg/dL in the absence of T2DM and hypertension [15].

Other inflammatory markers (CRP or degree of leukocytosis) have been suggested for inclusion in the definition of MHO [16,17].

An additional marker that is increasingly important in the context of the MHO phenotype is liver fat content. The prevalence of non-alcoholic fatty liver disease appears to be significantly lower in patients with MHO compared with MUO individuals [12]. According to our current knowledge, the classification of "metabolically benign obesity" or "metabolically healthy obesity" only refers to metabolic or cardiovascular complications and does not consider that obesity may be associated with other non-metabolic complications such as orthopedic problems, pulmonary complications, or other physiological conditions. Considering that the descriptions of MHO are inconsistent, the elucidation of the factors or mechanisms underlying this protective profile is far from complete although some works are trying to establish a standard definition of MHO [18].

3. Underlying Mechanisms That Explain the Existence of MHO

3.1. Subclinical Inflammation

Inflammation promotes insulin resistance. Greater adipose tissue inflammation is closely associated with increased metabolic risk for T2DM, cardiovascular disease, and fatty liver disease, whereas obese adults without adipose tissue inflammation exhibit reduced metabolic risk.

There is growing evidence to suggest that subclinical inflammation may be the underlying mechanism that determines whether or not an individual is MHO [16]. Subclinical inflammation is associated with insulin resistance, and CRP has emerged as one of the best predictors of vascular inflammation, metabolic syndrome and cardiovascular disease [19]. There is a strong correlation between circulating CRP levels and anthropometric markers and body composition, and CRP has been proposed as a screening tool to assess the risk of the metabolic syndrome in youth [20]. In adulthood, the MHO phenotype is associated with low levels of complement component 3, CRP, alpha necrosis tumor factor (TNF-α), interleukin 6 (IL-6), and a low number of white blood cells, supporting the concept of a more favorable inflammatory state compared to non-MHO subjects [21].

On the other hand, anti-inflammatory adipokines, such as adiponectin, IL-4, IL-10, IL-13, IL-1 receptor antagonist, and transforming growth factor beta are abundant within the adipose tissues of lean individuals, whereas obese adipose tissue is dominated by the release of pro-inflammatory adipokines, including leptin, resistin, TNF-a, IL-6, IL-18, retinol-binding protein 4, lipocalin 2, angiopoietin-like protein 2, CC-chemokine ligand 2, CXC-chemokine ligand 5, and nicotinamide phosphoribosyltransferase [22].

Other systemic inflammation markers or adipose tissue inflammation markers are free fatty acids (FFA) and the number and activation status of peripheral leukocytes. Thus obese patients with T2DM have higher circulating levels of IL-6, FFA and glycerol and a greater absolute number of peripheral leukocytes compared with non-diabetic obese subjects [23,24]. Similarly, our group found that morbidly obese subjects without metabolic disease had a low degree of insulin resistance and identical adipose tissue inflammation markers as those of non-obese subjects, with no infiltration of macrophages and elevated values of TNF-α and IL-6 expression in visceral adipose tissue [25]. All these results suggest that MUO patients show a higher degree of both systemic and local fat inflammation compared with MHO individuals [23].

3.2. Expansion Capacity of Adipose Tissue

Previously, to explain the transition from normal adipose tissue to that which leads to metabolic abnormalities, studies proposed the "adipose tissue expandability hypothesis". This postulated that once adipocytes reached a threshold capacity for storage, they begin to promote insulin resistance with lipotoxicity and adipokine release. This was supported by knockout studies with PPARγ, lipodystrophy models, and alterations in adipokine secretion following saturation of adipose tissue. Investigating this fact led to further characterization of genetic contributors to the pathways of adipogenesis (SFRP1, Wnt, S14), apoptosis (TRAIL, TWEAK, BCL2, CASP3/7), and angiogenesis (VEGF-A, -B,-C,-D). To improve the understanding of adipose tissue in the context of MHO patients, Tinahones *et al.* looked at genes associated with both lipolysis and lipogenesis and BMI, insulin, and HOMA-IR. They found a positive correlation in PPARγ, DGAT1, AQP7, GK, ATGL, HSL, and perilipin and BMI, insulin, and HOMA-IR in both subcutaneous and visceral fat tissues. Additionally, they demonstrated a negative correlation between genes—ACC1, PEPCK, ACSS2, FABP4—and the aforementioned measures of metabolic risk.

A fairly solid theory attributes the differences between MHO and MUHO subjects to the different capacity for adaptation to excess energy in adipose tissue [26]. When increased fat storage is required, fat tissue needs to increase its storage capacity and can increase the size of adipocytes or increase their number [27]. In addition, this increase in the overall amount of fat must be accompanied by increased vascularization [28]. In those subjects in whom adipose tissue has difficulty expanding in the healthiest way, which is increasing cellularity, metabolic disease does appear [29]. That is what we see in MHO who keep the proper storage capacity. But the loss of expansion capacity can even occur in patients with normal weight, so this theory would explain the existence of metabolically unhealthy lean subjects [30]. Furthermore, the lack of expansion capacity of adipose tissue has been linked to the loss of its main lipogenic function, and the appearance of lipotoxic products in adipose tissue [31].

Traditionally it was thought that there was little cell turnover in adipose tissue in adulthood. Today it is known that adipose tissue is capable of hyperplasia throughout life, and stem/progenitor cells are responsible for this adipose tissue hyperplasia [27,32,33]. Pre-adipocytes found in the vascular stroma are progenitor cells that differentiate into mature adipocytes through a complex program of gene expression [33–36]. Another variable that is directly related to the total number of fat cells is cell death, which may occur by necrosis, autophagy or apoptosis [37,38]. These studies have also alluded to reduced adipocyte hypertrophy, fibrosis and stress as potential contributors to this presentation. Therefore, there are four factors that are directly related to the ability for adipose tissue expansion and functionality: (1) lipogenesis; (2) adipogenesis via the newly formed progenitor cells; (3) apoptotic and anti-apoptotic pathways; and (4) angiogenesis.

Our group, in collaboration with other groups, has shown that metabolically healthy subjects have higher lipogenic [39,40] and angiogenic [41,42] capacity than metabolically unhealthy patients. Furthermore, there is also considerable evidence that adipogenesis and the functionality of mesenchymal cells to become new adipocytes is higher in metabolically healthy subjects because they exhibit mesenchymal cells in the stroma of adipose tissue with a greater capacity to differentiate both bone and fat tissue and a lower senescence [36]. This increased ability to form new adipocytes in the MHO individuals is an observation contributed by our group which clearly shows that the apoptosis of adipocytes increases with obesity, and this has a direct relationship with the degree of adipose tissue inflammation [43].

Adipose tissue is a key regulator of inflammation, and inflammation is involved in the onset and development of atherosclerosis, metabolic syndrome, and T2DM. Although the results of these initial studies suggest that MHO is characterized by a lower inflammatory cytokine environment than MUO, further studies are necessary to better identify the adipose tissue hormones that promote a healthy metabolic profile in obese adults.

There are several adipose tissue compartments and they have different connections with metabolic diseases. Visceral and intrahepatic fat has a direct association with obesity, while subcutaneous fat is not associated with metabolic disease [44]. A plausible hypothesis is that the healthiest way to accumulate fat is through subcutaneous fat expansion but when this capacity is decreased or lost it must resort to other compartments and metabolic diseases occur. Could the MHO phenotype be defined as a group of obese patients with predominantly subcutaneous fat deposits and with little or no visceral and intrahepatic fat? These questions and more still need to be answered.

3.3. Other Possible Mechanisms

A new potential factor to explain the differences between MHO and MUO could be circulating microRNA [45]. Insulin resistance in peripheral organs, such as the liver, can develop due to toxic stimulus, initiating secretion of microRNAs associated with insulin resistance, which are incorporated into muscle and fat cells, inducing insulin resistance in these tissues [46].

A study revealed that 20% of patients with a BMI above 40 kg/m^2 had adiponectin levels above the average of subjects with normal BMI, and these adiponectin levels above a certain threshold increase the probability of being metabolically healthy, even after correcting for the confounding effects of age, insulin and waist circumference [15]. This suggests that adiponectin plays a crucial role in the pathogenesis of metabolic complications associated with obesity as patients with the MHO phenotype have similar levels of adiponectin as those found in normal-weight subjects [15]. Furthermore, individuals with the MHO phenotype have a lower visceral fat, liver fat, and muscle fat content than obese subjects without MHO or obese people with insulin resistance, suggesting that the MHO phenotype is associated with improved ability to capture FFA in adipose tissue [12]. These differences in body composition between MHO patients and non-MHO patients are consistent between genders [3].

Finally, lifestyle factors such as level of physical activity or cardiorespiratory condition also appear to play a key role in distinguishing whether or not an individual is MHO. MHO subjects show higher levels of physical activity compared to MUO individuals and have a more favourable lifestyle [14,47,48]. Likewise, occupational physical activity or leisure time physical activity also appears to be important, since the two exercise regimens are differentially associated with obesity and insulin resistance [49].

4. Do Metabolically Healthy Obese Subjects Improve after an Intervention?

The decisive feature of MHO is the absence of visceral fat accumulation. Until definitive data emerges linking genetic predisposition to MHO, currently recommended lifestyle modifications appear beneficial. Thus, promoting lifestyle modifications directed at minimizing visceral fat accumulation is a fundamental public health measure.

However, it is not completely clear if obese subjects with a MHO phenotype would benefit from traditional lifestyle interventions, which focus on dietary therapy and/or increased physical exercise. Few studies have analyzed the metabolic effects of lifestyle modifications with a restrictive diet and/or exercise in MHO subjects, and their results have been contradictory [50,51]. Supporting the theory that MHO and non-MHO individuals could require a different treatment approach, Karelisy *et al.* showed that MHO individuals reacted differently, from a metabolic viewpoint, to a six-month calorie restricted diet compared to "at-risk" obese people despite achieving similar weight loss [52]. There are some studies that showed combining a Mediterranean diet with moderate to high intensity aerobic training is more effective at improving body composition [53,54]. Although the public health message for all obese patients should continue to promote healthy lifestyle habits, the controversial results of lifestyle interventions in MHO individuals would justify prioritizing, for cost-efficacy reasons, the intensive interventions in metabolically abnormal obese individuals and monitoring MHO subjects for early detection of the development of metabolic abnormalities [55].

Currently, bariatric surgery remains among the best options for patients suffering from severe obesity, with excellent results regarding long-term weight loss and decreases in peripheral and visceral fat depot sizes [56]. More research is needed to study the effects of different therapeutic approaches on the metabolic profile of healthy but obese individuals. Results in this area are essential for understanding the pathophysiology and to implement appropriate metabolically healthy obese and healthy non-obese intervention strategies.

5. Do Metabolically Healthy Obese Subjects Stay Healthy as the Years Pass?

Debate continues concerning whether individuals with MHO are truly healthy. The literature differs regarding the relative risk of disease among this population. MHO individuals are at decreased risk for developing cardiovascular disease compared with MUO individuals [57]. Long-term studies have suggested that MHO is a transient state. For example, among a group of Japanese Americans with MHO, two-thirds developed metabolic syndrome during 10 years of observation, and the metabolic abnormality was independently associated with visceral fat accumulation, female sex, higher fasting plasma insulin concentration, and lower serum HDL associated cholesterol concentration [58]. Consistent with this report, among the 1051 participants in the Pizarra Study, the prevalence of MHO decreased during 11 years of observation [59].

Individuals with MHO are not at increased risk for developing cardiovascular disease compared to metabolically healthy normal weight [MHNW] individuals [60–63]. Studies with longer follow-up periods (>15 years) have reported that MHO individuals were at an increased risk for major cardiovascular disease events as compared to MHNW individuals [64,65]. Recently, analysts conducting a systematic review of the associations between BMI and metabolic status with total mortality and cardiovascular events reported that MHO individuals appear to be at increased risk for cardiovascular events, as compared to MHNW individuals [66]. These researchers concluded that obese individuals are at increased risk for adverse long-term outcomes, even in the absence of metabolic abnormalities, compared with MHNW individuals.

A recent study evaluated the prevalence of elevated plasma high sensitivity CRP (hs-CRP) concentrations and hepatic steatosis in MHO, MHNW, and in metabolically unhealthy normal-weight (MUNW) individuals [67]. They observed that both elevated plasma hs-CRP concentrations and hepatic steatosis are more prevalent among MHO and MUNW individuals than they are among MHNW individuals. However, they are most prevalent among individuals with MHO, suggesting that obesity in the absence of metabolic risk factors is not entirely benign but is associated with subclinical vascular inflammation. Another recent study reported that 42% of their subjects with MHO developed the metabolic syndrome within 10 years [68], again suggesting that MHO is not without increased health risks. However, the identification of predictors, biological determinants, and mechanisms underlying MHO, determining whether MHO represents a transient phenotype that is affected by aging, behavioral, and environmental factors, and accurately calculating the true health risks associated with MHO remain viable topics for diligent study through properly designed and conducted longitudinal studies.

The Bogalusa Heart Study examined 1098 individuals, both children (5–17 years) and adults (24–43 years), who participated in the study between 1997 and 2002. Participants with the MHO phenotype during childhood were more likely to maintain MHO status in adulthood. Despite the level of obesity and fat mass continuing to increase throughout childhood and adulthood, this group of MHO individuals showed a generally comparable cardiometabolic profile with non-obese children and adults. In addition, the carotid intima-media thickness did not differ in adulthood among previous MHO children and non-obese children. These results are very important because they show that the MHO phenotype that starts in childhood and continues into adulthood may have a very favourablecardiometabolic risk profile [69]. Even more importantly, there is increasing evidence showing that the metabolic profile of MHO individuals is almost indistinguishable from that of lean individuals [4,7,70].

To date it is not at all clear whether the MHO phenotype decreases morbidity and mortality associated with obesity. MHO patients have a lower prevalence of risk factors for the development of certain diseases. For example, the intima-media thickness as a risk marker of atherosclerosis is significantly different between individuals with the MHO phenotype and metabolically healthy non-obese patients [5,12,70]. However, a recent meta-analysis has evaluated eight studies comparing mortality data from any cause or cardiovascular events in six groups of patients defined by BMI category (n = 61,386) and metabolic comorbidities, with a 10-year follow up. Analyses revealed that MHO individuals had an increased risk (relative risk (RR): 1.24) compared with MHNW subjects, but this was only detected in studies of 10 or more years of follow-up. In addition, all metabolically unhealthy subjects, regardless of their weight, had an increased risk compared with healthy lean individuals. Curiously in metabolically unhealthy patients, the normal-weight individuals had a higher risk (RR: 3.13), followed by overweight (RR: 2.70) and finally obese subjects (RR: 2.65) [71]. Similar results were published, indicating that both MHO and MUO individuals ultimately had a higher risk of mortality [72].

This evidence, too, is conflicting, with the underlying question being whether MHO presentations simply represent an early snapshot along the timeline of metabolic health. One group found that nearly 50% of MHO patients transitioned to metabolically unhealthy phenotypes when followed longitudinally for 10 years. Therefore, at present, it is not clear whether MHO individuals will remain such with the passage of time, or if their cardiovascular morbidity and mortality is comparable to that of non-obese subjects.

6. Conclusions

MHO is common among the obese population and constitutes a unique subset of characteristics that reduce metabolic and cardiovascular risk factors despite the presence of excessive fat mass. The protective factors that grant a healthier profile to individuals with MHO are being elucidated.

Despite the knowledge that visceral fat deposition is the seminal factor that ultimately causes insulin resistance and the detrimental inflammatory and hormonal profile that contributes to increased risk for cardiovascular disease, it remains unknown whether MHO has genetic predisposing factors, and whether MHO ultimately succumbs to insulin resistance and the metabolic syndrome.

Acknowledgments: This work was supported in part by grants from Instituto de Salud Carlos III (PI12/0235) and Consejería de Innovacion, Ciencia y Empresa de la Junta de Andalucía (CTS-8181). This study has been co-funded by FEDER funds. A.M.G. is the recipient of a postdoctoral grant (Rio Hortega CM 14/00078) from the Spanish Ministry of Economy and Competitiveness. All sources of funding of the study should be disclosed.

Author Contributions: A.M.G. and F.T. wrote the manuscript. I.C.P. helped with final revisions and writing the manuscript. M.R. reviewed the manuscript.

Conflicts of Interest: The authors declare no conflict of interest.

References

1. Sims, E. Are there persons who are obese, but metabolically healthy? *Metabolism* **2001**, *50*, 1499–1504. [CrossRef] [PubMed]
2. Roberson, L.; Aneni, E.; Maziak, W.; Agatston, A.; Feldman, T.; Rouseff, M.; Tran, T.; Blaha, M.J.; Santos, R.D.; Sposito, A.; *et al.* Beyond BMI: The "Metabolically healthy obese" phenotype & its association with clinical/subclinical cardiovascular disease and all-cause mortality—A systematic review. *BMC Public Health* **2014**, *14*, 1–12.

3. Wildman, R.; Muntner, P.; Reynolds, K.; McGinn, A.; Rajpathak, S.; Wylie-Rosett, J.; Sowers, M.R. The obese without cardiometabolic risk factor clustering and the normal weight with cardiometabolic risk factor clustering: Prevalence and correlates of 2 phenotypes among the US population (NHANES 1999–2004). *Arch. Intern. Med.* **2008**, *168*, 1617–1624. [CrossRef] [PubMed]

4. Pajunen, P.; Kotronen, A.; Korpi-Hyövälti, E.; Keinänen-Kiukaanniemi, S.; Oksa, H.; Niskanen, L.; Saaristo, T.; Saltevo, J.T.; Sundvall, T.; Vanhala, M.; *et al.* Metabolically healthy and unhealthy obesity phenotypes in the general population: The FIN-D2D survey. *BMC Public Health* **2011**, *1*, 754–762. [CrossRef] [PubMed]

5. Shea, J.; Randell, E.; Sun, G. The prevalence of metabolically healthy obese subjects defined by BMI and dual-energy X-ray absorptiometry. *Obesity (Silver Spring)* **2011**, *19*, 624–630. [CrossRef] [PubMed]

6. Van Vliet-Ostaptchouk, J.; Nuotio, M.; Slagter, S.; Doiron, D.; Fischer, K.; Foco, L.; Gaye, A.; Gögele, M.; Heier, M.; Hiekkalinna, T.; *et al.* The prevalence of metabolic syndrome and metabolically healthy obesity in Europe: A collaborative analysis of ten large cohort studies. *BMC Endocr. Disord.* **2014**, *14*, 9–22. [CrossRef] [PubMed]

7. Karelis, A. Metabolically healthy but obese individuals. *Lancet* **2008**, *372*, 1281–1283. [CrossRef]

8. Blüher, M. The distinction of metabolically 'healthy' from 'unhealthy' obese individuals. *Curr. Opin. Lipidol.* **2010**, *21*, 38–43. [CrossRef] [PubMed]

9. Brochu, M.; Tchernof, A.; Dionne, I.; Sites, C.K.; Eltabbakh, G.H.; Sims, E.A.; Poehlman, E.T. What are the physical characteristics associated with a normal metabolic profile despite a high level of obesity in postmenopausal women? *J. Clin. Endocrinol. Metab.* **2001**, *86*, 1020–1025. [PubMed]

10. Karelis, A.; Faraj, M.; Bastard, J.; St-Pierre, D.; Brochu, M.; Prud'homme, D.; Rabasa-Lhoret, R. The metabolically healthy but obese individual presents a favorable inflammation profile. *J. Clin. Endocrinol. Metab.* **2005**, *90*, 4145–4150. [CrossRef] [PubMed]

11. Kantartzis, K.; Machann, J.; Schick, F.; Rittig, K.; Machicao, F.; Fritsche, A.; Häring, H.-U.; Stefan, N. Effects of a lifestyle intervention in metabolically benign and malign obesity. *Diabetologia* **2011**, *54*, 864–868. [CrossRef] [PubMed]

12. Stefan, N.; Kantartzis, K.; Machann, J.; Schick, F.; Thamer, C.; Rittig, K.; Balletshofer, B.; Machicao, F.; Fritsche, A.; Häring, H.U. Identification and characterization of metabolically benign obesity in humans. *Arch. Intern. Med.* **2008**, *168*, 1609–1616. [CrossRef] [PubMed]

13. Camhi, S.M.; Katzmarzyk, P.T. Differences in body composition between metabolically healthy obese and metabolically abnormal obese adults. *Int. J. Obes. (Lond.)* **2014**, *38*, 1142–1145. [CrossRef] [PubMed]

14. Bobbioni-Harsch, E.; Pataky, Z.; Makoundou, V.; Laville, M.; Disse, E.; Anderwald, C.; Konrad, T.; Golay, A. Frommetabolic normality to cardiometabolic risk factors in subjects with obesity. *Obesity (Silver Spring)* **2012**, *20*, 2063–2069. [CrossRef] [PubMed]

15. Aguilar-Salinas, C.; García, E.; Robles, L.; Riaño, D.; Ruiz-Gomez, D.; García-Ulloa, A.; Melgarejo, M.A.; Zamora, M.; Guillen-Pineda, L.E.; Mehta, R.; *et al.* High adiponectin concentrations are associated with the metabolically healthy obese phenotype. *J. Clin. Endocrinol. Metab.* **2008**, *93*, 4075–4079. [CrossRef] [PubMed]

16. Karelis, A.; Rabasa-Lhoret, R. Obesity: Can inflammatory status define metabolic health? *Nat. Rev. Endocrinol.* **2013**, *9*, 694–695. [CrossRef] [PubMed]

17. Hamer, M.; Stamatakis, E. Metabolically healthy obesity and risk of all-cause and cardiovascular disease mortality. *J. Clin. Endocrinol. Metab.* **2012**, *97*, 2482–2488. [CrossRef] [PubMed]

18. Phillips, C.M.; Dillon, C.; Harrington, J.M.; McCarthy, V.J.C.; Kearney, P.M.; Fitzgerald, A.P.; Perry, I.J. Defining metabolically healthy obesity: Role of dietary and lifestyle factors. *PLoS ONE* **2013**, *8*, e76188. [CrossRef] [PubMed]

19. Sutherland, J.; McKinley, B.; Eckel, R. The metabolic syndrome and inflammation. *Metab. Syndr. Relat. Disord.* **2004**, *2*, 82–104. [CrossRef] [PubMed]

20. DeBoer, M. Obesity, systemic inflammation, and increased risk for cardiovascular disease and diabetes among adolescents: A need for screening tools to target interventions. *Nutrition* **2013**, *29*, 379–386. [CrossRef] [PubMed]

21. Phillips, C.; Perry, I. Does inflammation determine metabolic health status in obese and nonobese adults? *J. Clin. Endocrinol. Metab.* **2013**, *98*, E1610–E1619. [CrossRef] [PubMed]

22. Ouchi, N.; Parker, J.L.; Lugus, J.J.; Walsh, K. Adipokines in inflammation and metabolic disease. *Nat. Rev. Immunol.* **2011**, *11*, 85–97. [CrossRef] [PubMed]

23. VanBeek, L.; Lips, M.; Visser, A.; Pijl, H.; Ioan-Facsinay, A.; Toes, R.; Berends, F.J.; van Dijk, K.W.; Koning, F.; van Harmelen, V. Increased systemic and adipose tissue inflammation differentiates obese women with T2DM from obese women with normal glucose tolerance. *Metabolism* **2014**, *63*, 492–501. [CrossRef] [PubMed]

24. Blüher, S.; Schwarz, P. Metabolically healthy obesity from childhood to adulthood-does weight status alone matter? *Metabolism* **2014**, *63*, 1084–1092. [CrossRef] [PubMed]

25. Barbarroja, N.; López-Pedrera, R.; Mayas, M.D.; García-Fuentes, E.; Garrido-Sánchez, L.; Macías-González, M.; Bekay, R.; Vidal-Puig, A.; Tinahones, F.J. The obese healthy paradox: Is inflammation the answer? *Biochem. J.* **2010**, *430*, 141–149. [CrossRef] [PubMed]

26. Lionetti, L.; Mollica, M.P.; Lombardi, A.; Cavaliere, G.; Gifuni, G.; Barletta, A. From chronic overnutrition to insulin resistance: The role of fat-storing capacity and inflammation. *Nutr. Metab. Cardiovasc. Dis.* **2009**, *19*, 146–152. [CrossRef] [PubMed]

27. De Ferranti, S.; Mozaffarian, D. The perfect storm: obesity, adipocyte dysfunction, and metabolic consequences. *Clin. Chem.* **2008**, *54*, 945–955. [CrossRef] [PubMed]

28. Ledoux, S.; Queguiner, I.; Msika, S.; Calderari, S.; Rufat, P.; Gasc, J.M.; Corvol, P.; Larger, E. Angiogenesis associated with visceral and subcutaneous adipose tissue in severe human obesity. *Diabetes* **2008**, *57*, 3247–3257. [CrossRef] [PubMed]

29. Arner, E.; Westermark, P.O.; Spalding, K.L.; Britton, T.; Rydén, M.; Frisén, J.; Bernard, S.; Arner, P. Adipocyte turnover: Relevance to human adipose tissue morphology. *Diabetes* **2010**, *59*, 105–109. [CrossRef] [PubMed]

30. Virtue, S.; Vidal-Puig, A. It's not how fat you are, it's what you do with it that counts. *PLoS Biol.* **2008**, *6*, e237. [CrossRef] [PubMed]

31. Barbarroja, N.; Rodriguez-Cuenca, S.; Nygren, H.; Camargo, A.; Pirraco, A.; Relat, J.; Cuadrado, I.; Pellegrinelli, V.; Medina-Gomez, G.; Lopez-Pedrera, C.; *et al.* Increased dihydroceramide/ceramide ratio mediated by defective expression of degs1 impairs adipocyte differentiation and function. *Diabetes* **2015**, *64*, 1180–1192. [CrossRef] [PubMed]

32. Spalding, K.L.; Arner, E.; Westermark, P.O.; Bernard, S.; Buchholz, B.A.; Bergmann, O.; Blomqvist, L.; Hoffstedt, J.; Näslund, E.; Britton, T.; *et al.* Dynamics of fat cell turnover in humans. *Nature* **2008**, *453*, 783–787. [CrossRef] [PubMed]

33. Baglioni, S.; Francalanci, M.; Squecco, R.; Lombardi, A.; Cantini, G.; Angeli, R.; Gelmini, S.; Guasti, D.; Benvenuti, S.; Annunziato, F.; *et al.* Characterization of human adult stem-cell populations isolated from visceral and subcutaneous adipose tissue. *FASEB J.* **2009**, *23*, 3494–3505. [CrossRef] [PubMed]

34. Isakson, P.; Hammarstedt, A.; Gustafson, B.; Smith, U. Impaired preadipocyte differentiation in human abdominal obesity: role of Wnt, tumor necrosis factor-alpha, and inflammation. *Diabetes* **2009**, *58*, 1550–1557. [CrossRef] [PubMed]

35. Cleveland-Donovan, K.; Maile, L.A.; Tsiaras, W.G.; Tchkonia, T.; Kirkland, J.L.; Boney, C.M. IGF-I activation of the AKT pathway is impaired in visceral but not subcutaneous preadipocytes from obese subjects. *Endocrinology* **2010**, *151*, 3752–3763. [CrossRef] [PubMed]

36. Roldan, M.; Macias-Gonzalez, M.; Garcia, R.; Tinahones, F.J.; Martin, M. Obesity short-circuits stemness gene network in human adipose multipotent stem cells. *FASEB J.* **2011**, *25*, 4111–4126. [CrossRef] [PubMed]

37. Sorisky, A.; Gagnon, A.M. Clinical implications of adipose tissue remodelling: Adipogenesis and apoptosis. *Can. J. Diabetes* **2002**, *26*, 232–240.

38. Arner, P.; Spalding, K.L. Fat cell turnover in humans. *Biochem. Biophys. Res. Commun.* **2010**, *396*, 101–104. [CrossRef] [PubMed]

39. Ortega, F.J.; Mayas, D.; Moreno-Navarrete, J.M.; Catalán, V.; Gómez-Ambrosi, J.; Esteve, E.; Rodriguez-Hermosa, J.I.; Ruiz, B.; Ricart, W.; Peral, B.; *et al.* The gene expression of the main lipogenic enzymes is downregulated in visceral adipose tissue of obese subjects. *Obesity* **2010**, *18*, 13–20. [CrossRef] [PubMed]

40. Clemente-Postigo, M.; Queipo-Ortuño, M.I.; Fernandez-Garcia, D.; Gomez-Huelgas, R.; Tinahones, F.J.; Cardona, F. Adipose tissue gene expression of factors related to lipid processing in obesity. *PLoS ONE* **2011**, *6*, e24783. [CrossRef] [PubMed]

41. Cao, Y. Adipose tissue angiogenesis as a therapeutic target for obesity and metabolic diseases. *Nat. Rev. Drug Discov.* **2010**, *9*, 107–115. [CrossRef] [PubMed]

42. Tinahones, F.J.; Coín-Aragüez, L.; Mayas, M.D.; Garcia-Fuentes, E.; Hurtado-Del-Pozo, C.; Vendrell, J.; Cardona, F.; Calvo, R.M; Obregon, M.J.; Bekay, E.L.R. Obesity-associated insulin resistance is correlated to adipose tissue vascular endothelial growth factors and metalloproteinase levels. *BMC Physiol.* **2012**, *12*. [CrossRef] [PubMed]

43. Tinahones, F.J.; Coín-Aragüez, L.; Murri, M.; Oliva-Olivera, W.; Mayas Torres, M.D.; Barbarroja, N.; Gomez-Huelgas, R.; Malagón, M.M.; Bekay, E.L.R. Caspase induction and BCL2 inhibition in human adipose tissue: A potential relationship with insulin signaling alteration. *Diabetes Care* **2013**, *36*, 513–521. [CrossRef] [PubMed]

44. Bluher, S.; Markert, J.; Herget, S.; Yates, T.; Davis, M.; Muller, G.; Waldow, T.; Schwarz, P.E. Who should we target for diabetes prevention and diabetes risk reduction? *Curr. Diabetes Rep.* **2012**, *12*, 147–156. [CrossRef] [PubMed]

45. Mitchell, P.S.; Parkin, R.K.; Kroh, E.M.; Fritz, B.R.; Wyman, S.K.; Pogosova-Agadjanyan, E.L.; Peterson, A.; Noteboom, J.; O'Briant, K.C.; Allen, A.; *et al.* Circulating microRNAs as stable blood-based markers for cancer detection. *Proc. Natl. Acad. Sci. USA* **2008**, *105*, 10513–10518. [CrossRef] [PubMed]

46. Zhang, T.; Lv, C.; Li, L.; Chen, S.; Liu, S.; Wang, C.; Su, B. Plasma miR-126 is a potential biomarker for early prediction of type 2 diabetes mellitus in susceptible individuals. *BioMed Res. Int.* **2013**, *2013*, 6. [CrossRef] [PubMed]

47. Ortega, F.; Lee, D.; Katzmarzyk, P.; Ruiz, J.; Sui, X.; Church, T. The intriguing metabolically healthy but obese phenotype: Cardiovascular prognosis and role of fitness. *Eur. Heart J.* **2013**, *34*, 389–397. [CrossRef] [PubMed]

48. Katzmarzyk, P.; Church, T.; Janssen, I.; Ross, R.; Blair, S. Metabolic syndrome, obesity, and mortality: Impact of cardiorespiratory fitness. *Diabetes Care* **2005**, *28*, 391–397. [CrossRef] [PubMed]

49. Larsson, C.; Krøll, L.; Bennet, L.; Gullberg, B.; Råstam, L.; Lindblad, U. Leisure time and occupational physical activity in relation to obesity and insulin resistance: A population-based study from the Skaraborg Project in Sweden. *Metabolism* **2012**, *61*, 590–598. [CrossRef] [PubMed]

50. Arsenault, B.J.; Côté, M.; Cartier, A.; Lemieux, I.; Després, J.P.; Ross, R.; Earnest, C.P.; Blair, S.N.; Church, T.S. Effect of exercise training on cardiometabolic risk markers among sedentary, but metabolically healthy overweight or obese post-menopausal women with elevated blood pressure. *Atherosclerosis* **2009**, *207*, 530–533. [CrossRef] [PubMed]

51. Janiszewski, P.M.; Ross, R. Effects of weight loss among metabolically healthy obese men and women. *Diabetes Care* **2010**, *33*, 1957–1959. [CrossRef] [PubMed]

52. Karelis, A.; Messier, V.; Brochu, M.; Rabasa-Lhoret, R. Metabolically healthy but obese women: Effect of an energy-restricted diet. *Diabetologia* **2008**, *51*, 1752–1754. [CrossRef] [PubMed]

53. Martínez-González, M.A.; Salas-Salvadó, J.; Estruch, R.; Corella, D.; Fitó, M.; Ros, E. PREDIMED INVESTIGATORS. Benefits of the Mediterranean diet: Insights from the PREDIMED Study. *Prog. Cardiovasc. Dis.* **2015**, *58*, 50–60.

54. Dalzill, C.; Nigam, A.; Juneau, M.; Guilbeault, V.; Latour, E.; Mauriège, P.; Gayda, M. Intensive lifestyle intervention improves cardiometabolic and exercise parameters in metabolically healthy obese and metabolically unhealthy obese in dividuals. *Can. J. Cardiol.* **2014**, *30*, 434–440. [CrossRef] [PubMed]

55. Samaropoulos, X.F.; Hairston, K.G.; Anderson, A.; Haffner, S.M.; Lorenzo, C.; Montez, M. A metabolically healthy obese phenotype in Hispanic participants in the IRAS family study. *Obesity (Silver Spring)* **2013**, *21*, 2303–2309. [CrossRef] [PubMed]

56. Buchwald, H.; Avidor, Y.; Braunwald, E.; Jensen, M.D.; Pories, W.; Fahrbach, K. Bariatric surgery: A systematic review and meta-analysis. *JAMA* **2004**, *292*, 1724–1737. [CrossRef] [PubMed]

57. Hinnouho, G.M.; Czernichow, S.; Dugravot, A.; Nabi, H.; Brunner, E.J.; Kivimaki, M. Metabolically healthy obesity and the risk of cardiovascular disease and type 2 diabetes: The Whitehall II cohort study. *Eur. Heart J.* **2015**, *36*, 551–559. [CrossRef] [PubMed]

58. Hwang, Y.C.; Hayashi, T.; Fujimoto, W.Y.; Kahn, S.E.; Leonetti, D.L.; McNeely, M.J. Visceral abdominal fat accumulation predicts the conversion of metabolically healthy obese subjects to an unhealthy phenotype. *Int. J. Obes.* **2015**, *39*, 1365–1370. [CrossRef] [PubMed]

59. Soriguer, F.; Gutierrez-Repiso, C.; Rubio-Martin, E.; Garcia-Fuentes, E.; Almaraz, M.C.; Colomo, N. Metabolically healthy but obese, a matter of time? Findings from the prospective Pizarra study. *J. Clin. Endocrinol. Metab.* **2013**, *98*, 2318–2325. [CrossRef] [PubMed]

60. Song, Y.; Manson, J.E.; Meigs, J.B.; Ridker, P.M.; Buring, J.E.; Liu, S. Comparison of usefulness of body mass index *versus* metabolic risk factors in predicting 10-year risk of cardiovascular events in women. *Am. J. Cardiol.* **2007**, *100*, 1654–1658. [CrossRef] [PubMed]

61. Meigs, J.B.; Wilson, P.W.; Fox, C.S.; Vasan, R.S.; Nathan, D.M.; Sullivan, L.M. Body mass index, metabolic syndrome, and risk of type 2 diabetes or cardiovascular disease. *J. Clin. Endocrinol. Metab.* **2006**, *91*, 2906–2912. [CrossRef] [PubMed]

62. Calori, G.; Lattuada, G.; Piemonti, L.; Garancini, M.P.; Ragogna, F.; Villa, M. Prevalence, metabolic features, and prognosis of metabolically healthy obese Italian individuals: The Cremona Study. *Diabetes Care* **2011**, *34*, 210–215. [CrossRef] [PubMed]

63. Ogorodnikova, A.D.; Kim, M.; McGinn, A.P.; Muntner, P.; Khan, U.; Wildman, R.P. Incident cardiovascular disease events in metabolically benign obese individuals. *Obesity (Silver Spring)* **2012**, *20*, 651–659. [CrossRef] [PubMed]

64. Arnlov, J.; Ingelsson, E.; Sundstrom, J.; Lind, L. Impact of body mass index and the metabolic syndrome on the risk of cardiovascular disease and death in middle-aged men. *Circulation* **2010**, *121*, 230–236. [CrossRef] [PubMed]

65. Flint, A.J.; Hu, F.B.; Glynn, R.J.; Caspard, H.; Manson, J.E.; Willett, W.C. Excess weight and the risk of incident coronary heart disease among men and women. *Obesity (Silver Spring)* **2010**, *18*, 377–383. [CrossRef] [PubMed]

66. Kramer, C.K.; Zinman, B.; Retnakaran, R. Are metabolically healthy overweight and obesity benign conditions? A systematic review and meta-analysis. *Ann. Intern. Med.* **2013**, *159*, 758–769. [CrossRef] [PubMed]

67. Shaharyar, S.; Roberson, L.L.; Jamal, O.; Younus, A.; Blaha, M.J.; Ali, S.S. Obesity and metabolic phenotypes (metabolically healthy and unhealthy variants) are significantly associated with prevalence of elevated C-reactive protein and hepatic steatosis in a large healthy Brazilian population. *J. Obes.* **2015**, *2015*, 178526. [CrossRef] [PubMed]

68. Eshtiaghi, R.; Keihani, S.; Hosseinpanah, F.; Barzin, M.; Azizi, F. Natural course of metabolically healthy abdominal obese adults after 10 years of follow-up: The Tehran Lipid and Glucose Study. *Int. J. Obes.* **2015**, *39*, 514–519. [CrossRef] [PubMed]

69. Li, S.; Chen, W.; Srinivasan, S.; Xu, J.; Berenson, G. Relation of childhood obesity/cardiometabolic phenotypes to adult cardiometabolic profile: The Bogalusa Heart Study. *Am. J. Epidemiol.* **2012**, *176*, S142–S149. [CrossRef] [PubMed]

70. Dvorak, R.; DeNino, W.; Ades, P.; Poehlman, E. Phenotypic characteristics associated with insulin resistance in metabolically obese but normal-weight young women. *Diabetes* **1999**, *48*, 2210–2214. [CrossRef] [PubMed]

71. Park, J.; Kim, S.; Cho, G.; Baik, I.; Kim, N.; Lim, H. Obesity phenotype and cardiovascular changes. *J. Hypertens.* **2011**, *29*, 1765–1772. [CrossRef] [PubMed]

72. Khan, U.; Wang, D.; Thurston, R.; Sowers, M.; Sutton-Tyrrell, K.; Matthews, K. Burden of subclinical cardiovascular disease in "metabolically benign" and "at-risk" overweight and obese women: The Study of Women's Health Across the Nation (SWAN). *Atherosclerosis* **2011**, *217*, 179–186. [CrossRef] [PubMed]

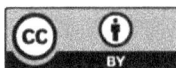

© 2016 by the authors. Licensee MDPI, Basel, Switzerland. This article is an open access article distributed under the terms and conditions of the Creative Commons Attribution (CC BY) license (http://creativecommons.org/licenses/by/4.0/).

nutrients

MDPI

Article

The Distribution of Obesity Phenotypes in HIV-Infected African Population

Kim Anh Nguyen [1,2], Nasheeta Peer [1,2], Anniza de Villiers [1], Barbara Mukasa [3], Tandi E. Matsha [4], Edward J. Mills [5] and Andre Pascal Kengne [1,2,*]

[1] Non-Communicable Diseases Research Unit, South African Medical Research Council, Cape Town 7505, South Africa; Kim.Nguyen@mrc.ac.za (K.A.N.); nasheeta.peer@mrc.ac.za (N.P.); Anniza.DeVilliers@mrc.ac.za (A.d.V.)
[2] Department of Medicine, University of Cape Town, Cape Town 7935, South Africa
[3] United Nations Population Fund (UNFPA), Mildmay Uganda PO Box 24985, Lweza, Uganda; barbara.mukasa@mildmay.or.ug
[4] Department of Biomedical Sciences, Faculty of Health and Wellness Science, Cape Peninsula University of Technology, Cape Town 7535, South Africa; matshat@cput.ac.za
[5] Global Evaluation Science, Vancouver, BC V6H 3X4, Canada; emills@redwoodoutcomes.com
* Correspondence: andre.kengne@mrc.ac.za; Tel.: +27-21-938-0841

Received: 21 March 2016; Accepted: 29 April 2016; Published: 2 June 2016

Abstract: The distribution of body size phenotypes in people with human immunodeficiency virus (HIV) infection has yet to be characterized. We assessed the distribution of body size phenotypes overall, and according to antiretroviral therapy (ART), diagnosed duration of the infection and CD4 count in a sample of HIV infected people recruited across primary care facilities in the Western Cape Province, South Africa. Adults aged $\geq$ 18 years were consecutively recruited using random sampling procedures, and their cardio-metabolic profile were assessed during March 2014 and February 2015. They were classified across body mass index (BMI) categories as normal-weight (BMI < 25 kg/m^2), overweight (25 $\leq$ BMI < 30 kg/m^2), and obese (BMI $\geq$ 30 kg/m^2), and further classified according to their metabolic status as "metabolically healthy" *vs.* "metabolically abnormal" if they had less than two *vs.* two or more of the following abnormalities: high blood glucose, raised blood pressure, raised triglycerides, and low HDL-cholesterol. Their cross-classification gave the following six phenotypes: normal-weight metabolically healthy (NWMH), normal-weight metabolically abnormal (NWMA), overweight metabolically healthy (OvMH), overweight metabolically abnormal (OvMA), obese metabolically healthy (OMH), and obese metabolically abnormal (OMA). Among the 748 participants included (median age 38 years (25th–75th percentiles: 32–44)), 79% were women. The median diagnosed duration of HIV was five years; the median CD4 count was 392 cells/mm^3 and most participants were on ART. The overall distribution of body size phenotypes was the following: 31.7% (NWMH), 11.7% (NWMA), 13.4% (OvMH), 9.5% (OvMA), 18.6% (OMH), and 15.1% (OMA). The distribution of metabolic phenotypes across BMI levels did not differ significantly in men *vs.* women (p = 0.062), in participants below *vs.* those at or above median diagnosed duration of HIV infection (p = 0.897), in participants below *vs.* those at or above median CD4 count (p = 0.447), and by ART regimens (p = 0.205). In this relatively young sample of HIV-infected individuals, metabolically abnormal phenotypes are frequent across BMI categories. This highlights the importance of general measures targeting an overall improvement in cardiometabolic risk profile across the spectrum of BMI distribution in all adults with HIV.

Keywords: obesity phenotype; metabolic abnormalities; HIV infection

1. Introduction

People living with HIV infection constitute a sizable proportion of the world population and the number is increasing [1]. The advent and uptake of antiretroviral therapy (ART) has turned HIV infection from a highly fatal infectious disease into a chronic manageable condition [2]. Consequently, the lifespan of HIV infected patients receiving ART is now close to that of the general population [3]. This has led to a rise in chronic and age-related conditions such as cardio-metabolic disorders in HIV-infected people [4,5], that is contributing substantially to the overall morbidity and mortality in this population [6,7].

A major contributor to cardio-metabolic diseases is the global obesity epidemic with 52% (1.9 millions) of the worldwide adult population being either overweight or obese in 2014 [8]. Obesity contributes to cardio-metabolic abnormalities by impairing metabolic functions that promote dyslipidemia, insulin resistance, as well as chronic inflammation [9]. Consequently, concepts such as "metabolically healthy" and "metabolically abnormal" have been used to characterize individuals across the distribution of body mass index (BMI) as a function of the underlying burden of metabolic abnormalities [10].

The changes in body fat distribution associated with HIV infection are well-described [11]. The advanced stage of untreated HIV infection is associated with changes in body fat content and distribution, which are partially and perhaps non-optimally restored following treatment with ART [12]. ART extends the lifespan of HIV-infected people by reducing the viral load with a subsequent strengthening of the immune system; notably, it does not eliminate the HIV infection. Hence, chronic inflammation persists and there is incomplete restoration of the immune system [13]. Additionally, various metabolic abnormalities are associated with HIV infection and its related treatments [14,15]. These include dyslipidemia, insulin resistance, and abnormal blood pressure levels, [13], which contribute to cardiovascular diseases (CVDs) and type 2 diabetes mellitus (T2DM) [13,16].

While obesity and HIV infection have been extensively researched separately, there is a dearth of data on the distribution of obesity phenotypes in HIV-infected people [17]. Therefore, in the current study, we assessed the distribution of obesity phenotypes, and the effects if any, of ART and other major distinctive characteristics of HIV infection, in a representative sample of people with HIV recruited across primary healthcare facilities in the Western Cape Province, South Africa.

2. Materials and Methods

2.1. Study Design and Sampling Procedure

A cross-sectional survey was conducted from March 2014 to February 2015 in a random sample of HIV-infected adults aged 18 years and older being treated at public healthcare facilities across the Western Cape Province in South Africa. Permission to conduct the survey was obtained from Health Research Office of the Western Cape Department of Health, and the relevant healthcare facilities.

The healthcare facilities considered for this study needed to provide ART to at least 325 HIV-infected patients per month to ensure adequate recruitment within a reasonable period. Thus, the sample frame comprised a total of 62 healthcare facilities with 42 across Cape Town and 20 in the surrounding rural municipalities. Of these, 17 facilities, including four rural, were randomly selected for inclusion in this study. At each participating healthcare facility, 15–60 patients were randomly sampled.

The study was approved by the South African Medical Research Council Ethics Committee and conducted in accordance with the principles of the Declaration of Helsinki.

2.2. Data Collection

A team of trained clinicians, nurses, and field workers collected data by administering questionnaires, clinical measurements, and biochemical analyses. Data were captured on electronic case report forms, which were available on personal digital assistants (PDAs), with built-in checks for quality control. Data were encrypted at the point of collection and sent via mobile connection to a dedicated server, from which it was further checked, downloaded, and stored for future use. The interviews and the physical assessments were conducted on the day of recruitment while the blood specimens were drawn the following day after the participant had fasted overnight.

2.2.1. Interviews

Socio-demographic data and medical history were obtained using a structured interviewer-administered questionnaire adapted from the World Health Organization's STEPwise approach to Surveillance (STEPS) tool. Self-reported data included duration of being diagnosed HIV infection and CD4 counts, whereas information on HIV treatment was obtained by capturing medications brought to by the participants.

2.2.2. Physical Examination

Anthropometric parameters including height, weight, and waist circumference (WC) were measured using standardized techniques. Height was measured to the nearest millimeter using a Leicester Height Scale (Seca, Liverpool, UK) with the participant barefoot and in the upright position. Weight was measured to the nearest gram using A&D Personal Scale (Model UC-321, Toshima-Ku, Tokyo, Japan) with the participant in light clothes, and without shoes. WC, recorded to the nearest millimeter, was taken at the level of umbilicus. After the participant was seated in a resting position for at least five minutes, blood pressure (BP) was measured in mmHg on the right arm, using a digital automatic BP monitor (Omron, M6 Comfort, Hoofddorp, The Netherland); three measurements were taken three minutes apart.

2.2.3. Laboratory Measurements

Biochemical parameters were analyzed at an ISO 15189 accredited pathology laboratory (PathCare, Reference Laboratory, Cape Town, South Africa) which had no access to participants' clinical information. All analyses were performed on venous blood samples collected after an overnight fast of at least eight hours. Serum cholesterol and triglycerides were measured by enzymatic colorimetric methods; ultrasensitive C-reactive protein was read; plasma glucose was measured by hexokinase method; all implemented using a Beckman Coulter AU 500 spectrophotometer. Insulin concentrations were measured by the Chemiluminesecence Immunoassay method while HbA1c level was determined using high-performance liquid chromatography technique. The homeostatic model assessment of insulin resistance (HOMA-IR) was calculated as the product of insulin (mIU/L) and glucose (mmol/L) by 22.5 [18].

2.3. Definitions

2.3.1. Socio-Demographic Characteristics

Education level was distinguished into primary education and secondary education or above. Smoking status was categorized as never-smoker, past-smoker (stopped smoking during the past 12 months), and current-smoker. Alcohol intake behavior was classified as non-heavy drinker (consumed <5 standard alcoholic drinks for men and < 4 standard alcoholic drinks for women in a row during the past 30 days), and heavy-drinker (consumed $\geqslant$5 standard alcoholic drinks for men and $\geqslant$4 standard alcoholic drinks for women in a row during the past 30 days). A standard alcoholic drink was corresponding to one can (340 mL) of beer, one glass (125 mL) wine, or one shot (25 mL) of spirits. Duration of diagnosed HIV infection was the time since being diagnosed with HIV. ARTs were categorized as first line ART, second line ART, and other regimens [19].

2.3.2. Body Size Phenotype

Body mass index (BMI) was calculated as weight (kg)/height $\times$ height (m^2). BMI was used to classify participants into three categories: normal weight (BMI < 25 kg/m^2), overweight (BMI $\geqslant$ 25 kg/m^2 and BMI < 30 kg/m^2) and obese (BMI $\geqslant$ 30 kg/m^2). There is no consensus on the definition and number of cardio-metabolic abnormalities to use when characterizing obesity phenotypes [20]. In the current study, we considered the following four abnormalities: (1) elevated BP determined using the average of the second and third BP measurements (systolic BP $\geqslant$ 130 mmHg or diastolic BP $\geqslant$ 85 mmHg or known hypertension on treatment); (2) high triglycerides ($\geqslant$1.69 mmol/L); (3) low high-density lipoprotein cholesterol (HDL-C $\leqslant$ 1.0 mmol/L in men; $\leqslant$1.3 mmol/L in women); (4) high blood glucose (fasting plasma glucose (FPG) $\geqslant$ 5.6 mmol/L or known diabetes mellitus). In secondary analysis, in a subset of participants with data available on insulin levels, we included insulin resistance as a fifth metabolic abnormality, by classifying as insulin resistant all participants with HOMA-IR above the data specific 90th percentile. Considering the lack of consensus on waist circumference (or waist-to-hip ratio) threshold to define abdominal obesity in African populations, the criteria of abdominal obesity which has been included in about 30% of studies on obesity phenotype [20] was not included in our panel of metabolic abnormalities.

Participants were then classified for metabolic status as "metabolically healthy" if they had none or one metabolic abnormality, and as "metabolically abnormal" if they had two or more metabolic abnormalities. Cross-classification of participants by BMI and metabolic status led to the following six phenotypes: (1) normal weight and metabolically healthy (NWMH); (2) normal weight and metabolically abnormal (NWMA); (3) overweight and metabolically healthy (OvMH); (4) overweight and metabolically abnormal (OvMA); (5) obese and metabolically healthy (OMH); and (6) obese and metabolically abnormal (OMA).

2.4. Statistical Analysis

Participants' characteristics are summarized as means (standard deviation, SD) and medians (25th to 75th percentiles) for continuous variables, and as count (percentages) for categorical variables. Comparison of baseline characteristics across BMI categories, by metabolic status, and by HIV-related characteristics were done using chi-square tests, fisher-exact test, *t*-tests or Kruskal-wallis tests for non-parametric data or Analysis of Variance test (ANOVA) where appropriate. The linear trends across BMI categories overall and by metabolic status were examined using the Cochrane-Armitage trend tests and Brown-Forsythe Levene procedures. The two-way interactions between BMI categories and metabolic status (B $\times$ M), and metabolic status and gender (M $\times$ G) were tested using linear and logistic regression models, by incorporating in the same model the main effects of the variables of interest as well as their interaction term.

To assess the association between each continuous metabolic trait and BMI categories, multinomial logistic regressions models (age and sex adjusted) were used to derive the odds ratio (OR) and 95% confidence interval for a unit higher level of each metabolic trait in relation with overweight and obesity risk, always using normal weight are reference category. The McFadden's R^2 [21] was then used as a measure of the overall performance of models containing age, gender, and each metabolic trait of interest. A two-side *p*-value < 0.05 indicates a statistical significance. All analyses were performed using the R statistical software version 3.0.3 (the R Foundation for Statistical Computing Platform, Vienna, Austria. For a *z*-value of 1.96 (corresponding to a 95% confidence interval), and an effective sample size of 748 participants, our study had a margin of error of 0.05% to detect a prevalence of normal weight metabolically abnormal phenotype of 1% in the total sample. The acceptable margin of error is 5%, indicating that our study was well-powered for the overall and subgroup analyses.

3. Results

3.1. Socio-Demographic Characteristics

Of the 831 participants who were interviewed and clinically assessed, 754 (91%) returned for biochemical measurements. Blood samples from six participants were inadequate for analyses resulting in 748 (99%) participants being included in the study. This comprised 591 women and 157 men who had complete data on the variables of interest.

The median age (25th–75th percentiles) was 38 (32–44) years overall, 41 (35–47) years in men, and 37 (31–43) years in women ($p < 0.001$). As shown in Table 1, most participants (84.9%) had secondary education or higher with a lower prevalence in men (75.8%) than in women (87.3%) ($p < 0.001$). About half of the participants (54.6%) were employed with similar rates in men and women (49.7% *vs.* 55.9%, $p = 0.162$). Current smoking was more prevalent in men than in women (58.8% *vs.* 16.1%, $p < 0.001$) but heavy alcohol consumption was similar (34.1% *vs.* 34.1%, $p = 0.975$).

Table 1. Characteristics of the HIV/AIDS patients (n (%), or median (25th–75th percentiles)).

Characteristics	Overall, (n = 748)	Men, (n = 157)	Women, (n = 591)	p
Age, year	38 (32–44)	41 (35–47)	37 (31–43)	<0.001
Education level, n (%)				<0.001
Primary	113/746 (15.1)	38/157 (24.2)	75/589 (12.7)	
Secondary and above	633/746 (84.9)	119/157 (75.8)	514/589 (87.3)	
Employed, n (%)	408/747 (54.6)	78/157 (49.7)	330/590 (55.9)	0.162
Smoking habit, n (%)				<0.001
Never smoke	461/718 (64.7)	34/156 (22.2)	427/562 (76.4)	
Current smoker	187/718 (25.3)	93/156 (58.8)	90/562 (16.1)	
Past smoker	70/718 (13.3)	29/156 (45.3)	42/562 (9.0)	
Heavy drinker, n (%)	64/187 (34.2)	22/64 (34.4)	42/123 (34.1)	0.975
HIV duration, years	5 (2–9)	4 (2–7)	5 (2.5–9)	<0.001
CD4, cells/mm^3	392(240–604)	272(193–448)	410(253–627)	0.001
ART treatment, n (%)				0.005
Non-ART	46/699 (6.6)	7/149 (4.7)	39/550 (7.1)	
first line	426/699 (60.9)	78/149 (52.3)	348/550 (63.3)	
second line	79/699 (11.3)	17/149 (11.4)	62/550 (11.3)	
Others	148/699 (21.2)	47/149 (31.5)	101/550 (18.3)	
Body mass index (kg/m^2)				
Median (P25–P75)	26.3 (22.1–32)	21.4 (19.8–22.4)	28.3 (23.8–28.9)	<0.001
<25, n (%)	325 (43.4)	126 (80.3)	199 (33.7)	
25.0–29.9, n (%)	171 (22.9)	21 (13.4)	150 (25.4)	
⩾30, n (%)	252 (33.7)	10 (6.4)	242 (40.9)	
Waist circumference, cm	88 (77.5–98)	78.9 (73.9–88.3)	90 (79.5–100.8)	<0.001
Systolic BP, mmHg	117 (107–129.5)	123.5 (114.5–140)	115 (105.8–127)	<0.001
Diastolic BP, mmHg	82 (75–90.5)	83 (76–94)	81.5 (74.8–89.8)	0.129
Total cholesterol, mmol/L	4.3 (3.7–5.1)	4.2 (3.5–5.0)	4.4 (3.8–5.1)	0.009
HDL-cholesterol, mmol/L	1.27 (1.03–1.5)	1.2 (1.0–1.5)	1.29 (1.08–1.52)	0.010
LDL-cholesterol, mmol/L	2.5 (2.0–3.1)	2.3 (1.7–3.0)	2.5 (2.0–3.1)	0.012
Triglycerides, mmol/L	1.0 (0.74–1.34)	1.12 (0.75–1.27)	0.97 (0.74–1.28)	0.023
Fasting glucose, mmol/L	5.0 (4.6–5.4)	5.1 (4.8–5.5)	4.9 (4.6–5.4)	0.010
HOMA-IR	1.36 (0.84–2.24)	0.94 (0.53–1.64)	1.49 (0.93–2.37)	<0.001
C-reactive protein, mg/L	5.6 (2.4–12)	5.0 (2.1–16.2)	5.6 (2.4–14.2)	0.728
Treated hypertension, n (%)	110 (14.7)	11 (7)	99 (16.8)	0.002
Treated diabetes, n (%)	28 (3.7)	8 (5.1)	20 (3.4)	0.432

ART, antiretroviral; BP, blood pressure; HDL, high density lipoprotein; HIV, human immunodeficiency virus; AIDS, acquired immunodeficiency syndrome; HOMA-IR, homeostatic model assessment of insulin resistance; LDL, low density lipoprotein.

3.2. Profile of HIV Infection

The median duration of diagnosed HIV infection was five years (25th–75th percentiles: 2–9) with no difference by gender ($p = 0.223$). The median CD4 count was 392 cells/mm^3 (25th–75th percentiles:

240–604) with higher levels in women than in men (410 cells/mm^3 *vs.* 272 cells/mm^3, $p = 0.002$). Most participants were receiving ART (93.4%) with the majority on first line ART (63.9%), while 11.8% received second line ART and 17.4% were on other ART regimens. Interestingly, there were significant differences in the distribution by gender ($p = 0.005$).

3.3. Profile of Cardio-Metabolic Abnormalities

The mean BMI was 26.3 kg/m^2 overall with significantly lower levels in men compared with women (21.4 kg/m^2 *vs.* 28.3 kg/m^2, $p < 0.001$). Overall, 43.4% of participants had normal BMI levels while 22.9% were overweight and 33.7% obese with significant differences by gender ($p < 0.001$). Women compared to men had larger WCs (90 cm *vs.* 79 cm, $p < 0.001$), higher HOMA-IR indices (1.49 *vs.* 0.94, $p < 0.001$), and total cholesterol levels (4.4 *vs.* 4.2 mmol/L, $p = 0.009$). However, they had lower levels of triglycerides (0.97 *vs.* 1.12 mmol/L, $p = 0.023$), fasting glucose (4.9 *vs.* 5.1 mmol/L, $p = 0.010$) and systolic BP (115 *vs.* 124 mmHg, $p < 0.001$). Furthermore, HDL-cholesterol levels (1.29 *vs.* 1.2 mmol/L, $p = 0.010$) and prevalent treated hypertension (16.8% *vs.* 7.0%, $p = 0.002$) were higher in women than men. Diastolic BP, hs-CRP, as well as prevalent treated diabetes were similar in both genders (all $p \geqslant 0.129$) (Table 1).

3.4. Distribution of Body Size Phenotypes

The proportion of $\geqslant 2$ metabolic abnormalities across normal-weight (27.1%), overweight (41.5%), and obese (44.8%) categories increased significantly in a linear trend (p-trend = 0.001). The distribution of body size phenotypes in the overall sample was 31.7% (NWMH), 11.7% (NWMA), 13.4% (OvMH), 9.5% (OvMA), 18.6% (OMH), and 15.1% (OMA), Figure 1.

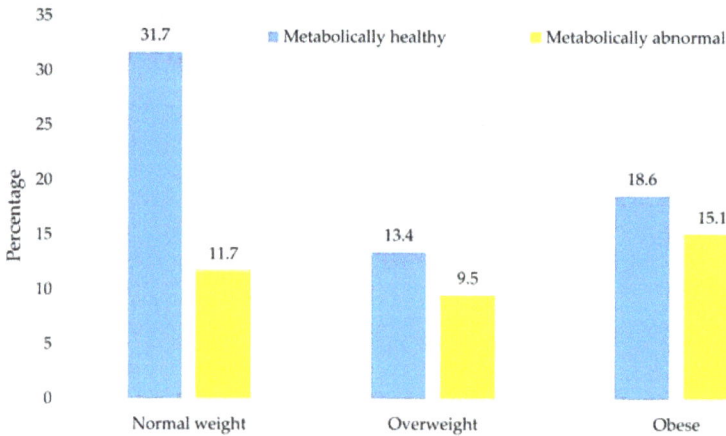

Figure 1. Distribution of metabolic phenotypes across body mass index categories. Each vertical bar represents the proportion of participants in the total sample with the corresponding combination of body size (normal-weight, overweight, or obese) and metabolic phenotype (healthy or abnormal). The accompanying proportions are shown at the tip of each bar.

In men, the majority (54.1%) were NWMH, just over a quarter (26.1%) were NWMA, while few fell into the other categories: 6.4% (OvMH), 7% (OvMA), 0.7% (OMH), and 5.7% (OMA). In contrast, the distribution in women was as follows: 25.7% (NWMH), 8% (NWMA), 15.2% (OvMH), 10.1% (OvMA), 23.4% (OMH), and 17.6% (OMA) (Figure 2). There was no statistically significant interaction by gender in the distribution of body size phenotypes (p-interaction = 0.062).

The distribution of metabolic phenotypes across BMI categories was not significantly different by longer or shorter duration of diagnosed HIV infection (median five years, p-interaction = 0.897)

(Figure 3a), higher or lower CD4 count (median 392 cells/mm^3, *p*-interaction = 0.447) (Figure 3b) or across the three ART regimens (*p*-interaction = 0.205) (Figure 3c). The proportion of ≥ 2 metabolic abnormalities tended to increase significantly and linearly across BMI categories within most of the latter subgroups except for lower CD4 count and the second line ART regimen.

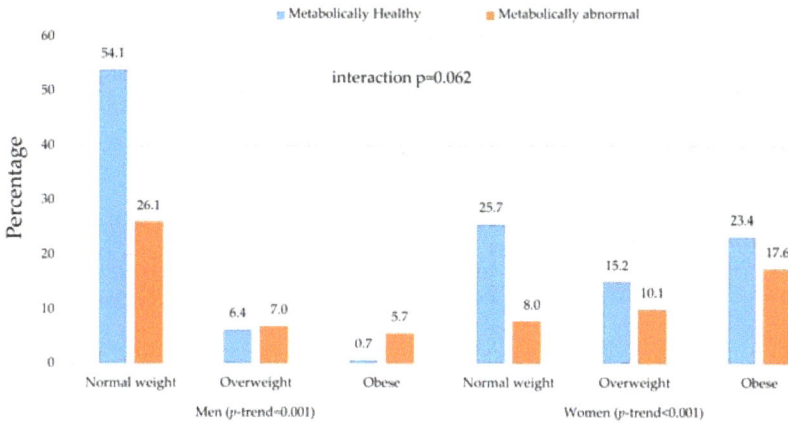

Figure 2. Distribution of metabolic phenotypes across body mass index categories in men and women. Each vertical bar represents the proportion of participants in the total gender-specific sub-sample with the corresponding combination of body size (normal-weight, overweight, or obese) and metabolic phenotype (healthy or abnormal). The accompanying gender-specific proportions are shown at the tip of each bar. The *p*-value for the interaction by gender in the distribution are shown, together with the *p*-value for le linear trend (*p*-trend) in the distribution of metabolic phenotypes across body mass index categories, seperately in men and women.

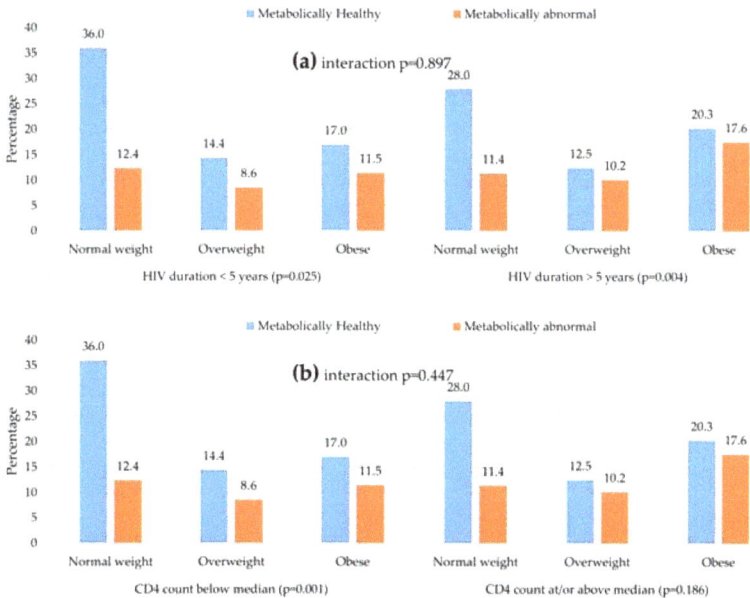

Figure 3. *Cont.*

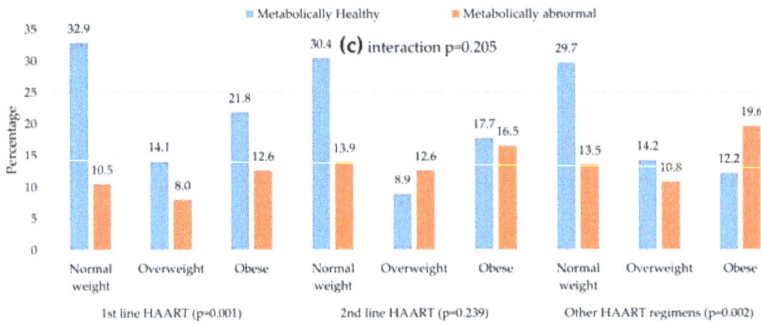

Figure 3. Distribution of body size phenotypes by major HIV predictive characteristics: (**a**) Distribution of metabolic phenotype across body mass index categories in participants below, and those at or above the median of diagnosed duration of HIV infection; (**b**) Distribution of metabolic phenotype across body mass index categories in participants below, and those at or above the median CD4 count; (**c**) Distribution of metabolic phenotype across body mass index categories in participants on different antiretroviral treatment regimens. For each figure panel, the *p*-values for the interactionb (interaction *p*) in the distribution across complementary subgroups are, together with the *p*-value for linear trend in the distribution of metabolic phenotype across body mass index categories within each subgroup (*p*-value attached to the name of the subgroup). Each vertical bar represents the proportion of participants in the subgroup specific sample with the corresponding combination of body size (normal-weight, overweight, or obese) and metabolic phenotype (healthy or abnormal). The accompanying proportions are shown at the tip of each bar.

3.5. Distribution of Metabolic Phenotypes within and Across BMI Categories

Within BMI categories, in addition to the expected differences in the levels of cardio-metabolic risk factors, participants with metabolically abnormal phenotypes tended to be older (all $p \leqslant 0.001$) and unemployed, although differences were significant only among normal weight and overweight (all $p \leqslant 0.002$), but not among obese participants (both $p \geqslant 0.215$). Furthermore, metabolically abnormal obese participants were likely to be men (8.0% *vs.* 0.7%, $p = 0.006$) and included fewer participants on first line ART ($p = 0.009$).

Age and level of education across BMI categories increased linearly overall (both $p \leqslant 0.012$), driven by a significant linear trend in metabolically healthy participants (both $p \leqslant 0.005$) but not in the metabolically abnormal (both $p \geqslant 0.396$), with however no evidence of statistical interaction (both p-interaction $\geqslant 0.065$). The proportion of men who were current smokers decreased linearly overall across increasing BMI categories ($p < 0.001$ for linear trend), and within both metabolic phenotype groups (p-trend = 0.001), with no evidence of statistical interaction (both interactions $p > 0.759$), Table 2.

Median WC, HOMA-IR, and HDL-C levels across BMI categories increased significantly overall (p-trend $\leqslant 0.001$) and within the metabolic phenotype groups (all p-trend $\leqslant 0.024$), without evidence of statistical interaction (all p-interaction $\geqslant 0.560$). Fasting glucose, triglycerides, and prevalence of hypertension also increase across increasing BMI categories, but only on the total cohort (p-trend $\leqslant 0.038$). Interaction analyses found BMI categories and metabolic status interacted to affect the distribution of fasting glucose (p-interaction = 0.044) whereas metabolic status interacted with gender to influence triglycerides distributions across BMI categories (p-interaction = 0.002).

Moreover, when further analyses in the subgroup of participants with data on insulin level ($n = 711$) that included insulin resistance (HOMA-IR in 90th) as a fifth metabolic abnormality. The prevalence $\geqslant 2$ risk factors was found to increase slightly across BMI categories: NWMA (12.8%), OvMA (9.3%), and OMA (16.6%), but the patterns within and across subgroups were mostly similar (Figure 4).

Table 2. Characteristics of participants across body mass index (BMI) categories and metabolic status [n (%), or median (25th–75th percentiles)].

BMI Categories	Normal Weight (n = 325)			Overweight (n = 171)			Obese (n = 252)			p-Trend			p-Interaction	
Metabolic Status	Healthy	Abnormal	p	Healthy	Abnormal	p	Healthy	Abnormal	p	Overall	Healthy	Abnormal	B × M	M × G
Prevalence, n (%)	237 (31.7)	88 (11.7)		100 (13.4)	71 (9.5)		139 (18.6)	113 (15.1)		<0.001	<0.001	<0.001	-	-
Men, n (%)	85 (35.9)	41 (46.6)	0.078	10 (10.0)	11 (15.5)	0.281	1 (0.7)	9 (8.0)	0.006	<0.001	<0.001	0.396	0.759	0.34
Age, years	36 (30–44)	42 (34–49)	<0.001	36 (31–42)	43 (36–47.5)	<0.001	37 (31.5–41)	39 (34–47)	0.001	0.002	<0.001	0.617	0.065	0.067
>7 school-years, n (%)	190/236 (80.5)	71/88 (80.7)	0.972	89/100 (89.0)	58/100 (92.1)	0.249	128/139 (92.1)	97/113 (85.8)	0.111	0.012	0.005	0.617	0.532	0.061
Unemployed, n (%)	84/236 (35.6)	48/88 (54.5)	0.002	38/100 (38.0)	47/71 (66.2)	<0.001	64/139 (46.0)	58/113 (51.3)	<0.001	0.081	0.131	0.132	0.056	0.238
Smoking habit, n (%)			0.523			0.327			0.144				0.925	
Never	105/230 (45.7)	33/85 (38.8)		78/96 (81.3)	49/68 (72.0)		111/132 (84.1)	85/107 (79.4)						
Current smoker	99/230 (43.0)	40/85 (47.1)		12/96 (12.5)	11/68 (16.2)		15/132 (11.4)	10/107 (9.3)						
Past smokers	26/230 (11.3)	12/85 (14.1)		6/96 (6.2)	8/68 (11.8)		6/132 (4.5)	12/107 (11.2)						
Heavy drinkers, n (%)	26/74 (35.1)	8/27 (29.6)	0.643	7/25 (28.0)	8/19 (42.1)	0.356	7/22 (31.8)	8/20 (40.0)	0.748	0.973	0.801	0.638	0.518	0.766
HIV diagnosed duration, years	4 (2–7.8)	5 (2–8)	0.577	4.3 (2–8)	6 (2–9)	0.149	5 (3–10)	6 (4–10)	0.334	0.413	0.435	0.436	0.820	>0.999
Median CD4 count, /mm³	311 (172–473)	350 (232–544)	0.448	433 (187–630)	395 (252–626)	0.201	452 (297–677)	434 (267–699)	0.009	0.335	0.213	0.627	0.77	0.430
Antiretroviral regimens, n (%)										0.947	0.386	0.963	0.363	0.179
First line	140/208 (67.3)	45/76 (59.2)		60/88 (68.3)	34/60 (56.6)		93/125 (74.4)	54/96 (56.2)						
Second line	24/208 (11.5)	11/76 (14.5)		7/88 (8.0)	10/60 (16.7)		14/125 (11.2)	13/96 (13.5)						
Others	44/208 (21.2)	20/76 (26.3)		21/88 (23.7)	16/60 (26.7)		18/125 (14.4)	29/96 (30.2)						
Waist circumference, cm	77 (72–80)	78 (72–86)	0.016	89 (85–92)	93 (86–95)	0.005	101 (95–108)	104 (99–111)	0.005	<0.001	<0.001	0.016	0.560	0.780
Systolic blood pressure, mmHg	114 (105–125)	128 (116–145)	<0.001	112 (104–124)	125 (117–140)	<0.001	113 (106–119)	124 (114–138)	<0.001	0.230	0.136	0.560	0.620	0.610
Diastolic blood pressure, mmHg	78 (72–85)	88 (81–92)	<0.001	81 (73–85)	88 (82–97)	<0.001	81 (75–85)	88 (80–96)	<0.001	0.954	0.771	0.819	0.230	0.510
Fasting glucose, mmol/L	4.9 (4.6–5.2)	5.3 (4.6–6.3)	<0.001	4.9 (4.6–5.2)	5.2 (4.7–5.7)	0.001	4.9 (4.6–5.4)	5.6 (5.0–6.4)	<0.001	0.010	0.583	0.049	0.044	0.510
Median HOMA-IR	0.85 (0.57–1.27)	1.16 (0.82–1.79)	<0.001	1.31 (0.93–1.81)	1.76 (1.05–2.49)	<0.001	1.9 (1.33–2.44)	2.52 (1.54–4.67)	<0.001	<0.001	0.001	0.006	0.630	0.290
Diabetes [a], n (%)	2/227 (0.9)	21/87 (24.1)	<0.001	1/96 (1.0)	10/68 (14.7)	0.001	2/128 (1.6)	27/110 (24.6)	<0.001	0.077	0.839	0.252	0.148	0.752
Hypertension [b], n (%)	52 (21.9)	50 (56.8)	<0.001	20 (20.0)	43 (60.6)	<0.001	35 (25.2)	70 (62.0)	<0.001	0.038	0.615	0.757	0.841	0.107

Table 2. *Cont.*

BMI Categories	Normal Weight (n = 325)			Overweight (n = 171)			Obese (n = 252)			p-Trend			p-Interaction	
Metabolic Status	Healthy	Abnormal	p	Healthy	Abnormal	p	Healthy	Abnormal	p	Overall	Healthy	Abnormal	B × M	M × G
Triglycerides, mmol/L	0.9 (0.7–1.2)	1.2 (1.0–1.9)	<0.001	0.9 (0.7–1.2)	1.2 (1.0–1.9)	<0.001	0.9 (0.7–1.2)	1.4 (1.0–1.9)	<0.001	0.033	0.647	0.472	0.720	0.002
HDL-cholesterol, mmol/L	1.4 (1.1–1.7)	1.2 (0.9–1.3)	<0.001	1.4 (1.2–1.7)	1.1 (1.0–1.2)	<0.001	1.4 (1.2–1.6)	1.1 (1.0–1.2)	<0.001	0.001	0.021	0.024	0.790	0.640
LDL-cholesterol, mmol/L	2.2 (1.8–2.9)	2.5 (1.9–3.1)	0.181	2.4 (2.0–3.0)	2.5 (2.0–3.3)	0.423	2.6 (2.2–3.1)	2.8 (2.3–3.4)	0.019	0.867	0.769	0.713	0.910	0.330
Total cholesterol, mmol/l	4.2 (3.6–5.0)	4.3 (3.5–4.9)	0.483	4.3 (3.7–5.1)	4.2 (3.6–4.9)	0.665	4.5 (3.9–5.1)	4.5 (4.0–5.2)	0.208	0.126	0.350	0.438	>0.999	0.710
C-reactive protein, mg/L	4.2 (1.5–12.1)	5.2 (2.5–16.1)	0.102	4.4 (2.3–10.4)	4.4 (2.0–8.5)	0.959	7.8 (3.5–15.8)	8.0 (3.8–16.6)	0.590	0.803	0.523	0.236	0.770	0.130

[a] Diabetes as FPG ≥ 7.0 mmol/L or on treatment; [b] hypertension as blood pressure (BP) ≥ 140/90 mmHg or on treatment.

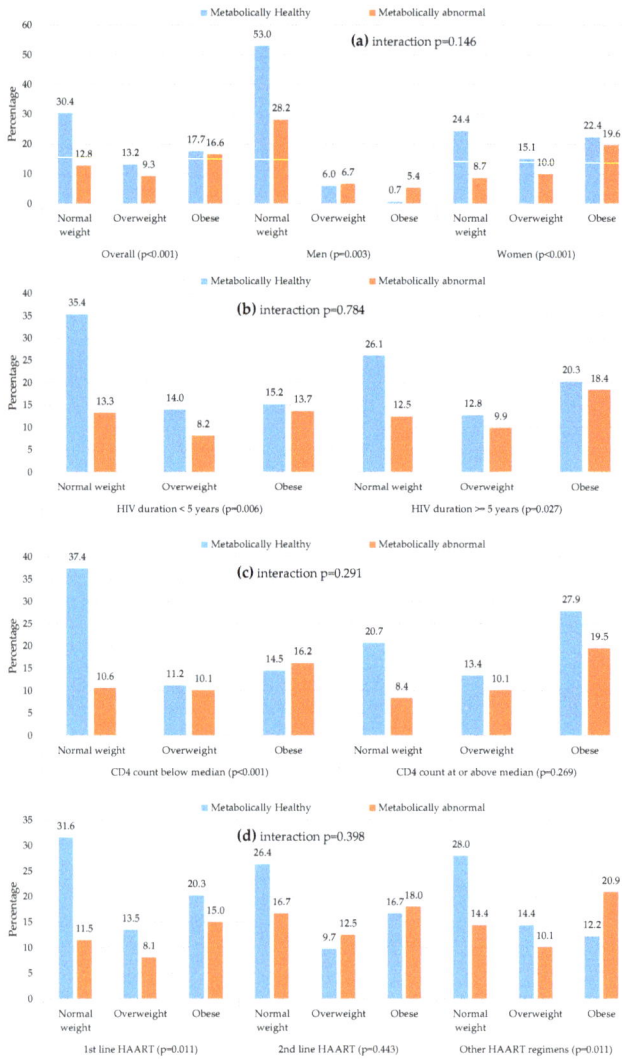

Figure 4. Distribution of metabolic phenotypes across body mass index by major characteristics: (**a**) Overall and in men and women; (**b**) in participants below, and those at or above the median of diagnosed duration of HIV infection; (**c**) in participants below and those at or above the median CD4 count; (**d**) in participants on different antiretroviral treatment regimens. Metabollically abnormal phenotype is based on the presence of any two of the following five abnormalities: elevated blood pressure or known hypertension; high triglycerides; low HDL-cholesterol, high blood glucose, or known diabetes; insulin resistance. For each figure panel, the *p*-values for the interaction (interaction *p*) in the distribution across complementary subgroups are, together with the *p*-value for linear trend in the distribution of metabolic phenotype across body mass index categories within each subgroup (*p*-value attached to the name of the subgroup). Each vertical bar represents the proportion of participants in the subgroup specific sample with the corresponding combination of body size (normal-weight, overweight, or obese) and metabolic phenotype (healthy or abnormal). The accompanying proportions are shown at the tip of each bar.

3.6. Prediction of Body Mass Index Categories by the Continuous Metabolic Traits

In multinomial logistic regression models, mutually adjusted for each other and using normal weight as a reference, male sex was associated with 81% (95% confidence interval: 68%–89%) lower odds of overweight and 94% (89%–97%) lower odds of obesity; while each year of older age was associated with 2% (0%–4%) higher odds of overweight and a non-significant 1% (−1% to 4%) higher odds of obesity. The McFadden R^2 for the overall performance of this basic model was 0.081. In the presence of age and sex, all metabolic trait with the exception of systolic blood pressure (for both overweight and obesity) and fasting plasma glucose (for overweight only) were significantly associated with odds of overweight and obesity (Table 3). The direction of the effect with increasing metabolic traits levels was always positive, except for HDL-cholesterol where increasing levels were associated with decreasing odds of overweight and obesity. The highest R^2 for the overall performance of resulting models was recorded for the model containing HOMA-IR (R^2 = 0.183); and ranged from 0.083 (for the model containing systolic blood pressure) to 0.103 (for the model containing either triglycerides or HDL-cholesterol), Table 3.

Table 3. Odds ratios (OR) and 95% confidence intervals (95% CI) from multinomial age and sex adjusted multinomial logistic regression models, showing the association of metabolic traits with body mass index categories.

Predictors	Normal Weight	Overweight		Obese		R^2
	Reference	OR (95% CI)	*p*-Value	OR (95% CI)	*p*-Value	
Age, per year	1.00	1.02 (1.00–1.04)	0.093	1.01 (0.99–1.04)	0.195	0.081
Sex, men	1.00	0.19 (0.11–0.32)	<0.001	0.06 (0.03–0.11)	<0.001	
Systolic blood pressure, per mmHg	1.00	1.01 (1.00–1.02)	0.204	1.01 (1.00–1.02)	0.167	0.083
Diastolic blood pressure, per mmHg	1.00	1.02 (1.00–1.04)	0.012	1.02 (1.01–1.04)	0.005	0.087
Triglycerides, per mmol/L	1.00	2.06 (1.41–3.02)	<0.001	2.70 (1.86–3.92)	<0.001	0.102
HDL-Cholesterol, per mmol/L	1.00	0.40 (0.24–0.66)	<0.001	0.27 (0.16–0.44)	<0.001	0.102
LDL-cholesterol, per mmol/L	1.00	1.15 (0.92–1.45)	<0.001	1.56 (1.26–1.93)	<0.001	0.092
Fasting plasma glucose, per mmol/L	1.00	0.93 (0.79–1.10)	0.417	1.18 (1.04–1.32)	0.007	0.090
HOMA-IR	1.00	1.42 (1.19–1.70)	<0.001	1.77 (1.49–2.10)	<0.001	0.183

R^2 is the McFadden pseudo-R^2 for the overall performance of the model containing age, sex, and the metabolic trait of interest.

4. Discussion

Although there have been rigorous reports on fat distribution and obesity in individuals with HIV infection, to our knowledge, this is one of the first studies to document the distribution of cardio-metabolic abnormalities in relation with body size in an HIV-infected population. Metabolically abnormal phenotypes, defined as the presence of ≥2 cardio-metabolic risk factors, were high across all BMI categories. Even in normal weight participants, over a quarter (27.1%) had metabolically abnormal phenotypes with this rising to 41.5% and 44.8% in the overweight and the obese, respectively. This suggests the likely influence of multiple factors in the development of cardio-metabolic abnormalities in this population. The high prevalence in normal weight HIV-infected individuals suggests the possible contribution of HIV-related factors and underscores the need to examine for cardio-metabolic abnormalities even in the absence of overweight and obesity.

In contrast, the much higher prevalence demonstrated with increasing adiposity may be attributable to the greater role of this conventional risk factor in the development of cardio-metabolic abnormalities in the HIV-infected population. This highlights the fine balance that needs to be maintained between ensuring adequate nutrition and optimal weight in the HIV-infected while simultaneously monitoring and guarding against excess weight gain. Thus, there is a need for holistic management of these co-morbidities that may indirectly be associated with HIV infection.

The prevalence of overweight and obesity, at 13.4% and 6.4% in men and 25.4% and 40.9% in women in this study approximated the adiposity distribution reported in South African National Health and Nutrition Survey (SANHANES-1) [22]. The overweight and obesity rates in the SANHANES-1 were 20.1% (95% CI: 13.7–26.4) and 11.6% (95% CI: 7.5–15.7) in men and 26.4% (95% CI: 21.7–31.0) and 44.8% (95% CI: 38.8–50.8) in women, respectively. Similar findings have been reported in the United States where obesity levels in HIV-infected men (19%) and women (42%) were comparable to the general population (men: 24.7%, women: 37%) [17]. It is thus important to assess adiposity in HIV-infected individuals and to implement appropriate management strategies for weight reduction, similar to general populations. Notably, that the distribution of overweight and obesity in this study mirrors that of the general population in the country is testimony of the successful implementation of ART strategies in this community.

Although the prevalence of the metabolically abnormal phenotypes by the BMI categories described in this study were significant at 11.7% (NWMA), 9.5% (OvMA), and 15.1% (OMA), a substantial proportion of participants were obese but metabolically healthy (18.6%). This agrees with the 6%–75% estimate of OMH in general populations globally and is likely because BMI is a proxy marker of cardiovascular risk. BMI measures general fat distribution and not visceral adipose tissue specifically, which is linked closely to insulin resistance and cardio-metabolic abnormalities. A better proxy for visceral adipose tissue is WC and, unsurprisingly, within BMI categories, participants with compared to without metabolic abnormalities had greater WC and elevated HOMA-IR index, a proxy measure of insulin resistance. Similar findings have also been reported in other studies [20,23–25]. Recent studies in Caucasians that have included insulin resistance among abnormal metabolic traits, have reported high prevalence of metabolically abnormal phenotypes both in obese and non-obese people [26,27].

The distribution of body size phenotypes in our study is comparable with results of local studies conducted in the general population in South Africa [24,28]. Our previous community-based study in mixed-ancestry adults in Cape Town applying the same definition criteria found OMH and NWMA to be present respectively 16.5% and 5% of the sample [24]. Furthermore, among normal-weight participants (17.1% of the sample), 29.1% were classified as metabolically abnormal, while among obese participants (53.7% of the sample), 30.8% were classified as metabolically healthy [24]. In another study in 103 normal-weight and 122 obese premenopausal urban black South African women, Jennings and co-workers found that 22% of the normal-weight participants were metabolically abnormal (defined by the presence of insulin resistance), while 38% of obese women were metabolically healthy (*i.e.*, did not have insulin resistance) [28]. There are no recent reports available from Africa for comparison of the metabolically abnormal phenotypes that include insulin resistance. Nevertheless, data from a study conducted almost two decades ago in Cameroon revealed a much lower prevalence of metabolic abnormalities with 1.4% (NWMA), 1.6% (OvMA), and 1.7% (OMA) [23]. This highlights the epidemiological transition under way in Sub-Saharan Africa with the majority of this study's participants having normal weight (61%) in the year 1994, unlike more recent reports, and the expected lower prevalence of cardio-metabolic risk factors compared with the present study [23]. Interestingly, there was no significant difference in the distribution of metabolic abnormalities across BMI groups by duration of diagnosed HIV infection, CD4 count levels or ART regimens. There have been diverse reports on the effects of HIV-specific factors on body fat de-arrangement, dyslipidemia, hyperglycemia, and metabolic syndrome. However, results from a recent systematic review and meta-analysis indicated that HIV-related characteristics had minor, if any, influence on the presence of metabolic syndrome [29]. Nevertheless, longitudinal studies are ideally required to pronounce on the absence or presence, if any, of a relationship between specific HIV-related factors and the development of cardio-metabolic abnormalities by body size phenotype.

The relationship of gender, smoking status, and alcohol consumption on the distribution of body size phenotypes remains inconclusive in studies conducted in general populations [10,30,31]. The findings of this study accorded with reports that showed little or no effect of smoking status and alcohol use on the distribution of body size phenotypes [26]. However, a few studies showed a higher prevalence of OMH in women than in men [26,32].

Limitations and Strengths

The cross-sectional design of this study precludes inferences of causal associations between the variables of interest and the development of cardio-metabolic abnormalities. The inclusion of an HIV-uninfected and HIV-infected ART-naïve comparative groups would have strengthened our analyses. Seeing that this was a clinic-based study limits its generalizability since it did not include HIV-infected individuals not attending healthcare facilities. However, these limitations are inevitable because the present project is part of a broad intervention study, which aims to explore the utilization of HIV-care infrastructure as a gateway to detect, manage, and control non-communicable diseases in HIV-infected populations in Africa. The relatively fewer men compared to women in the study, characteristic of epidemiological studies in the country, might overestimate the prevalence of obesity phenotypes. In the absence of detailed information on dietary habits/food consumption and data on ethnicity, we could not explore possible effects of lifestyle factors and ethnicity on the distribution of body size phenotypes among the participants. Nevertheless, differences in MHO prevalence according to ethnicity have been reported, although this recent meta-analysis did not include any studies based on African cohorts [33]. There are reports indicating that overall dietary intake was not associated with healthy obesity in both Europeans and African Americans [27,34]. In addition to lifestyle and ethnicity, data was not available on the pharmacological compounds included in the ART regimens of the participants as well as the duration of treatment with those compounds, precluding detailed analyses by potency of pharmacological compounds and duration of treatments.

Nonetheless, the inclusion of participants from 17 healthcare facilities, including both urban and rural sites strengthens the representativeness in terms of the characteristics assessed. Furthermore, this study is among the first to describe the high prevalence of metabolically abnormal phenotypes across BMI categories in a relatively young HIV-infected population. The study findings underscore the need for further research, particularly longitudinal studies, to understand the development of cardio-metabolic abnormalities in the local HIV-infected population and the differential role played by conventional risk factors as opposed to HIV-related influences.

5. Conclusions

The high prevalence of metabolically abnormal phenotypes across all BMI categories, notably in a relatively young HIV-infected population, highlights the importance of holistic management in HIV-infected individuals. Ideally, cardio-metabolic assessments/screenings should be done at baseline and at regular intervals thereafter, particularly in high-risk groups. Furthermore, considering the high prevalence of overweight and obesity in the HIV-infected, lifestyle measures for weight reduction need to be encouraged. This is a captive audience who present regularly to healthcare facilities and the opportunity should be used to raise greater awareness on cardiovascular disease prevention. Such a strategy, targeting all HIV-infected patients, may contribute to a general improvement in cardiovascular health across the spectrum of BMI distribution. If proven successful, it may possibly have wider applicability in the general population.

Acknowledgments: Grand Challenge Canada, through the Global Alliance on Chronic Diseases initiative. KAN is supported by the NRF Innovation Doctoral Research Scholarship, Doctoral Scholarship, and Yeoman Bequest Bursary through the University of Cape Town. The funding bodies did not make provision for cost of open access publications.

Author Contributions: A.P.K., E.J.M., and B.M. conceived the study and acquired the funding. A.d.V. operationalized and supervised data collection in collaboration with T.E.M. and K.A.N., N.P. analyzed the data and drafted the manuscript. All co-authors substantially revised the manuscript and approved the submission.

Conflicts of Interest: The authors declare no conflict of interest.

Abbreviations

The following abbreviations are used in this manuscript:

ANOVA	analysis of variance
ART	antiretroviral therapy
AIDS	acquired immunodeficiency syndrome
BMI	body mass index
B × M	interaction between BMI and metabolic status
BP	blood pressure
CVD	cardiovascular disease
DBP	diastolic blood pressure
FPG	fasting plasma glucose
HDL-C	high density lipoprotein cholesterol
HIV	human immunodeficiency virus
HOMA-IR	homeostatic model assessment of insulin resistance
Hs-CRP	high sensitivity-C reactive protein
LDL-C	low density lipoprotein cholesterol
M × G	interaction between metabolic status and gender
NWMH	normal-weight metabolically healthy
NWMA	normal weight metabolically abnormal
OvMH	overweight metabolically healthy
OvMA	overweight metabolically abnormal
OMH	obese metabolically healthy
OMA	obese metabolically abnormal
PDA	personal digital assistant
SBP	systolic blood pressure
SD	standard deviation
T2DM	type 2 diabetes mellitus
WC	waist circumference

References

1. Murray, C.J.; Ortblad, K.F.; Guinovart, C.; Lim, S.S.; Wolock, T.M.; Roberts, D.A.; Dansereau, E.A.; Graetz, N.; Barber, R.M.; Brown, J.C.; *et al.* Global, regional, and national incidence and mortality for HIV, tuberculosis, and malaria during 1990–2013: A systematic analysis for the global burden of disease study 2013. *Lancet* **2014**, *384*, 1005–1070. [CrossRef]
2. World Health Organisation. Millennium Development Goals (mdgs) 6: Combat HIV/AIDS, Malaria and Other Diseases. Available online: http://www.who.int/topics/millennium_development_goals/diseases/en/ (accessed on 21 March 2016).
3. Samji, H.; Cescon, A.; Hogg, R.S.; Modur, S.P.; Althoff, K.N.; Buchacz, K.; Burchell, A.N.; Cohen, M.; Gebo, K.A.; Gill, M.J.; *et al.* Closing the gap: Increases in life expectancy among treated HIV-positive individuals in the United States and Canada. *PLoS ONE* **2013**, *8*, e81355. [CrossRef] [PubMed]
4. Boodram, B.; Plankey, M.W.; Cox, C.; Tien, P.C.; Cohen, M.H.; Anastos, K.; Karim, R.; Hyman, C.; Hershow, R.C. Prevalence and correlates of elevated body mass index among HIV-positive and HIV-negative women in the women's interagency HIV study. *AIDS Patient Care STDS* **2009**, *23*, 1009–1016. [CrossRef] [PubMed]
5. Crum-Cianflone, N.; Roediger, M.P.; Eberly, L.; Headd, M.; Marconi, V.; Ganesan, A.; Weintrob, A.; Barthel, R.V.; Fraser, S.; Agan, B.K. Increasing rates of obesity among HIV-infected persons during the HIV epidemic. *PLoS ONE* **2010**, *5*, e10106. [CrossRef] [PubMed]
6. Weber, R.; Ruppik, M.; Rickenbach, M.; Spoerri, A.; Furrer, H.; Battegay, M.; Cavassini, M.; Calmy, A.; Bernasconi, E.; Schmid, P.; *et al.* Decreasing mortality and changing patterns of causes of death in the swiss HIV cohort study. *HIV Med.* **2013**, *14*, 195–207. [CrossRef] [PubMed]

7.   Palella, F.J., Jr.; Baker, R.K.; Moorman, A.C.; Chmiel, J.S.; Wood, K.C.; Brooks, J.T.; Holmberg, S.D. Mortality in the highly active antiretroviral therapy era: Changing causes of death and disease in the HIV outpatient study. *J. Acquir. Immune Defic. Syndr.* **2006**, *43*, 27–34. [CrossRef] [PubMed]

8.   World Health Organisation. *Global Status Report on Noncommunicable Diseases 2014*; WHO: Geneva, Switzerland, 2014; p. 298.

9.   Cornier, M.A. The metabolic syndrome. *Endocr. Rev.* **2008**, *29*, 777–822. [CrossRef] [PubMed]

10.   Wildman, R.P.; Muntner, P.; Reynolds, K.; McGinn, A.P.; Rajpathak, S.; Wylie-Rosett, J.; Sowers, M.R. The obese without cardiometabolic risk factor clustering and the normal weight with cardiometabolic risk factor clustering: Prevalence and correlates of 2 phenotypes among the US population (NHANES 1999–2004). *Arch. Intern. Med.* **2008**, *168*, 1617–1624. [CrossRef] [PubMed]

11.   Van Wijk, J.P.H.; Cabezas, M.C. Hypertriglyceridemia, metabolic syndrome, and cardiovascular disease in HIV-infected patients: Effects of antiretroviral therapy and adipose tissue distribution. *Int. J. Vasc. Med.* **2012**, *2012*. [CrossRef] [PubMed]

12.   Giralt, M.; Domingo, P.; Guallar, J.P.; de la Concepcion, M.L.R.; Alegre, M.; Domingo, J.C.; Villarroya, F. HIV-1 infection alters gene expression in adipose tissue, which contributes to HIV-1/haart-associated lipodystrophy. *Antivir. Ther.* **2006**, *11*, 729–740. [PubMed]

13.   Grinspoon, S.; Carr, A. Cardiovascular risk and body-fat abnormalities in HIV-infected adults. *N. Engl. J. Med.* **2005**, *352*, 48–62. [CrossRef] [PubMed]

14.   Anuurad, E.; Bremer, A.; Berglund, L. HIV protease inhibitors and obesity. *Curr. Opin. Endocrinol. Diabetes Obes.* **2010**, *17*, 478–485. [CrossRef] [PubMed]

15.   Worm, S.W.; Lundgren, J.D. The metabolic syndrome in HIV. *Best Pract. Res. Clin. Endocrinol. Metab.* **2011**, *25*, 479–486. [CrossRef] [PubMed]

16.   Stanley, T.L.; Grinspoon, S.K. Body composition and metabolic changes in HIV-infected patients. *J. Infect. Dis.* **2012**, *205*, S383–S390. [CrossRef] [PubMed]

17.   Thompson-Paul, A.M.; Wei, S.C.; Mattson, C.L.; Robertson, M.; Hernandez-Romieu, A.C.; Bell, T.K.; Skarbinski, J. Obesity among HIV-infected adults receiving medical care in the United States: Data from the cross-sectional medical monitoring project and national health and nutrition examination survey. *Medicine* **2015**, *94*. [CrossRef] [PubMed]

18.   Matthews, D.R.; Hosker, J.P.; Rudenski, A.S.; Naylor, B.A.; Treacher, D.F.; Turner, R.C. Homeostasis model assessment: Insulin resistance and beta-cell function from fasting plasma glucose and insulin concentrations in man. *Diabetologia* **1985**, *28*, 412–419. [CrossRef] [PubMed]

19.   South African National Department of Health. *National Consolidated Guidelines for the Prevention of Mother-to-Child Transmission of HIV (Pmtct) and the Management of HIV in Children, Adolescents and Adults*; National Department of Health of Republic of South Africa: Pretoria, South Africa, 2015.

20.   Rey-Lopez, J.P.; de Rezende, L.F.; Pastor-Valero, M.; Tess, B.H. The prevalence of metabolically healthy obesity: A systematic review and critical evaluation of the definitions used. *Obes. Rev.* **2014**, *15*, 781–790. [CrossRef] [PubMed]

21.   McFadden, D.L. Conditional logit analysis of qualitative choice behavior. In *Frontiers in Econometrics*; Zarembka, P., Ed.; Academic Press: New York, NY, USA, 1973; pp. 105–142.

22.   Shisana, O.; Labadarios, D.; Rehle, T.; Simbayi, L. *South African National Health and Nutrition Examination Survey (Sanhanes-1)*; Human Science Research Council (HSRC) Press: Cape Town, South Africa, 2013.

23.   Mbanya, V.N.; Echouffo-Tcheugui, J.B.; Akhtar, H.; Mbanya, J.C.; Kengne, A.P. Obesity phenotypes in urban and rural cameroonians: A cross-sectional study. *Diabetol. Metab. Syndr.* **2015**, *7*, 21. [CrossRef] [PubMed]

24.   Matsha, T.E.; Hartnick, M.D.; Kisten, Y.; Eramus, R.T.; Kengne, A.P. Obesity phenotypes and subclinical cardiovascular diseases in a mixed-ancestry South African population: A cross-sectional study. *J. Diabetes* **2014**, *6*, 267–270. [CrossRef] [PubMed]

25.   Beraldo, R.A.; Meliscki, G.C.; Silva, B.R.; Navarro, A.M.; Bollela, V.R.; Schmidt, A.; Foss-Freitas, M.C. Comparing the ability of anthropometric indicators in identifying metabolic syndrome in HIV patients. *PLoS ONE* **2016**, *11*, e0149905. [CrossRef] [PubMed]

26.   Velho, S.; Paccaud, F.; Waeber, G.; Vollenweider, P.; Marques-Vidal, P. Metabolically healthy obesity: Different prevalences using different criteria. *Eur. J. Clin. Nutr.* **2010**, *64*, 1043–1051. [CrossRef] [PubMed]

27. Phillips, C.M.; Dillon, C.; Harrington, J.M.; McCarthy, V.J.; Kearney, P.M.; Fitzgerald, A.P.; Perry, I.J. Defining metabolically healthy obesity: Role of dietary and lifestyle factors. *PLoS ONE* **2013**, *8*, e76188. [CrossRef] [PubMed]

28. Jennings, C.L.; Lambert, E.V.; Collins, M.; Joffe, Y.; Levitt, N.S.; Goedecke, J.H. Determinants of insulin-resistant phenotypes in normal-weight and obese black african women. *Obesity* **2008**, *16*, 1602–1609. [CrossRef] [PubMed]

29. Nguyen, K.A.; Peer, N.; Mills, E.J.; Kengne, A.P. A meta-analysis of the metabolic syndrome prevalence in the global HIV-infected population. *PLoS ONE* **2016**, *11*, e0150970. [CrossRef] [PubMed]

30. Lopez-Garcia, E.; Guallar-Castillon, P.; Leon-Muñoz, L.; Rodriguez-Artalejo, F. Prevalence and determinants of metabolically healthy obesity in Spain. *Atherosclerosis* **2013**, *231*, 152–157. [CrossRef] [PubMed]

31. Lee, K. Metabolically obese but normal weight (MONW) and metabolically healthy but obese (MHO) phenotypes in Koreans: Characteristics and health behaviors. *Asia Pac. J. Clin. Nutr.* **2009**, *18*, 280–284. [PubMed]

32. Hirigo, A.T.; Tesfaye, D.Y. Influences of gender in metabolic syndrome and its components among people living with HIV virus using antiretroviral treatment in Hawassa, Southern Ethiopia. *BMC Res. Notes* **2016**, *9*, 145. [CrossRef] [PubMed]

33. Wang, B.; Zhuang, R.; Luo, X.; Yin, L.; Pang, C.; Feng, T.; You, H.; Zhai, Y.; Ren, Y.; Zhang, L.; *et al.* Prevalence of metabolically healthy obese and metabolically obese but normal weight in adults worldwide: A meta-analysis. *Horm. Metab. Res.* **2015**, *47*, 839–845. [CrossRef] [PubMed]

34. Kimokoti, R.W.; Judd, S.E.; Shikany, J.M.; Newby, P.K. Metabolically healthy obesity is not associated with food intake in white or black men. *J. Nutr.* **2015**, *145*, 2551–2561. [CrossRef] [PubMed]

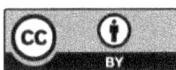

© 2016 by the authors. Licensee MDPI, Basel, Switzerland. This article is an open access article distributed under the terms and conditions of the Creative Commons Attribution (CC BY) license (http://creativecommons.org/licenses/by/4.0/).

nutrients

MDPI

Article

Mother and Infant Body Mass Index, Breast Milk Leptin and Their Serum Leptin Values

Francesco Savino [1,*,†], Allegra Sardo [1,†], Lorenza Rossi [1,†], Stefania Benetti [1,†], Andrea Savino [1,†] and Leandra Silvestro [2]

[1]   Department of Pediatrics, Regina Margherita Children' Hospital, Città della Salute e della Scienza di Torino, Piazza Polonia 94, Torino I-10126, Italy; allegra.sardo@gmail.com (A.S.); lory_rossi@hotmail.it (L.R.); stefy_benetti@virgilio.it (S.B.); andrea.savino817@edu.unito.it (A.S.)
[2]   Department of Public Health and Pediatric Sciences, University of Turin I-10126, Italy; leandra.silvestro@unito.it
*   Correspondence: francesco.savino@unito.it; Tel.: +39-113-135-257; Fax: +39-011-677-082
†   These authors contributed equally to this work.

Received: 17 May 2016; Accepted: 17 June 2016; Published: 21 June 2016

Abstract: Purpose: This study investigates correlations between mother and infant Body Mass Index (BMI), their serum leptin values and breast milk leptin concentration in early infancy. Subjects and Methods: We determined serum leptin values in 58 healthy infants and leptin values in their mothers' breast milk, using radioimmunoassay (RIA). Infant and maternal anthropometrics were measured. Results: Median leptin concentration was 3.9 ng/mL (interquartile range (IQR): 2.75) in infant serum, 4.27 ng/mL (IQR: 5.62) in maternal serum and 0.89 ng/mL (IQR: 1.32) in breast milk. Median maternal BMI and weight were 24 kg/m^2 (IQR: 4.41) and 64 kg (IQR: 15). Median infant BMI was 15.80 kg/cm^2 (IQR: 4.02), while average weight was 5.130 kg (IQR: 1.627). Infants serum leptin values positively correlated with infants' BMI ($p = 0.001$; $r = 0.213$) and breast milk leptin ($p = 0.03$; $r = 0.285$). Maternal serum leptin values positively correlated with maternal BMI ($p = 0.000$, $r = 0.449$) and breast milk leptin ones ($p = 0.026$; $r = 0.322$). Conclusion: Breast milk leptin and maternal BMI could influence infant serum leptin values. Further studies are needed to better elucidate the role of genetics and environment on infant leptin production and risk of obesity later in life.

Keywords: mothers; serum leptin; BMI; breast milk; infancy

1. Introduction

Leptin is a polypeptide hormone, made of 167 amino acids and discovered by Zhang *et al.* in 1994 thanks to studies on ob/ob gene in mice [1]. This hormone is the product of the ob gene, located on chromosome 7q31.3. It circulates in plasma free or bound to proteins and it exerts its action through the soluble-OB (s-OB) receptor [2]. The primary function of this hormone is to inhibit food intake and to promote energy expenditure by regulating neuronal activity in hypothalamic arcuate nuclei: leptin, in fact, activates anorectic Pro-opiomelanocortin/ Cocaine-and amphetamine-regulated-transcript (POMC/CART) neurons and hinders the activity of those which stimulate food intake Neuropeptide Y/Agouti-related protein (NPY/AgRP) [3].

There are increasing data that environmental factors in early life predict later health. The early adiposity rebound recorded in most obese subjects suggests that factors promoting body fat development operate in the first years of life [4]. It has been shown that higher serum leptin values correlate with lower body mass index (BMI) in childhood and with lower predisposition to develop metabolic disorders in adolescence and adulthood [5].

Schuster *et al.* suggest that milk leptin could provide a link between maternal body composition and infant growth and development and also plays a role in regulating infant appetite and food intake during early infancy [6].

Increased maternal body mass index is a well-established risk factor for later infant obesity [7–9] and prevalence of obesity women is increasing worldwide [10]. Evidence suggests that human milk may decrease the transmission of obesity from mothers to their children, for example exerting its effects on early growth of the infant microbiome, as recently proposed by Lemas *et al.* [11].

It is known that leptin is mainly produced by white adipose tissue; this is the reason why serum leptin values directly correlate with body fat stores. During fasting or weight loss, leptin levels decrease, while during overeating, they increase [12]. Leptin is also released by the hypothalamus, pituitary gland, skeletal muscle, stomach, liver, placenta and mammary gland [13,14].

Leptin is found in breast milk and, interestingly, it is not only related with infants' body fat mass, but also with that of their mothers [15]. It is produced by mammary epithelial cells and it is associated with fat globules. Studies conducted on mice have shown that this hormone is transferred from maternal blood to breast milk and that it is then transferred from milk to mice puppies' bloodstream. Interestingly, the presence of leptin receptors has been found on gastric and intestinal epithelial cells of both humans and rats, suggesting that leptin may play a role in the regulation of GI functions [16]. It could be assumed that leptin taken by children with breast milk can directly pass into their bloodstream through gut since leptin receptor isoform has been found in brush border, basolateral membrane, and cytoplasm of enterocytes [17].

The amount of different adipokines in human breast milk is supposed to affect energy intake of the infant. [18] It is not well determined whether only leptin plays a causal role in early life fat deposition prevention since recently it has been reported that also sOB receptor values could have a part in the regulation of infant energy intake and infant growth and development [19].

The aim of this study is to measure leptin in mother and infant serum and in breast milk in order to look for correlations between mother and infant BMI, their serum leptin values and breast milk leptin concentration in early infancy.

2. Materials and Methods

2.1. Subjects

2.1.1. Infants

We enrolled 58 AGA healthy term infants who were admitted to the Department of Pediatrics of the University of Turin, Regina Margherita Children's Hospital, between June 2013 and July 2015. The infants underwent blood tests during routine outpatient examinations. The study protocol was approved by the local Ethical Committee at Ospedale Mauriziano—Ospedale Infantile Regina Margherita (Ethical approval code: 4698, Protocol Version 1.0., 23 May 2013)—S. Anna Torino, and infants' parents gave their written consent.

Criteria for enrollment were as follows:

Age: children from 10 days of life to 6 months and 15 days of life;
Gestational age: from 38 to 40 weeks;
Birth characteristics: birth weight from 2500 g to 4500 g, APGAR equal or above 7 and absence of neonatal diseases;
Nutrition: infants were fed with breast milk and they had not been weaned;
Clinical condition: at the time of blood sampling, infants did not have acute diseases and were afebrile.

At the time of sampling, infants were exclusively breastfed and they had not received any complementary feeding.

2.1.2. Mothers

Fifty-eight caucasian mothers belonging to a rural or urban setting were enrolled with their children. Regarding delivery, 19 mothers underwent a Caesarian section, while 39 had a spontaneous delivery. Criteria for enrollment were as follows:

Mothers who delivered infants at 38 to 40 weeks' gestation;
Mothers who were planning to exclusively breastfeed;

Mothers who signed written informed consent. Eligibility criteria for mothers were no maternal medical complications, non-smoking mothers, normal response to a glucose tolerance test, no mastitis, no prescribed medication, no digestive disorders.

2.2. BMI Measurement

Anthropometric measures were collected by two trained medical doctors with high intra-observer and inter-observer reliability.

Infants were weighed with an electronic integrating scale (SECA, model 757, Vogel & Halke, Hamburg, Germany), were measured in length with a stat meter and BMI was calculated as the ratio of body weight (kg) to the square of length (m^2). Mothers were weighed with a scale (Wunder, Italy), measured in height with a stat meter (Holtain Limited, Crymych, Dyfed, UK) and BMI was calculated as above.

2.3. Blood Sampling and Hormone Analysis

For the evaluation of leptin in serum, infants underwent four hours fasting before blood testing usually at 8.00 in the morning. The sample was stored in a refrigerator for 60 min and was then put in the refrigerated centrifuge at 4 °C at 4000 revolutions/min for 10 min. The serum obtained was divided into 2 test tubes and was stored in a freezer at −30 °C. The same procedure was carried out for mothers.

Hormone analysis was conducted with a commercially available radioimmunoassay (RIA) kit (LEP R-40, Multispecie-Leptin-RIA-Sensitive, Mediagnost, Reutlingen, Germany) with a sensitivity of 0.04 ng/mL (0.01 ng/mL with the procedure for increased sensitivity). The intra-assay variation was less than 5%, and the inter-assay variation did not exceed 7.6%.

2.4. Breast Milk Sampling and Hormone Analysis

About 5 mL of foremilk samples were collected from the lactating women by hand expression between 07:00 and 09:00. All milk samples were collected in tubes containing protease inhibitors (Sigma-Aldrich Company Ltd., Dorset, England) and immediately frozen at −20 °C. Samples were thawed at 4–6 °C overnight and centrifuged at 2500 revolutions at 4 for 20 min to separate the fat milk. Like serum leptin, 2 mL of skimmed breast milk leptin was analyzed with a RIA kit (LEP R-40, Multispecie-Leptin-RIA-Sensitive, Mediagnost, Reutlingen, Germany) with a sensitivity of 0.04 ng/mL (0.01 ng/mL with the procedure for increased sensitivity).

2.5. Statistical Analysis

Statistical analyses were conducted using SPSS software (version 21.0, SPSS, Inc., Chicago, IL, USA). First, we performed univariate descriptive analysis. The normal distribution of the variables was tested by the Shapiro-Wilk test. Continuous variables were expressed as median and interquartile range (IQR). Data that were not normally distributed were analysed with the Mann-Whitney U test and the Kruskal-Wallis test. Correlations are expressed by the Spearman correlation coefficient. All tests were done with two tails, with a fixed significance alpha =5%.

3. Results

Median leptin concentration was 3.9 ng/mL (IQR: 2.75) in infant serum, 4.27 ng/mL (IQR: 5.62) in maternal serum and 0.89 ng/mL (IQR: 1.32) in breast milk (Tables 1 and 2). Statistical significance was set at $p < 0.05$ and correlations were assessed using Spearman's rho.

Table 1. Infant anthropometric parameters and serum leptin values (median + interquartile range (IQR)).

Parameters	Infants
	n = 58
Age (days)	61 (76.5)
Gestational Age (weeks)	39 (1.5)
Birth Weight (kg)	3.275 (0.622)
Birth Length (cm)	49.45 (2.2)
Birth Cranial Circumference (cm)	34.05 (1.5)
Weight (kg)	5.130 (1.269)
Height (cm)	55 (3.25)
Cranial Circumference (cm)	39 (3)
BMI (kg/m^2)	15.80 (2.47)
Serum Leptin (ng/mL)	3.9 (2.75)

Table 2. Maternal anthropometric parameters, serum leptin and Breast Milk (BM) leptin values (median + IQR).

Parameters	Mothers
	n = 58
Age (years)	28.5 (8)
Weight (kg)	64 (12.59)
Height (cm)	164 (0.064)
BMI (kg/m^2)	24 (4.52)
Serum Leptin (ng/mL)	4.27 (5.62)
Breast Milk Leptin (ng/mL)	0.89 (1.32)

We evaluated the impact of potential confounders on breast milk leptin values and maternal and infant serum leptin values. Particularly, we analyzed the effect of infant age and gender on leptin concentrations.

Regarding infant age, we divided our cohort into three age groups at enrollment. We obtained a median (IQR) leptin concentration of 2.87 (2.53) ng/mL in infant serum, 3.27 (5.38) ng/mL in maternal serum and 0.83 (1.17) ng/mL in breast milk in group 1 (<2 months; $n = 30$), of 4.54 (9.89) ng/mL in infant serum, 2.46 (1.49) ng/mL in maternal serum and 1.18 (1.29) ng/mL in breast milk in group 2 (<4 months; $n = 18$) and of 4.85 (7.51) ng/mL in infant serum, 3.21 (2.25) ng/mL in maternal serum and 0.87 (3.55) ng/mL in breast milk in group 3 (4–6 months; $n = 10$). No significant differences in breast milk and infant and serum leptin values were detected among the three groups ($p > 0.05$).

We divided patients by gender into two groups: as concernes males ($n = 26$), the median (IQR) leptin concentration was 2.83 (2.16) ng/mL in infant serum, 3.27 (5.13) ng/mL in maternal serum and 0.83 (1.32) ng/mL in breast milk; in females ($n = 32$), the median (IQR) leptin concentration was 4.79 (8.46) ng/mL in infant serum, 2.84 (2.14) ng/mL in maternal serum and 0.93 (2.59) ng/mL in breast milk. With reference to gender, we did not observe any statistical differences in breast milk leptin values and maternal and infant serum leptin values ($p > 0.05$).

3.1. Infant Serum Leptin Values and Infant BMI

Serum leptin values positively correlated with infants' weight ($p = 0.002$; $r = 0.2$) and BMI ($p = 0.001$; $r = 0.213$), as shown in Figure 1.

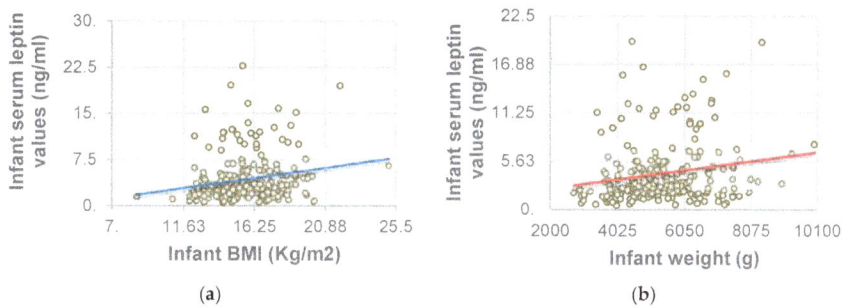

Figure 1. Correlation between infant serum leptin values and infant Body Mass Index (BMI) and weight. (**a**) Association between serum leptin values and BMI; (**b**) Association between serum leptin values and weight.

The positive correlation between infant serum leptin values and both infant BMI and weight suggests that leptin concentrations are directly related to body fat stores. This hormone is primarily released by adipocytes in adipose white tissue [15]. This is the reason why infants with higher BMI have higher serum leptin values [20].

3.2. Maternal Serum Leptin Values, Maternal BMI and Breast Milk Leptin

Maternal BMI positively correlated with maternal serum leptin levels ($p = 0.000$; $r = 0.449$) and breast milk leptin ($p = 0.004$; $r = 0.368$) as illustrated in Figure 2. We found a significant correlation between breast milk leptin and maternal serum leptin values ($p = 0.026$; $r = 0.322$) as shown in Figure 3.

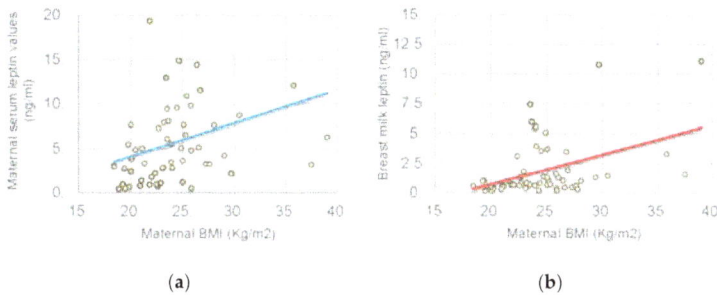

Figure 2. Correlation between maternal BMI and maternal serum leptin and breast milk leptin. (**a**) Association between maternal BMI and maternal serum leptin values; (**b**) Association between maternal BMI and breast milk leptin.

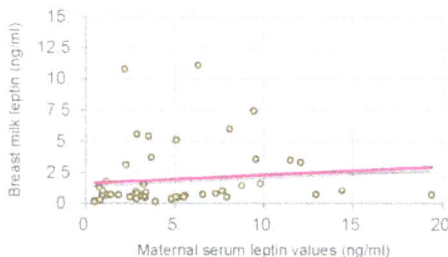

Figure 3. Correlation between maternal serum leptin and breast milk leptin.

We found a positive and significant correlation between BMI and serum leptin values. As shown for infants, mothers with higher BMI have higher serum leptin values, suggesting that leptin concentration is directly proportional to body fat mass percentage [20].

Regarding breast milk, it is interesting that a positive correlation exists between maternal BMI and leptin levels in breast milk [21]. It could be that not only breast milk leptin depends on the amount produced by mammary epithelial cells, but also on the amount released from maternal body fat stores.

A significant correlation was observed between maternal serum leptin values and breast milk leptin [22]. Also Weyermann *et al.* [23] observed that leptin concentration in breast milk correlated positively with leptin in maternal serum.

3.3. Infant Serum Leptin Values, Maternal Serum Leptin Values and Breast Milk Leptin

We did not find any significant correlation between maternal and infant serum leptin values ($p > 0.05$), suggesting that further studies are required to investigate the possible role of maternal leptin in the regulation of infant metabolism [24]. Regarding breast milk leptin and infant serum leptin values, we obtained a positive correlation, as illustrated in Figure 4 ($p = 0.03$; $r = 0.285$).

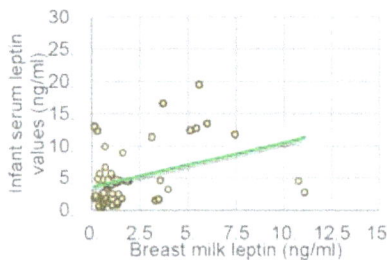

Figure 4. Correlation between breast milk leptin and infant serum leptin values.

The higher the breast milk leptin concentration is, the higher infant serum leptin values are. These findings suggest a possible association between breast milk components and infant adiposity [18].

4. Discussion

This study presents data of a positive correlation between breast milk leptin and infant serum leptin values. Furthermore, our study is strengthened by the fact that we found that breast milk leptin directly correlates with maternal serum leptin values. Actually, we did not obtain a significant association between maternal and infant serum leptin values. Regarding maternal and infant BMI, we showed that breast milk leptin and maternal serum leptin values directly correlate with materal BMI. In addition, we demonstrated a positive association between infant BMI and infant serum leptin values. We evaluated the possible impact of infant age and gender on infant and maternal serum leptin values and breast milk leptin concentrations. We did not obtain any significant differences in leptin values among the created groups.

4.1. Serum Leptin Values and BMI

Leptin is mainly produced by adipocytes; thus its levels are strictly associated to body fat mass percentage. During fasting, this hormone decreases; on the other hand, in overeating, its levels increase [25]. Both in infants and their mothers, we found that this hormone correlates with BMI and weight. Higher BMI correlates with higher serum leptin levels. It is known that people with an elevated BMI have high serum leptin levels not only because they have a larger amount of fat mass, but also because their adipocytes are bigger. What is more, Dusserre *et al.* showed that leptin values vary according to the type of adipose tissue that releases them: omental adipocytes express leptin mRNA less than subcutaneous adipocytes [26].

4.2. Breast Milk Leptin and Maternal Serum Leptin Values

Casabiell *et al.* showed that leptin is transferred from maternal bloodstream to breast milk in mice [16]. We found a positive correlation between breast milk leptin values and maternal serum leptin ones. It is thus possible that leptin in breast milk depends not only on the amount produced by mammary epithelial cells, but also on the amount in maternal bloodstream. It would be interesting to evaluate if maternal leptin values represent a predictor for infant obesity [27].

4.3. Breast Milk Leptin and Infant Serum Leptin Values

Leptin receptors have been found on gastrointestinal epithelial cells, suggesting that this hormone could be absorbed from infant mucosa and then transferred to infant bloodstream. The significant correlation that we found between breast milk leptin and infant serum leptin values could indicate that leptin in children is influenced by both infant fat stores and breast milk leptin. In previous studies, we demonstrated that formula fed infants have lower leptin levels than breast milk fed ones [28]. Data on the presence of leptin in infant formula are still controversial [29], however more investigations are needed to detect if hormones present in breast milk have a beneficial effect on obesity later in life [30,31].

4.4. Study Limitations

This study has several limitations. We could not assess the influence of leptin circadian variations since we do not have daily access to serum leptin samples, nor were we able to assess daily changes in breast milk leptin.

Moreover, we did not measure serum leptin at the same age time in all subjects enrolled.

However, baseline characteristics were similar among the infants in the study group.

Further, we were unable to measure fat mass at the same time of leptin sampling in mothers and infants.

Finally, since this study is observational it is important to interpret our correlations with caution.

Our findings are consistent with the possibility that breast milk leptin affects infant health later in life and opens new implications for research such as the role of breastfeeding and infant metabolic response.

Therefore, a follow-up of our patients, based on these results, will help us build a stronger overall evidence base and fill the gap in knowledge.

It is known that early nutrition plays an important role in the development of metabolic diseases in adolescence and adulthood. It has been shown that breastfed infants are at lower risk to become obese than formula-fed ones [32]. The positive correlation observed between maternal serum leptin concentration and maternal BMI is strictly linked to breast milk leptin values, suggesting that the amount of leptin in breast milk is influenced not only by mammary gland, but also by leptin released from maternal fat storages [33]. Interestingly, in a previous study, we demonstrated that infant serum leptin values are correlated to maternal BMI, thus showing that infants breast-fed by mothers with high BMI receive higher amounts of leptin [34]. Children with obese mothers seem to be at higher risk to become obese themselves [35]. The protective effect of breastfeeding against early childhood obesity may differ with race and ethnicity [36].

Many factors related to breastfeeding may influence childhood weight outcomes and obesity such as breastfeeding duration [37]; however, it should be considered that, ingesting high amounts of leptin, infants with obese mothers become leptin resistant and have alterations in appetite regulation [7,9,38]. In animal models it has been shown that obese phenotype can be transmitted by mothers to the following generations [39]. Since recently it has been observed that higher perinatal leptin is associated with lower adiposity at 3 years of life [40], leptin could be a key to understand the relationship between maternal BMI and infant growth and development. Intersting data showed that breast feeding affects infant's self-regulation of milk intake during late infancy [41].

5. Conclusions

Understanding the determinants of infant body mass index is relevant for the study of childhood obesity and the related risk of obesity in adulthood.

The existing data of the effects of breast milk leptin on infant growth and adiposity are controversial. Growing evidence suggests that human milk may reduce the transfer of obesity from mother to progenies and leptin is one of the possible factors involved.

In this study we investigated the possible correlations between maternal and infant serum leptin values, breast milk leptin concentrations and infant and maternal BMI. We demonstrated a positive correlation between infants' serum leptin concentrations and both maternal and infant BMI.

Regarding breast milk leptin values, we obtained a positive association not only with maternal BMI but also with maternal and infant serum leptin values.

There was no association between infant and maternal serum leptin concentrations.

Leptin is a peptide hormone produced by both adipocytes and mammary gland and it could be considered a marker that may signify excess fat accumulation.

Overall, our findings show that breast feeding and maternal BMI could influence infant serum leptin values. Further studies are needed to better elucidate the role of genetics on infant leptin production and risk of obesity later in life.

Acknowledgments: We are grateful to Sapienza, D. for perfoming hormone assays at the Laboratory analysis "Baldi and Riberi", Molinette—Città della Salute e della Scienza di Torino, Italy.

Author Contributions: F.S. conceived the study and designed the research, and wrote the manuscript. A.S. performed the experiments and wrote the manuscript. L.R. performed the experiments; analyzed the data. A.S. searched references and revised the manuscript. L.S. conceived the study and revised the manuscript. All authors read and approved the final manuscript.

Conflicts of Interest: The authors declare no conflict of interest.

References

1. Zhang, Y.; Proenca, R.; Maffei, M.; Barone, M.; Leopold, L.; Friedman, J.M. Positional cloning of the mouse obese gene and its human homologue. *Nature* **1994**, *372*, 425–432. [CrossRef] [PubMed]

2. Tartaglia, L.; Dembski, M.; Weng, X.; Deng, N.; Culpepper, J.; Devos, R.; Richards, G.J.; Campfield, L.A.; Clark, F.T.; Deeds, J.; *et al.* Identification and expression cloning of a leptin receptor. *Cell* **1995**, *83*, 1263–1271. [CrossRef]

3. Spanswick, D.; Smith, M.; Groppi, V.E.; Logan, S.; Ashford, M.L. Leptin inhibits hypothalamic neurons by activation of ATP-sensitive potassium channels. *Nature* **1997**, *390*, 521–525. [PubMed]

4. Rolland-Cachera, M.F.; Akrout, M.; Péneau, S. Nutrient intakes in early life and risk of obesity. *Int. J. Environ. Res. Public Health* **2012**, *13*, 564. [CrossRef] [PubMed]

5. Savino, F.; Liguori, S.; Benetti, S.; Sorrenti, M.; Fissore, M.F.; di Montezemolo, L.C. High serum leptin levels in infancy can potentially predict obesity in childhood, especially in formula-fed infants. *Acta Paediatr. Int. J. Paediatr.* **2013**. [CrossRef] [PubMed]

6. Miralles, O.; Sánchez, J.; Palou, A.; Picó, C. A physiological role of breast milk leptin in body weight control in developing infants. *Obesity* **2006**, *14*, 1371–1377. [CrossRef] [PubMed]

7. Andreas, N.; Hyde, M.; Gale, C.; Parkinson, J.; Jeffries, S.; Holmes, E.; Modi, N. Effect of maternal body mass index on hormones in breast milk: A systematic review. *PLoS ONE* **2014**. [CrossRef] [PubMed]

8. Bider-Canfield, Z.; Martinez, M.P.; Wang, X.; Yu, W.; Bautista, M.P.; Brookey, J.; Page, K.A.; Buchanan, T.A.; Xiang, A.H. Maternal obesity, gestational diabetes, breastfeeding and childhood overweight at age 2 years. *Pediatr. Obes.* **2016**. [CrossRef] [PubMed]

9. Gruszfeld, D.; Kułaga, Z.; Wierzbicka, A.; Rzehak, P.; Grote, V.; Martin, F.; Poncelet, P.; Closa-Monasterolo, R.; Escribano, J.; Verduci, E.; *et al.* Leptin and adiponectin serum levels from infancy to school age: Factors influencing tracking. *Child Obes.* **2016**, *12*, 179–187. [CrossRef] [PubMed]

10. NCD Risk Factor Collaboration (NCD-RisC). Trends in adult body-mass index in 200 countries from 1975 to 2014: A pooled analysis of 1698 population-based measurement studies with 19.2 million participants. *Lancet* **2016**, *387*, 1377–1396.

11. Lemas, D.J.; Young, B.E.; Baker, P.R., II; Tomczik, A.C.; Soderborg, T.K.; Hernandez, T.L. Alterations in human milk leptin and insulin are associated with early changes in the infant intestinal microbiome. *Am. J. Clin. Nutr.* **2016**, *103*, 1291–1300. [CrossRef] [PubMed]

12. Havel, P.; Townsend, R. High-fat meals reduce 24-h circulating leptin concentrations in women. *Diabetes* **1999**, *48*, 334–341. [CrossRef] [PubMed]

13. Hassink, S.; de Lancey, E.; Sheslow, D.V.; Smith-Kirwin, S.M.; O'Connor, D.M.; Considine, R.V.; Opentanova, I.; Dostal, K.; Spear, M.L.; Leef, K.; *et al.* Placental leptin: An important new growth factor in intrauterine and neonatal development? *Pediatrics* **1997**. [CrossRef]

14. Bado, A.; Levasseur, S.; Attoub, S.; Kermorgant, S.; Laigneau, J.P.; Bortoluzzi, M.N.; Moizo, L.; Lehy, T.; Guerre-Millo, M.; le Marchand-Brustel, Y.; *et al.* The stomach is a source of leptin. *Nature* **1998**, *394*, 790–793. [PubMed]

15. Houseknecht, K.; McGuire, M.; Portocarrero, C.P.; McGuire, M.A.; Beerman, K. Leptin is present in human milk and is related to maternal plasma leptin concentration and adiposity. *Biochem. Biophys. Res. Commun.* **1997**, *240*, 742–747. [CrossRef] [PubMed]

16. Casabiell, X.; Piñeiro, V.; Tomé María, A.; Peinó, R.; Diéguez, C.; Casanueva, F. Presence of leptin in colostrum and/or breast milk from lactating mothers: A potential role in the regulation of neonatal food intake. *J. Clin. Endocrinol. Metab.* **1997**, *82*, 4270–4273. [CrossRef] [PubMed]

17. Barrenetxe, J.; Villaro, C.; Guembe, L.; Pascual, I.; Muñoz-Navas, M.; Barber, A.; Lostao, M.P. Distribution of the long leptin receptor isoform in brush border, basolateral membrane, and cytoplasm of enterocytes. *Gut* **2002**, *50*, 797–802. [CrossRef] [PubMed]

18. Fields, D.A.; Schneider, C.R.; Pavela, G. A narrative review of the associations between six bioactive components in breast milk and infant adiposity. *Obesity* **2016**, *24*, 1213–1221. [CrossRef] [PubMed]

19. Zepf, F.D.; Rao, P.; Moore, J.; Stewart, R.; Ladino, Y.M.; Hartmann, B.T. Human breast milk and adipokines—A potential role for the soluble leptin receptor (sOb-R) in the regulation of infant energy intake and development. *Med. Hypothesis* **2016**, *86*, 53–55. [CrossRef] [PubMed]

20. Sinha, M.; Caro, J. Clinical aspects of leptin. *Vitam. Horm.* **1998**, *54*, 1–30. [PubMed]

21. Uysal, F.; Onal, E.; Aral, Y.Z.; Adam, B.; Dilmen, U.; Ardiçolu, Y. Breast milk leptin: Its relationship to maternal and infant adiposity. *Clin. Nutr.* **2002**, *21*, 157–160. [CrossRef] [PubMed]

22. Schuster, S.; Hechler, C.; Gebauer, C.; Kiess, W.; Kratzsch, J. Leptin in maternal serum and breast milk: Association with infants' body weight gain in a longitudinal study over 6 months of lactation. *Pediatr. Res.* **2011**, *70*, 633–637. [CrossRef] [PubMed]

23. Weyermann, M.; Beermann, C.; Brenner, H.; Rothenbacher, D. Adiponectin and leptin in maternal serum, cord blood, and breast milk. *Clin. Chem.* **2006**, *52*, 2095–2102. [CrossRef] [PubMed]

24. Castagno, E.; Liguori, S.A.; Viola, S.; Lupica, M.M.; Oggero, R.; Savino, F. Serum leptin levels in breastfed infants in the first six months of life, in their mothers and in breast milk. *Dig. Liver Dis.* **2009**, *41*, S226. [CrossRef]

25. Ahima, R.; Prabakaran, D.; Mantzoros, C.; Qu, D.; Lowell, B.; Maratos-Flier, E.; Flier, J.S. Role of leptin in the neuroendocrine response to fasting. *Nature* **1996**, *382*, 250–252. [CrossRef] [PubMed]

26. Dusserre, E.; Moulin, P.; Vidal, H. Differences in mRNA expression of the proteins secreted by the adipocytes in human subcutaneous and visceral adipose tissues. *Biochim. Biophys.* **2000**, *1500*, 88–96. [CrossRef]

27. Misra, V.; Straughen, J.; Trudeau, S. Maternal serum leptin during pregnancy and infant birth weight: The influence of maternal overweight and obesity. *Obesity* **2013**, *21*, 1064–1069. [CrossRef] [PubMed]

28. Savino, F.; Liguori, S.A.; Petrucci, E.; Lupica, M.M.; Fissore, M.F.; Oggero, R.; Silvestro, L. Evaluation of leptin in breast milk, lactating mothers and their infants. *Eur. J. Clin. Nutr.* **2010**, *64*, 972–977. [CrossRef] [PubMed]

29. Lage, M.; Baldelli, R.; Camiña, J.P.; Rodriguez-Garci, J.; Peñalva, A.; Dieguez, C.; Casanueva, F.F. Presence of bovine leptin in edible commercial milk and infant formula. *J. Endocrinol. Invest.* **2002**, *25*, 670–674. [CrossRef] [PubMed]

30. Savino, F.; Fissore, M.; Liguori, S.A.; Oggero, R. Can hormones contained in mothers' milk account for the beneficial effect of breast-feeding on obesity in children? *Clin. Endocrinol.* **2009**, *81*, 757–765. [CrossRef] [PubMed]

31. Savino, F.; Liguori, S.; Fissore, M.; Oggero, R. Breast milk hormones and their protective effect on obesity. *Int. J. Pediatr. Endocrinol.* **2009**. [CrossRef]

32. Oddy, W. Infant feeding and obesity risk in the child. *Breastfeed. Rev.* **2012**, *20*, 7–12. [PubMed]

33. Savino, F.; Sorrenti, M.; Bennetti, S.; Lupica, M.M.; Liguori, S.A.; Oggero, R. Resistin and leptin in breast milk and infants in early life. *Early Hum. Dev.* **2012**, *88*, 779–782. [CrossRef] [PubMed]

34. Savino, F.; Liguori, S.A.; Oggero, R.; Silvestro, L.; Miniero, R. Maternal BMI and serum leptin concentration of infants in the first year of life. *Acta Paediatr.* **2006**, *95*, 414–418. [CrossRef] [PubMed]

35. Parsons, T.; Power, C.; Manor, O. Fetal and early life growth and body mass index from birth to early adulthood in 1958 British cohort: Longitudinal study. *BMJ* **2001**, *323*, 1331–1335. [CrossRef] [PubMed]

36. Ehrenthal, D.B.; Wu, P.; Trabulsi, J. Differences in the protective effect of exclusive breastfeeding on child overweight and obesity by mother's race. *Matern. Child Health J.* **2016**. [CrossRef] [PubMed]

37. Modrek, S.; Basu, S.; Harding, M.; White, J.S.; Bartick, M.C.; Rodriguez, E.; Rosenberg, K.D. Does breastfeeding duration decrease child obesity? An instrumental variables analysis. *Pediatr. Obes.* **2016**. [CrossRef] [PubMed]

38. Doneray, H.; Orbak, Z.; Yildiz, L. The relationship between breast milk leptin and neonatal weight gain. *Acta Paediatr.* **2009**, *98*, 643–647. [CrossRef] [PubMed]

39. Wang, H.; Ji, J.; Yu, Y.; Wei, X.; Chai, S.; Liu, D.; Huang, D.; Li, Q.; Dong, Z.; Xiao, X. Neonatal overfeeding in female mice predisposes the development of obesity in their male offspring via altered central leptin signalling. *J. Neuroendocrinol.* **2015**, *27*, 600–608. [CrossRef] [PubMed]

40. Boeke, C.E.; Mantzoros, C.S.; Hughes, M.D.; Rifas-Shiman, S.L.; Villamor, E.; Zera, C.A.; Gillman, M.W. Differential associations of leptin with adiposity across early childhood. *Obesity* **2013**, *21*, 1430–1437. [CrossRef] [PubMed]

41. Li, R.; Fein, S.B.; Grummer-Strawn, L.M. Do infants fed from bottles lack self-regulation of milk intake compared with directly breastfed infants? *Pediatrics* **2010**, *125*, 1386–1393. [CrossRef] [PubMed]

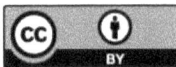

© 2016 by the authors. Licensee MDPI, Basel, Switzerland. This article is an open access article distributed under the terms and conditions of the Creative Commons Attribution (CC BY) license (http://creativecommons.org/licenses/by/4.0/).

nutrients

MDPI

Article

Association between Body Mass Index and All-Cause Mortality in Hypertensive Adults: Results from the China Stroke Primary Prevention Trial (CSPPT)

Wei Yang [1], Jian-Ping Li [1], Yan Zhang [1], Fang-Fang Fan [1], Xi-Ping Xu [2], Bin-Yan Wang [2], Xin Xu [2], Xian-Hui Qin [2], Hou-Xun Xing [3], Gen-Fu Tang [3], Zi-Yi Zhou [3], Dong-Feng Gu [4], Dong Zhao [5] and Yong Huo [1,*]

[1] Department of Cardiology, Peking University First Hospital, Beijing 100034, China;
    ywyy2008@163.com (W.Y.); lijianping@medmail.com.cn (J.-P.L.); drzhy1108@163.com (Y.Z.);
    fang9020@126.com (F.-F.F.)
[2] National Clinical Research Center for Kidney Disease, State Key Laboratory for Organ Failure Research,
    Renal Division, Nanfang Hospital, Southern Medical University, Guangzhou 510515, China;
    xipingxu126@126.com (X.-P.X.); binyanwang126@126.com (B.-Y.W.); xux007@163.com (X.X.);
    xianhuiqin@126.com (X.-H.Q.)
[3] Institute for Biomedicine, Anhui Medical University, Hefei 230032, China; ausachina@163.com (H.-X.X.);
    tanggenfu@163.com (G.-F.T.); zhouziyi19920319@126.com (Z.-Y.Z.)
[4] State Key Laboratory of Cardiovascular Disease, Fuwai Hospital, National Center
    for Cardiovascular Diseases, Chinese Academy of Medical Sciences and Peking Union Medical College,
    Beijing 100037, China; gudongfeng@vip.sina.com
[5] Department of Epidemiology, Beijing Anzhen Hospital, Capital Medical University,
    Beijing Institute of Heart, Lung and Blood Vessel Diseases, Beijing 100029, China; deezhao@vip.sina.com
* Correspondence: huoyong@263.net.cn; Tel.: +86-10-83572283

Received: 11 April 2016; Accepted: 15 June 2016; Published: 22 June 2016

Abstract: The association between elevated body mass index (BMI) and risk of death has been reported in many studies. However, the association between BMI and all-cause mortality for hypertensive Chinese adults remains unclear. We conducted a post-hoc analysis using data from the China Stroke Primary Prevention Trial (CSPPT). Cox regression analysis was performed to determine the significance of the association of BMI with all-cause mortality. During a mean follow-up duration of 4.5 years, 622 deaths (3.0%) occurred among the 20,694 participants aged 45–75 years. A reversed J-shaped relationship was observed between BMI and all-cause mortality. The hazard ratios (HRs) for underweight (<18.5 kg/m^2), overweight (24.0–27.9 kg/m^2), and obesity ($\geqslant 28.0$ kg/m^2) were calculated relative to normal weight (18.5–23.9 kg/m^2). The summary HRs were 1.56 (95% CI, 1.11–2.18) for underweight, 0.78 (95% CI 0.64–0.95) for overweight and 0.64 (95% CI, 0.48–0.85) for obesity. In sex-age-specific analyses, participants over 60 years of age had optimal BMI in the obesity classification and the results were consistent in both males and females. Relative to normal weight, underweight was associated with significantly higher mortality. Excessive weight was not associated with increased risk of mortality. Chinese hypertensive adults had the lowest mortality in grade 1 obesity.

Keywords: obesity; body mass index; mortality; hypertension; China

1. Introduction

Obesity is a global epidemic issue that is highly prevalent in both developed and developing countries; it affects people of both sexes and all ages, has adverse health consequences, accrues large economic costs, and has negative social implications [1]. Body mass index (BMI), defined as weight in kilograms divided by the square of the height in meters, is commonly used in clinical practice to screen for overweight and obesity and to guide weight loss recommendations. In China, an increasingly large proportion of the population has a BMI $\geqslant 25$ kg/m^2, the standard definition of overweight [2]. Although obesity has been demonstrated to be associated with multiple non-communicable diseases, including hypertension, type 2 diabetes, coronary heart disease, stroke and several cancers [3], the association between BMI and all-cause mortality remains controversial: a direct association, a J-shaped, a U-shaped, or a reversed J-shaped relationship have all been recently reported [4–8].

The World Health Organization (WHO) defines the following six categories based on BMI values: <18.5 kg/m^2 = underweight; 18.5 to 24.9 kg/m^2 = normal weight; 25.0 to 29.9 kg/m^2 = overweight; 30.0 to 34.9 kg/m^2 = grade 1 obesity; 35.0 to 39.9 kg/m^2 = grade 2 obesity; and $\geqslant 40$ kg/m^2 = grade 3 obesity [9]. These definitions of overweight and obesity are mainly based on criteria derived from studies that involved populations of European origin. It has been suggested that the associations of BMI with body composition and health outcomes may differ between Asian and European populations [10]. The BMI cut-off points for overweight and obesity should be lower for Asian populations than they are for European populations (suggested cut-off points for Asians are $\geqslant 23.0$ kg/m^2 for overweight and $\geqslant 27.5$ kg/m^2 for obesity) [10]. However, a consensus statement from the WHO concluded that the available data were not sufficient to support Asian-specific cut-off points [10]. The Ministry of Health of the People's Republic of China determined a reclassification of BMI for Chinese adults that differs from the WHO classification: underweight (<18.5 kg/m^2), normal weight (18.5–23.9 kg/m^2), overweight (24.0–27.9 kg/m^2) and obesity ($\geqslant 28.0$ kg/m^2) [11].

For decades, the prevalence of hypertension has been increasing in China, and by the year 2010 it reached 20% [12]. During the period of 2005–2009, about 42% of Chinese adults aged 35–70 years were hypertensive [12]. Although obesity is clearly regarded as a risk factor for developing hypertension, the optimal BMI for middle-aged or elderly hypertensive Chinese remains unclear. Therefore, the objective of this study was to evaluate the relationship between BMI and all-cause mortality in hypertensive Chinese adults.

2. Materials and Methods

2.1. Data Sources

This post-hoc analysis utilizes data from the China Stroke Primary Prevention Trial (CSPPT), which enrolled 20,702 subjects with primary hypertension in a multi-community, randomized, double-blind, controlled trial to assess whether enalapril maleate and folic acid supplementation was more effective in reducing risk of stroke than enalapril maleate supplementation alone. This study was conducted in accordance with the principles of the Declaration of Helsinki. The Human Subjects Committee at the Biomedical Institute of Anhui Medical University approved the study protocol. All patients provided written informed consent prior to data collection.

2.2. Participants and Treatment

The methods and primary results of the CSPPT trial have been reported elsewhere [13]. Briefly, the CSPPT was conducted from 19 May 2008 to 24 August 2013 in 32 communities in Jiangsu and Anhui Provinces in China. Eligible participants were men and women aged 45–75 years old who had hypertension, defined as seated resting systolic blood pressure (SBP) $\geqslant 140$ mmHg or diastolic blood pressure (DBP) $\geqslant 90$ mmHg at both the screening and recruitment visit, or who were on anti-hypertensive medication. The major exclusion criteria included history of physician-diagnosed stroke, myocardial infarction (MI), heart failure, post-coronary revascularization, or congenital heart disease.

The current analysis was designed to investigate the relationship between BMI and all-cause mortality in this cohort. All-cause mortality included death due to any reason. After excluding eight subjects with missing information on weight and height, the final analysis included 20,694 subjects.

Participants contributed person-years from the date of recruitment until date of death or end of follow-up (24 August 2013). BMI classifications as set according to the guidelines from the Ministry of Health of the People's Republic of China were used and included: underweight (<18.5 kg/m^2), normal weight (18.5–23.9 kg/m^2), overweight (24.0–27.9 kg/m^2) and obesity ($\geq$28.0 kg/m^2). At the initial study visit trained research staff measured and recorded height (to the nearest 0.1 cm) and weight (to the nearest 0.1 kg) for each participant. In addition, trained staff collected baseline demographic data, medical history, and medication use. Cigarette smoking was classified into never, former, and current smoker (defined as smoke at least one cigarette per day for more than one year). Alcohol drinking was stratified into never, former and current drinker (defined as drink alcohol at least twice weekly for more than one year). Education was categorized into illiterate (0 years of education), primary school (1–6 years), and secondary school (>6 years) or above. Stress was defined as mild, moderate or severe according to the participant's personal evaluation.

2.3. Follow-Up and Outcomes

Patients were evaluated every three months for an average of five years to assess blood pressure (BP), adherence to medication, and adverse outcomes including stroke, composite major cardiovascular (CV) events and resultant death, and all-cause death. The study outcomes were adjudicated according to standard criteria by a clinical end points committee.

2.4. Statistical Analysis

All participants were divided into four groups according to the Chinese classification for BMI (<18.5, 18.5–23.9, 24.0–27.9, $\geq$28.0 kg/m^2). Baseline characteristics of all participants were compared using the analysis of variance (ANOVA) for continuous variables and the χ^2 test for categorical variables. All-cause mortality was first assessed using the Kalpan-Meier method and log-rank tests, and then multivariable Cox proportional-hazards regression models were applied to calculate hazard ratios (HR) and 95% confidence intervals (CI) for the risk of all-cause mortality in each of the BMI groups. Potential confounders were adjusted including sex, age, center, baseline and on-treatment BP, smoking status, alcohol drinking, education, stress, fasting blood glucose (FBG), total cholesterol (TC), triglycerides (TG), serum creatinine (SCr), homocysteine (Hcy) and albumin. Further stratified analyses by subgroups including sex, age, center, smoking and alcohol drinking status, education, stress and albumin levels were also explored by Cox proportional-hazards regression models to test for consistency of results. All tests were two-sided, and *p*-values less than 0.05 were considered statistically significant. All analyses were performed by EmpowerStats [14] and the statistical package R [15].

3. Results

3.1. Patient Characteristics

Baseline characteristics of all patients are presented in Table 1. Of the 20,694 participants, 59.0% were female, and the mean age was 60.0 years (SD, 7.5 years), with a range from 45 to 75 years. The mean BMI was 25.0 kg/m^2 (SD, 3.4 kg/m^2). Men had a lower of BMI 24.2 kg/m^2 (SD, 3.7 kg/m^2) than women, who had a BMI of 25.4 kg/m^2 (SD, 3.4 kg/m^2). The percentages of underweight, normal weight, overweight and obese were 2.5%, 39.1%, 38.9% and 19.5%, respectively. Higher BMI categories were associated with younger age, female gender, better education, and higher levels of FBG, TC, TG, albumin, and baseline and on-treatment blood pressure measurements. Lower BMI categories were associated with higher HDL-C levels and current smoking status.

Table 1. Baseline characteristics of the study participants by BMI categories [1].

Variables	BMI Categories, kg/m^2					
	All Subjects	<18.5	18.5–23.9	24.0–27.9	⩾28.0	*p*-Value
Number (%)	20,694	526(2.5)	8083 (39.1)	8043 (38.9)	4042 (19.5)	
Age, mean (SD), years	60.0 (7.5)	64.6 (6.7)	61.3 (7.4)	59.3 (7.5)	58.2 (7.4)	<0.001
BMI, mean (SD), kg/m^2	25.0 (3.7)	17.5 (0.8)	21.8 (1.4)	25.8 (1.1)	30.4 (2.2)	<0.001
Male, No. (%)	8491 (41.0)	271 (51.5)	3863 (47.8)	3137 (39.0)	1220 (30.2)	<0.001
Center, No. (%)						<0.001
Anqing	5211 (25.2)	350 (66.5)	3119 (38.6)	1406 (17.5)	336 (8.3)	
Lianyungang	15,483 (74.8)	176 (33.5)	4964 (61.4)	6637 (82.5)	3706 (91.7)	
SBP, mean (SD), mmHg						
baseline	166.9 (20.4)	164.3 (17.9)	166.0 (20.0)	167.1 (20.4)	168.4 (21.4)	<0.001
on-treatment	139.4 (10.9)	138.8 (10.8)	138.9 (11.0)	139.4 (10.8)	140.4 (11.0)	<0.001
DBP, mean (SD),mmHg						
baseline	94.1 (11.9)	88.0 (11.4)	91.8 (11.7)	95.0 (11.6)	97.7 (11.9)	<0.001
on-treatment	82.9 (7.5)	78.9 (7.7)	81.5 (7.4)	83.5 (7.2)	85.3 (7.2)	<0.001
Pulse, mean (SD),bpm	73.6 (10.1)	74.0 (11.0)	73.6 (10.2)	73.5 (10.1)	73.8 (9.9)	0.53
Smoking status (%)						<0.001
never	14,252 (68.9)	293 (55.7)	5015 (62.1)	5791 (72.0)	3153 (78.0)	
former	1567 (7.6)	35 (6.7)	604 (7.5)	649 (8.1)	279 (6.9)	
current	4867 (23.5)	198 (37.6)	2459 (30.4)	1601 (19.9)	609 (15.1)	
Alcohol drinking (%)						<0.001
never	14,265 (69.0)	343 (65.2)	5155 (63.8)	5665 (70.5)	3102 (76.8)	
former	1458 (7.0)	52 (9.9)	609 (7.5)	540 (6.7)	257 (6.4)	
current	4960 (24.0)	131 (24.9)	2313 (28.6)	1836 (22.8)	680 (16.8)	
Education (%)						<0.001
illiterate	13,221 (63.9)	365 (69.4)	5261 (65.1)	4999 (62.2)	2596 (64.3)	
primary	3446 (16.7)	103 (19.6)	1468 (18.2)	1296 (16.1)	579 (14.3)	
secondary or above	4015 (19.4)	58 (11.0)	1347 (16.7)	1745 (21.7)	865 (21.4)	
Stress (%)						0.035
mild	12,578 (60.8)	289 (54.90)	4846 (60.0)	4960 (61.7)	2479 (61.4)	
moderate	6921 (33.4)	204 (38.8)	2765 (34.2)	2627 (32.7)	1323 (32.8)	
severe	1189 (5.7)	33 (6.3)	464 (5.7)	454 (5.6)	237 (5.9)	
FPG, mean (SD), mmol/L	5.8 (1.7)	5.3 (1.6)	5.6 (1.6)	5.9 (1.8)	6.1 (1.7)	<0.001
TC, mean (SD), mmol/L	5.5 (1.2)	5.0 (1.2)	5.4 (1.2)	5.6 (1.2)	5.7 (1.2)	<0.001
TG, mean (SD), mmol/L	1.7 (1.2)	1.2 (0.5)	1.4 (0.8)	1.8 (1.0)	2.0 (1.8)	<0.001
HDL-C, mean (SD), mmol/L	1.3 (0.4)	1.6 (0.4)	1.5 (0.4)	1.3 (0.3)	1.2 (0.3)	<0.001
SCr, mean (SD), umol/L	66.0 (19.3)	67.6 (16.7)	67.3 (19.6)	65.6 (20.5)	64.0 (16.3)	<0.001
Hcy, mean (SD), umol/L	14.5(8.4)	14.3 (7.7)	14.5 (8.1)	14.5 (8.4)	14.3 (8.9)	0.534
Albumin, mean (SD), g/L	49.0 (5.9)	47.57 (6.6)	48.57 (6.0)	49.34 (5.7)	49.34 (5.6)	<0.001
Treatment (%)						0.832
Enalapril	10,352 (50.0)	271 (51.5)	4053 (50.1)	4025 (50.0)	2003 (49.6)	
Enalapril-Folic Acid	10,342 (50.0)	255 (48.5)	4030 (49.9)	4018 (50.0)	2039 (50.4)	

[1] For the determination of *p*-values, two-sample *t*-tests for continuous variables, chi-square tests for categorical variables. SBP, systolic blood pressure; DBP, diastolic blood pressure; FBG, fasting blood glucose; TC, total cholesterol; TG, triglycerides; SCr, serum creatinine; Hcy, homocysteine.

3.2. BMI and Mortality

The relationship between BMI and overall mortality for all patients with hypertension is shown in Table 2. During a median follow-up period of 4.5 years (88,466.64 person-years), 622 deaths occurred. Specifically, with increasing BMI, the all-cause mortality rate in underweight, normal weight, overweight and obese groups was 7.8%, 3.9%, 2.4% and 1.8%, respectively. According to the BMI category, the all-cause mortality rate per 1000 person-years was 17.63, 8.93, 5.76 and 4.24, respectively. In a crude Cox proportional-hazards regression model, the HRs were 1.97 (95% CI, 1.42–2.73) for underweight, 0.64 (95% CI, 0.54–0.77) for overweight and 0.47 (95% CI, 0.37–0.61) for obesity compared with normal weight. In model II, after adjusting for sex, age, center, baseline and on-treatment BP, smoking status, alcohol drinking, education, stress and serum biochemical measurements, the HRs were 1.56 (95% CI, 1.11–2.18) for underweight, 0.78 (95% CI, 0.64–0.95) for overweight and 0.64 (95% CI, 0.48–0.85) for obesity compared with normal weight.

Table 2. Hazard ratios for all-cause mortality according to BMI status [1].

BMI kg/m^2	N	Event (%)	Curde Rate	All-Cause Mortality			
				Model 1	p-Value	Model 2	p-Value
Continuous	20,694	622 (3.0%)	7.03	0.90 (0.88, 0.92)	<0.001	0.94 (0.91, 0.96)	<0.001
<18.5	526	41 (7.8%)	17.63	1.97 (1.42, 2.73)	<0.001	1.56 (1.11, 2.18)	0.010
18.5–23.9	8083	312 (3.9%)	8.93	1		1	
24.0–27.9	8043	197 (2.4%)	5.76	0.64 (0.54, 0.77)	<0.001	0.78 (0.64, 0.95)	0.012
⩾28	4042	72 (1.8%)	4.24	0.47 (0.37, 0.61)	<0.001	0.64 (0.48, 0.85)	0.002

[1] Multivariable Cox proportional-hazards regression models were applied to calculate hazard ratios (HR) and 95% confidence intervals (CI) for the risk of all-cause mortality in each of the BMI groups. A BMI (kg/m^2) of 18.5–23.9 was used as the reference to estimate all HRs. Crude rates are all-cause mortality per 1000 person-years. Model 1: crude; Model 2: adjustment for sex, age, center, baseline and on-treatment BP, smoking status, alcohol drinking, education, stress, fasting blood glucose, total cholesterol, triglycerides, serum creatinine, homocysteine, albumin.

Figure 1 shows the Kaplan-Meier curves of the cumulative hazards of all-cause mortality stratified by BMI categories. All-cause mortality between each of the four BMI groups was significantly different (log-rank test, $p < 0.001$). With increased BMI, the cumulative mortality risk gradually decreased, rendering the underweight group with the maximum mortality risk.

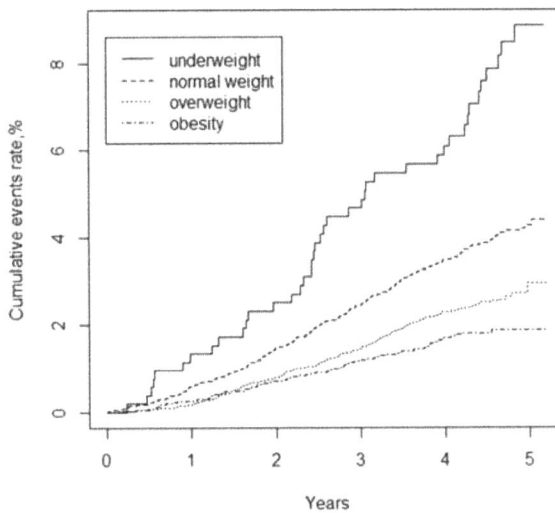

Figure 1. Kaplan-Meier curves of cumulative hazards of all-cause mortality stratified by BMI categories (underweight <18.5, normal weight 18.5–23.9, overweight 24.0–27.9, obesity ⩾28.0 kg/m^2). log-rank test, $p < 0.001$.

Further stratified analyses were performed by important covariables including gender, center, smoking status, alcohol drinking status, education, stress and albumin levels (Table 3). There were no significant interactions in any of the subgroups ($p > 0.05$ for all comparisons). The beneficial effect appeared to be more pronounced in participants older than 60 years.

We subsequently repeated the analysis using narrower BMI categories (<18.5, 18.5–19.9, 20.0–21.9, 22.0–23.9, 24.0–25.9, 26.0–27.9, 28.0–29.9, 30–34.9, ⩾35 kg/m^2) to delineate the relationship between BMI and mortality with greater precision. Compared to patients with normal BMI (between 22.0 and 23.9 kg/m^2), patients with grade 1 obesity (30–34.9 kg/m^2) had the lowest risk of all-cause mortality (Figure 2). However, all-cause mortality increased drastically for patients with severe obesity (⩾35 kg/m^2).

Table 3. Multivariable hazard ratios for mortality [1].

Variables	N	Death, n	%	BMI Categories(kg/m²)								Adjusted * p for Interaction
				<18.5		18.5–23.9		24.0–27.9		≥28		
				HR 95%CI	p-Value	HR 95%CI	p-Value	HR 95%CI	p-Value	HR 95%CI	p-Value	
All Participants	20,694	622	3.0	1.56 (1.10, 2.14)	0.012	1		0.80 (0.66, 0.97)	0.026	0.66 (0.49, 0.87)	0.003	
Sex												0.692
Females	12,203	258	2.1	1.24 (0.66, 2.33)	0.505	1		0.78 (0.58, 1.05)	0.097	0.60 (0.41, 0.89)	0.010	
Males	8491	364	4.3	1.74 (1.16, 2.58)	0.007	1		0.82 (0.63, 1.07)	0.144	0.71 (0.46, 1.09)	0.119	
Center												0.719
Anqing	5211	218	4.2	1.58 (1.04, 2.38)	0.030	1		0.72 (0.49, 1.05)	0.090	0.88 (0.45, 1.72)	0.709	
Lianyungang	15,483	404	2.6	1.59 (0.88, 2.88)	0.125	1		0.84 (0.67, 1.06)	0.153	0.65 (0.47, 0.90)	0.009	
Age												0.588
<60	10,469	172	1.6	1.82 (0.78, 4.25)	0.167	1		0.82 (0.56, 1.19)	0.302	0.84 (0.52, 1.34)	0.463	
≥60	10,225	450	4.4	1.62 (1.13, 2.34)	0.009	1		0.75 (0.60, 0.95)	0.016	0.53 (0.36, 0.76)	<0.001	
Smoking Status												0.298
Never	14,254	327	2.3	1.40 (0.83, 2.37)	0.208	1		0.80 (0.61, 1.04)	0.090	0.62 (0.43, 0.89)	0.009	
Former	1570	75	4.8	3.76 (1.64, 8.67)	0.002	1		1.37 (0.75, 2.49)	0.305	1.28 (0.56, 2.90)	0.558	
Current	4869	219	4.5	1.33 (0.79, 2.25)	0.281	1		0.70 (0.50, 1.00)	0.052	0.60 (0.33, 1.09)	0.095	
Alcohol												0.906
Never	14,265	355	2.5	1.54 (0.98, 2.43)	0.064	1		0.75 (0.58, 0.97)	0.026	0.63 (0.44, 0.89)	0.009	
Former	1458	80	5.5	2.51 (1.17, 5.42)	0.019	1		0.85 (0.48, 1.48)	0.559	0.50 (0.20, 1.28)	0.148	
Current	4960	186	3.8	1.27 (0.65, 2.47)	0.482	1		0.93 (0.65, 1.34)	0.695	0.84 (0.46, 1.55)	0.581	
Education												0.599
Illiterate	13,221	411	3.1	1.43 (0.95, 2.15)	0.087	1		0.75 (0.59, 0.96)	0.021	0.67 (0.48, 0.94)	0.022	
Primary	3446	116	3.3	1.52 (0.70, 3.31)	0.290	1		0.98 (0.63, 1.53)	0.935	0.49 (0.22, 1.09)	0.080	
Secondary or above	4015	94	2.3	2.18 (0.88, 5.40)	0.093	1		0.78 (0.47, 1.29)	0.330	0.68 (0.33, 1.39)	0.290	
Stress												0.506
Mild	12,574	391	3.1	1.26 (0.79, 2.00)	0.333	1		0.73 (0.57, 0.94)	0.013	0.66 (0.47, 0.94)	0.019	
Moderate	6919	202	2.9	1.89 (1.13, 3.17)	0.016	1		0.91 (0.64, 1.29)	0.602	0.58 (0.33, 1.01)	0.054	
Severe	1188	28	2.4	2.97 (0.59, 14.93)	0.187	1		1.29 (0.49, 3.42)	0.604	0.90 (0.24, 3.32)	0.869	
Albumin, g/L												0.527
<49	11,813	412	3.5	1.48 (1.00, 2.18)	0.051	1		0.73 (0.57, 0.93)	0.012	0.68 (0.48, 0.97)	0.033	
≥49	8876	210	2.4	1.87 (0.98, 3.56)	0.058	1		0.87 (0.63, 1.20)	0.394	0.56 (0.34, 0.90)	0.016	

[1] Cox proportional-hazards regression models to test interaction terms between BMI and other factors, but none were found to be significant. * Adjustment for sex, age, center, baseline and on-treatment BP, smoking status, alcohol drinking, education, stress, fasting blood glucose, total cholesterol, triglycerides, serum creatinine, homocysteine, albumin; sex, center, age, smoking status, alcohol, education, stress and albumin were not adjusted for in each corresponding subgroup analyses.

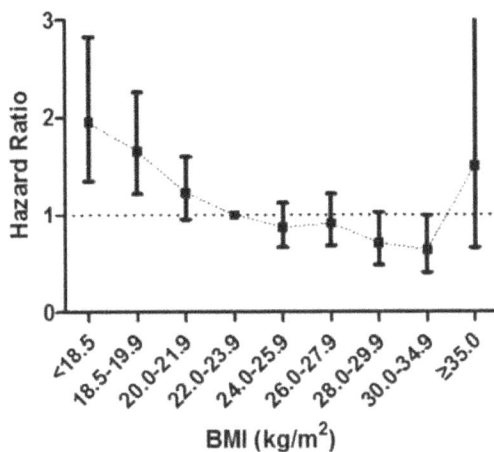

Figure 2. Hazard ratios for all-cause mortality according to narrower BMI categories. A BMI (in kg/m^2) of 22.0–23.9 was used as the reference to estimate all HRs. Adjustment for sex, age, center, baseline and on-treatment BP, smoking status, alcohol drinking, education, stress, fasting blood glucose, total cholesterol, triglycerides, serum creatinine, homocysteine, albumin.

4. Discussion

Our post-hoc analysis of this Chinese population with primary hypertension in the CSPPT showed the association between BMI and all-cause mortality followed a reversed J-shaped curve with increased risk at low and high BMI status. Even after adjusting for potential confounders, the results were similar. Compared to normal weight, the HRs were 1.56 (95% CI, 1.11–2.18) for underweight, 0.78 (95% CI, 0.64–0.95) for overweight and 0.64 (95% CI, 0.48, 0.85) for obesity. In this population, the optimal BMI was grade 1 obesity (30–34.9 kg/m^2). Stratified analyses were consistent in all important covariables. Moreover, overweight or obese patients older than 60 years showed the most benefit.

Many studies conducted on different populations showed a U-shaped or J-shaped association between BMI and all-cause mortality, which is consistent with our results when applied to the underweight participants only [4–8]. In these studies, the population age distribution and whether subgroup analyses were performed by age group might be two major reasons for the controversial results. Janssen *et al.* found that BMI was inversely associated with mortality risk in elderly Asians [16]. Compared to middle-aged adults, some previous studies found that the optimal BMI among the elderly shifted upwards [17,18]. This finding is similar to what has been observed in other Asian regions such as Taiwan [19], Hong Kong [20], India and Bangladesh [8], among others [4,5,7]. Many of the elderly participants from these studies were residents of live-in care facilities, and/or were diagnosed with a health ailment such as hypertension, or were from undeveloped communities compared with urban residents. However, the optimal range of BMI proposed among the elderly varies among studies. As the world's population ages and the number of hypertensive adults rises, our findings are important for health care professionals and policy-makers whose decisions affect elderly hypertensives.

Several potential explanations for the observed obesity paradox seen in our study exist. Firstly, reverse causality is a major problem in observational studies. For example, weight loss is classically experienced prior to death among the elderly who are ill. Secondly, socioeconomic status could confound the association between BMI and the risk of death, as people from less well-developed countries with a high BMI are more likely to have a higher socioeconomic status, allowing them better access to health care than those with a lower BMI [8]. However, the participants in our study are from rural communities, and a similar relation between BMI and socioeconomic status exists for them. Thirdly, in a meta-analysis of patients with existing coronary artery disease, those classified as

Nutrients **2016**, *8*, 384

overweight and obese had longer survival rates, potentially because of the benefit from the body's reservation of nutrition within the population of elderly suffering from illness [21]. Fourthly, intensive pharmacotherapy could play a large role in the reverse J-shaped relationship. It has been demonstrated that patients with intensive pharmacotherapy are more likely to reach targets for secondary prevention. In population studies conducted in the USA and Canada, obese patients are more likely to meet targets for BP, lipids, and glycemic control than normal-weight patients [22]. In addition, hypertensive participants are relatively less healthy compared to the general population, although in our study we excluded patients with stroke and MI. Mary *et al.* found that among elderly Chinese with poor health status, there was an inverse, dose-response relationship between BMI and mortality, and this relationship was more pronounced in the group with the most morbidity compared to subjects of normal weight [23]. Another interpretation is that BMI can be a marker of adiposity, fitness and muscle mass, so that BMI maintenance in older people serves as an overall marker of health. Song *et al.* accessed the sex-age-specific association between BMI and all-cause mortality in the general population, and showed that the optimal BMI increased according to age and the trend was consistent in both males and females [24]. Similarly, Woo *et al.* found that in older elderly (aged over 75 years), a higher BMI was a protection from mortality [17].

Our study also has several limitations. Firstly, our participants were all middle-aged or elderly hypertensives; therefore, the result of this study cannot be generalized to all populations. Secondly, with the strict exclusion of the history of cardiovascular disease, cardiovascular cause of death counted for only 14% of all-cause death, which is less than other studies conducted on Chinese hypertensive adults. The association between BMI and a specific cause of death cannot be analyzed. Thirdly, in the current study, relatively few elderly were $\geqslant 30$ kg/m^2 (10% of total subjects) and $\geqslant 35$ kg/m^2 (1%); thus, the impact of obesity cannot be adequately assessed. Moreover, although we have excluded subjects with a baseline diagnosis of coronary heart disease, stroke, cancer, or acquired organic diseases, some preexisting illness may modify the association between BMI and mortality risk. However, according to our investigation, after excluding those subjects with no history of disease at baseline and who survived the first two years of follow-up, the BMI and all-cause mortality association was consistent with all 4.5 years of this study.

5. Conclusions

In conclusion, this study revealed a reversed J-shaped association between BMI and all-cause mortality in Chinese hypertensive adults. Relative to normal weight, underweight was associated with significantly higher mortality. Excessive weight was not associated with increased risk of mortality. A BMI classification of grade 1 obesity for Chinese hypertensive adults without stroke or MI showed the lowest mortality. Additional large-scale prospective studies with well-controlled confounding factors are needed to further address this important public health issue.

Acknowledgments: This research was supported by the Ministry of Science and Technology of the People's Republic of China (2012zx 09101105); the Major State Basic Research Development Program of China (973 program, No. 2012CB517703); and Projects of National Natural Science Foundation of China (grants 81437052).

Author Contributions: Y.H.: study supervision, access to all data in the study, integrity of data, and accuracy of the data analysis; W.Y., F.F.F., X.P.X., Z.Y.Z. and Y.H.: study concept and design and statistical analysis; X.P.X., B.Y.W., X.X., X.H.Q., H.X.X., G.F.T. and Y.H.: acquisition of data; W.Y., F.F.F., X.P.X., B.Y.W., Z.Y.Z. and Y.H.: analysis and interpretation of data; W.Y. and Y.H.: drafting of the manuscript; X.P.X., D.F.G. and D.Z. provided a critical review of the content of the manuscript, and revised the manuscript for important intellectual content; J.P.L., Y.Z., X.P.X., B.Y.W., H.X.X., G.F.T. and Y.H.: administrative, technical, or material support; and all authors: critical revision of the manuscript for important intellectual content.

Conflicts of Interest: The authors declare no conflict of interest.

Abbreviations

The following abbreviations are used in this manuscript:

BMI	body mass index
BP	blood pressure
CI	confidence interval
CSPPT	China Stroke Primary Prevention Trial
CV	major cardiovascular
DBP	diastolic blood pressure
FBG	fasting blood glucose
Hcy	homocysteine
HR	hazard ratio
MI	myocardial infarction
SBP	systolic blood pressure
SCr	serum creatinine
TC	total cholesterol
TG	triglycerides
WHO	The World Health Organization

References

1. Yang, Z.; Hall, A.G. The Financial Burden of Overweight and Obesity among Elderly Americans: The Dynamics of Weight, Longevity, and Health Care Cost. *Health Serv. Res.* **2008**, *43*, 849–868. [CrossRef] [PubMed]

2. World Health Organization. WHO Global Infobase, 2014. Available online: http://www.who.int/gho/ncd/risk_factors/overweight_text/en/ (accessed on 22 December 2015).

3. World Health Organization. *Physical Status: The Use and Interpretation of Anthropometry*; Report of a WHO Expert Committee; WHO Technical Report Series No. 854; World Health Organization: Geneva, Switzerland, 1995.

4. Flegal, K.M.; Graubard, B.I.; Williamson, D.F.; Gail, M.H. Excess deaths associated with underweight, overweight, and obesity. *JAMA* **2005**, *293*, 1861–1867. [CrossRef] [PubMed]

5. Flegal, K.M.; Kit, B.K.; Orpana, H.; Graubard, B.I. Association of all-cause mortality with overweight and obesity using standard body mass index categories: A systematic review and meta-analysis. *JAMA* **2013**, *309*, 71–82. [CrossRef] [PubMed]

6. Hu, F.B.; Willett, W.C.; Li, T.; Stampfer, M.J.; Colditz, G.A.; Manson, J.E. Adiposity as Compared with Physical Activity in Predicting Mortality among Women. *N. Engl. J. Med.* **2004**, *351*, 2694–2703. [CrossRef] [PubMed]

7. Winter, J.E.; MacInnis, R.J.; Wattanapenpaiboon, N.; Nowson, C.A. BMI and all-cause mortality in older adults: A meta-analysis. *Am. J. Clin. Nutr.* **2014**, *99*, 875–890. [CrossRef] [PubMed]

8. Zheng, W.; McLerran, D.F.; Rolland, B.; Zhang, X.; Inoue, M.; Matsuo, K.; He, J.; Gupta, P.C.; Ramadas, K.; Tsugane, S.; *et al.* Association between body-mass index and risk of death in more than 1 million Asians. *N. Engl. J. Med.* **2011**, *364*, 719–729. [CrossRef] [PubMed]

9. Haslam, D.W.; James, W.P. Obesity. *Lancet* **2005**, *366*, 1197–1209. [CrossRef]

10. WHO Expert Consultation. Appropriate body-mass index for Asian populations and its implications for policy and intervention strategies. *Lancet* **2004**, *363*, 157–163.

11. Chen, C.; Lu, F.C. The guidelines for prevention and control of overweight and obesity in Chinese adults. *Biomed. Environ. Sci.* **2004**, *17*, 1–36. [PubMed]

12. Liu, L.S. 2010 Chinese guidelines for the management of hypertension. *Zhonghua Xin Xue Guan Bing Za Zhi* **2011**, *39*, 579–615. [PubMed]

13. Huo, Y.; Li, J.; Qin, X.; Huang, Y.; Wang, X.; Gottesman, R.F.; Tang, G.; Wang, B.; Chen, D.; He, M.; *et al.* Efficacy of Folic Acid Therapy in Primary Prevention of Stroke Among Adults With Hypertension in China. *JAMA* **2015**, *313*, 1325. [CrossRef] [PubMed]

14. EmpowerStats. Available online: http://www.empowerstats.com (accessed on 25 March 2016).

15. R Software, Version 3.2.1. Available online: http://www.R-project.org/ (accessed on 25 March 2016).

16. Janssen, I.; Mark, A.E. Elevated body mass index and mortality risk in the elderly. *Obes. Rev.* **2007**, *8*, 41–59. [CrossRef] [PubMed]

17. Woo, J.; Ho, S.C.; Sham, A. Longitudinal changes in body mass index and body composition over 3 years and relationship to health outcomes in Hong Kong Chinese age 70 and older. *J. Am. Geriatr. Soc.* **2001**, *49*, 737–746. [CrossRef] [PubMed]

18. Chung, W.; Ho, F.; Cheng, N.; Lee, M.; Yeh, C. BMI and all-cause mortality among middle-aged and older adults in Taiwan: A population-based cohort study. *Public Health. Nutr.* **2015**, *18*, 1839–1846. [CrossRef] [PubMed]

19. Lin, W.; Albu, J.; Liu, C.; Huang, H.; Pi-Sunyer, F.X.; Li, C.; Li, T.; Lin, C.; Huang, K. Larger Body Mass Index and Waist Circumference Are Associated with Lower Mortality in Chinese Long-Term Care Facility Residents. *J. Am. Geriatr. Soc.* **2010**, *58*, 2092–2098. [CrossRef] [PubMed]

20. Lee, J.S.W.; Auyeung, T.; Chau, P.P.H.; Hui, E.; Chan, F.; Chi, I.; Woo, J. Obesity Can Benefit Survival—A 9-Year Prospective Study in 1614 Chinese Nursing Home Residents. *J. Am. Med. Dir. Assoc.* **2014**, *15*, 342–348. [CrossRef] [PubMed]

21. Romero-Corral, A.; Montori, V.M.; Somers, V.K.; Korinek, J.; Thomas, R.J.; Allison, T.G.; Mookadam, F.; Lopez-Jimenez, F. Association of bodyweight with total mortality and with cardiovascular events in coronary artery disease: A systematic review of cohort studies. *Lancet* **2006**, *368*, 666–678. [CrossRef]

22. Chang, V.W.; Asch, D.A.; Werner, R.M. Quality of care among obese patients. *JAMA* **2010**, *303*, 1274–1281. [CrossRef] [PubMed]

23. Schooling, C.M.; Lam, T.H.; Li, Z.B.; Ho, S.Y.; Chan, W.M.; Ho, K.S.; Tham, M.K.; Cowling, B.J.; Leung, G.M. Obesity, physical activity, and mortality in a prospective Chinese elderly cohort. *Arch. Intern. Med.* **2006**, *166*, 1498–1504. [CrossRef] [PubMed]

24. Yi, S.; Ohrr, H.; Shin, S.; Yi, J. Sex-age-specific association of body mass index with all-cause mortality among 12.8 million Korean adults: A prospective cohort study. *Int. J. Epidemiol.* **2015**, *44*, 1696–1705. [CrossRef] [PubMed]

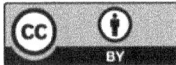

© 2016 by the authors. Licensee MDPI, Basel, Switzerland. This article is an open access article distributed under the terms and conditions of the Creative Commons Attribution (CC BY) license (http://creativecommons.org/licenses/by/4.0/).

nutrients

MDPI

Article

Relationship between the Balance of Hypertrophic/Hyperplastic Adipose Tissue Expansion and the Metabolic Profile in a High Glucocorticoids Model

María Guillermina Zubiría [1,2], Ana Alzamendi [1], Griselda Moreno [3], Andrea Portales [1,2], Daniel Castrogiovanni [1], Eduardo Spinedi [4] and Andrés Giovambattista [1,2,*]

[1]   Neuroendocrinology Laboratory, Multidisciplinary Institute of Cellular Biology (IMBICE, CICPBA-CONICET-UNLP), Calles 526 10 y 11, La Plata 1900, Argentina; gzubiria@imbice.gov.ar (M.G.Z.); aalzamendi@imbice.gov.ar (A.A.); andreaeportales@gmail.com (A.P.); dcastrogiovanni@yahoo.com (D.C.)
[2]   Biology Department, School of Exact Sciences, Universidad Nacional de La Plata, La Plata 1900, Argentina
[3]   Institute of Immunological and Physiopathological Research (IIFP, CONICET-UNLP), School of Exact Sciences, Universidad Nacional de La Plata, La Plata 1900, Argentina; gmoreno@iifp.laplata-conicet.gov.ar
[4]   Center of Experimental and Applied Endocrinology (CENEXA, UNLP-CONICET, PAHO/WHO Collaborating Center for Diabetes), La Plata Medical School, Universidad Nacional de La Plata, La Plata 1900, Argentina; spinedi@cenexa.org
*   Correspondence: agiovamba@imbice.gov.ar; Tel.: +54-221-421-0112

Received: 30 March 2016; Accepted: 14 June 2016; Published: 2 July 2016

Abstract: Adipose tissue (AT) expansion is the result of two processes: hyperplasia and hypertrophy; and both, directly or indirectly, depend on the adipogenic potential of adipocyte precursor cells (APCs). Glucocorticoids (GCs) have a potent stimulatory effect on terminal adipogenesis; while their effects on early stages of adipogenesis are largely unknown. In the present work, we study, in a model of high GC levels, the adipogenic potential of APCs from retroperitoneal AT (RPAT) and its relationship with RPAT mass expansion. We employed a model of hyper-adiposity (30- and 60-day-old rats) due to high endogenous GC levels induced by neonatal treatment with L-monosodium glutamate (MSG). We found that the RPAT APCs from 30-day-old MSG rats showed an increased adipogenic capacity, depending on the APCs' competency, but not in their number. Analyses of RPAT adipocyte diameter revealed an increase in cell size, regardless of the rat age, indicating the prevalence of a hypertrophic process. Moreover, functional RPAT alterations worsened in 60-day-old rats, suggesting that the hyperplastic AT expansion found in 30-day-old animals might have a protective role. We conclude that GCs chronic excess affects APCs' adipogenic capacity, modifying their competency. This change would modulate the hyperplastic/hypertrophic balance determining healthy or unhealthy RPAT expansion and, therefore, its functionality.

Keywords: retroperitoneal adipose tissue; adipogenesis; stromal vascular fraction cells; cell determination; adipogenic competency

1. Introduction

Glucocorticoids (GCs) have several effects on adipose tissue (AT) biology: among others, they regulate terminal adipocyte differentiation, AT endocrine function and lipogenic-lipolysis balance [1–3]. Some of these effects are more predominant on visceral (VAT) rather than on subcutaneous (SCAT) AT function [4]. One clear example is the Cushing's syndrome (CS) phenotype, mainly characterized by high GC levels in blood and increased VAT rather than SCAT mass [5]. Other features of CS, some of them shared by the human metabolic syndrome (MS) phenotype, are the presence of VAT hypertrophic adipocytes, altered lipid metabolism and impaired adipokine secretion [6]. The existence of these alterations suggests that GCs have a pivotal role in the pathogenesis of central obesity and the associated alterations seen in the CS phenotype.

Neonatal i.p. administration of the neurotoxin monosodium L-glutamate (MSG) in rodents causes neuronal loss, mainly at the hypothalamic arcuate nucleus level [7], triggering a failure in hypothalamus-pituitary-adrenal axis regulation, which results in high plasma GC levels [8]. Because of this reason, the MSG treatment has been widely used to generate animal models resembling that of the human CS phenotype. We have extensively used the MSG rat model, which is characterized by increased VAT mass with hypertrophic adipocytes and an altered peripheral pattern of adipokines [8,9].

It is generally accepted that the ability of an AT depot to expand its mass depends on two processes: the generation of new adipocytes (adipogenesis) and the hypertrophy of mature AT cells. It has been proposed [10] that at the AT level, hyperplasia contributes to maintaining a pool of small and functional adipocytes, thus preventing the development of metabolic alterations associated with hypertrophic obesity [11]. Indeed, adipocyte hypertrophy is associated with cell dysfunction, such as insulin resistance [12] and changes in the adipokine secretion pattern [13,14].

During the adipogenic process, adipose precursor cells (APCs) differentiate into mature adipocytes in two sequential steps: commitment of mesenchymal stem cells (MSCs) to APCs, acquiring their adipogenic potential and restricting them to the adipocyte linage, followed by terminal adipocyte differentiation [15]. CD34 is a cell surface antigen that distinguishes between adipogenic and non-adipogenic cell subpopulations in the stromal vascular fraction (SVF) of the AT [16]. This CD34+ subpopulation expresses almost exclusively the transcriptional factor Zinc finger protein 423 (Zfp423) [17], which in turn activates the basal expression of cell peroxisome proliferator-activated receptor (PPAR)-γ2, a key pro-adipogenic signal that assures APCs conversion into adipocytes [18]. The differential expression of both transcriptional factors determines the competency of APCs, that is, the cell's ability to differentiate into adipocytes after the addition of defined stimuli [15].

GCs are one of the most important cell differentiation inducers through their inhibitory effect on Preadipocyte Factor 1 (Pref-1) and Wingless-type MMTV integration site family member 10b (Wnt-10b) expression [19–21]. Both, Pref-1 and Wnt-10b, are highly expressed in preadipocytes and absent in mature adipocytes [22,23]. In vitro experiments with the preadipocyte cell line 3T3-L1 have shown that Pref-1 is an early target for dexamethasone (DXM) action and that its expression decreases with high DXM concentrations, at the same time that adipocyte differentiation increases [19]. Similarly, in vivo and in vitro studies demonstrated that the inhibition of the Wnt/b-catenin signaling pathway by methylprednisolone or DXM, respectively, can promote adipocyte differentiation [21,24]. Several studies show that GCs can affect adipogenesis through their binding to mineralocorticoid (MR) and/or glucocorticoid (GR) receptors [25–27], although the contribution of MR and GR in mediating GCs' adipogenic effect has not been fully understood.

While the activity of GCs on adipocyte terminal differentiation has been extensively studied, the effect of chronic GC exposure of SVF cells remains almost unexplored. Using adult male MSG rats, it has been previously demonstrated that adipogenesis is inhibited as a consequence of long-term GC exposure of SVF cells, thus contributing to hypertrophic retroperitoneal AT (RPAT) mass expansion [28]. The present study focuses on the APCs' adipogenic potential during in vivo RPAT mass expansion under an earlier chronic GCs circulating excess.

2. Materials and Methods

2.1. Animals and Treatment

Sprague-Dawley newborn pups were i.p. injected with either 4 mg/g of body weight (BW) MSG (Sigma Chemical CO., St. Louis, MO, USA) dissolved in sterile 0.9% NaCl or 10% NaCl (litter-mate controls; CTR) on alternate days between 2 and 10 days of age [9]. CTR and MSG male rats were used for experimentation at 30 days of age. Additional groups of rats at 60 days of age were used for a set of comparative experiments (SVF cell composition analysis by flow cytometry and adipocyte size measurements, as described below). Animals under non-fasting (basal) conditions (between 08:00 a.m. and 09:00 a.m.) were euthanized, and trunk blood was collected into Ethylenediaminetetraacetic acid (EDTA)-coated tubes. After centrifugation (3000 rpm for 15 min at 4 °C), plasma samples were kept frozen (-20 °C) until metabolite measurements. Retroperitoneal adipose tissue (RPAT) pads were aseptically dissected, placed into sterile conic tubes containing 10 mL sterile Dulbecco's Modified Eagle's Medium-Low Glucose (1 g/L) (DMEM) and immediately processed as describe below (Section 2.3). Animals were euthanized according to protocols for animal use, in agreement with the National Institutes of Health (NIH) Guidelines for the care and use of experimental animals. All experiments were approved by our Institutional Animal Care Committee (ID 03-05-12).

2.2. Plasma Measurements

Circulating levels of leptin (LEP), insulin (INS) and corticosterone (CORT) were determined by specific radioimmunoassays (RIAs) developed in our laboratory as previously validated and described [8]. LEP (standard curve 0.05–25 ng/mL) coefficients of variation (CV) intra- and inter-assay were 4%–7% and 9%–11%, respectively. INS (standard curve 0.08–10 ng/mL) CVs intra- and inter-assay were 3%–7% and 8%–11%, respectively. CORT (standard curve 0.05–50 μg/dL) CVs intra- and inter-assay were 4%–6% and 8%–10%, respectively. Peripheral glucose (Glu) and triglyceride (TG) levels were measured using commercial kits (Wiener Laboratory, Rosario, Argentina).

2.3. RPAT SVF Cell and Adipocyte Isolation

Fresh RPAT pads were dissected, weighed and digested with collagenase as previously reported [29]. Briefly, fat tissues were minced and digested using 1 mg/mL collagenase solution in DMEM (at 37 °C, for 1 h). After centrifugation (at 1000 rpm for 15 min), floating mature adipocytes were separated and reserved for adipocyte size analyses. The SVF cell-pellet was collected, filtered (in a 50-μm mesh nylon cloth) and washed with DMEM ($\times$3). SVF cells were then resuspended in DMEM supplemented with 10% (*vol/vol*) fetal bovine serum (FBS), 4-(2-hydroxyethyl)-1-piperazineethanesulfonic acid (HEPES, 20 nM), 100 IU/mL penicillin and 100 μg/mL streptomycin.

2.4. Adipocyte Size Analysis

The size of the isolated fat cells was measured as previously described [30], with minor changes. Briefly, a 50–150-μL aliquot from the top layer obtained as previously described (Section 2.3) was added to 450 μL DMEM. Five to ten microliters from the cell suspension were placed into the Neubauer chamber and coverslipped. Five representative pictures from each sample were taken using a Nikon Eclipse 50i microscope equipped with a camera (Nikon Digital Sight D5-U3, Melville, NY, USA). Cell diameters were measured with image analysis software (Image ProPlus6.0, Rockville, MD, USA). Values below 25 μm were discarded as they can be considered lipid droplets. The values were recorded and assigned to groups differing by 10 μm in diameter, creating a histogram with 10-μm bins. Histograms were used to determine whether the distribution of adipocyte diameters was normal or binomial and to assess the presence of different sized adipocyte subpopulations. We measured an average of 500–600 cells per site to calculate average adipocyte size.

2.5. SVF Cell Composition Analysis by Flow Cytometry

SVF cells from RPAT pads from CTR and MSG animals were isolated, and at least 2×10^5 cells (in 100 μL Phosphate-buffered saline (PBS)/0.5% Bovine Serum Albumin (BSA)) were incubated with fluorescent antibodies or respective isotype controls (1/50 diluted, for 1 h at 4 °C). After washing steps, flow cytometry was analyzed using a FACSCalibur flow cytometer (Becton Dickinson Biosciences, San Jose, CA, USA). A combination of cell surface markers was used to identify APCs as: $CD34^+/CD45^-/CD31^-$ [31]. The conjugated monoclonal antibodies used were: anti-rat

CD34:PE (PE: phycoerythrin), anti-rat CD45:FITC (FITC: fluorescein isothiocyanate) and anti-rat CD31:FITC (1 μg/1 × 10^6 cells, Santa Cruz Biotechnology Inc., Santa Cruz, CA, USA). Samples were analyzed using CellQuest Pro (Becton-Dickinson, San Jose, CA, USA) and FlowJo software (TreeStar, San Carlo, CA, USA).

2.6. RPAT SVF Cell Culture and Proliferation

RPAT SVF cells from CTR and MSG groups were seeded (2 × 10^4 cells/cm^2) in 24-well plates (Greiner Bio-One, Kremsmünster, Austria) and cultured in DMEM supplemented with 10% (v/v) FBS and antibiotics at 37 °C in a 5% CO_2-atmosphere [29]. Cells were left in culture to proliferate for up to 9 days (proliferation day: Pd 9). Every 24 h, cells (4 wells per day) were washed (×1) with PBS buffer, and 0.25% (w/v) trypsin solution (dissolved in PBS-EDTA) was added for 2–3 min at 37 °C; the cell suspension was then collected, and the cell number was determined in a Neubauer chamber.

2.7. Cell Differentiation Assay

Proliferating CTR and MSG SVF cells (having reached 70%–80% confluence after 5–6 days of culture) were induced to differentiate by the addition of a differentiation mix containing 5 μg/mL INS, 0.25 μM DXM, 0.5 mM 3-isobutyl-L-methylxanthine (IBMX) in DMEM-HEPES, supplemented with 10% FBS and antibiotics [29]. After 48 h, media were removed and replaced with fresh media containing 5 μg/mL INS, 10% FBS and antibiotics (DMEM + INS). Cell samples were harvested on different differentiation days (Dd) and processed for several determinations, as described below. Medium samples of Dd 10 were kept frozen at −20 °C until the measurement of LEP concentrations (Section 2.8.3).

2.8. Determinations

2.8.1. RNA Isolation and Real-Time Quantitative PCR

Total RNA was isolated from cells of both groups by the TRIzol extraction method (Invitrogen, Life Tech., Carlsbad, CA, USA). Total RNA was reverse-transcribed using random primers (250 ng) and RevertAid Reverse Transcriptase (200 U/μL, Thermo Scientific, Vilnius, Lithuania). Two microliters of cDNA were amplified with HOT FIRE Pol EvaGreen qPCR Mix Plus (Solis BioDyne, Tartu, Estonia) containing 0.5 μM of each specific primer, using the LightCycler Detection System (MJ Mini Opticon, Bio-Rad, CA, USA). PCR efficiency was near 1. Expression levels were analyzed for β-actin (ACTβ, reporter gene), adiponectin (Adipoq), GR, Leptin (Ob), MR, PPAR-γ2, CCAAT/enhancer binding protein alpha (C/EBPα), Pref-1, Wnt-10b and Zfp423 (the designed primers are shown in alphabetical order in Table 1). Relative changes in the expression level of one specific gene (ΔΔCt) were calculated by the ΔCt method.

2.8.2. Immunofluorescence Assay

CTR and MSG SVF cells were cultured in cover glasses and differentiated as mentioned before. On Dd 4, when it was previously detected that PPARγ2 reaches its highest expression [28], cells were fixed with 10% formalin (for 10–15 min), rinsed twice with PBS and treated with Triton 0.2% for 15 min. Subsequently, cells were incubated overnight with primary antibody PPAR-γ (2 μg/0.1 mL, Santa Cruz Biotechnology Inc., Santa Cruz, CA, USA). For visualization, we used secondary antibody Alexa-Fluor 594 labeled (Invitrogen Life Technologies, Carlsbad, CA, USA), and the nucleus staining was performed with Vectashield (Vector Laboratories, Burlingame, CA, USA) with 4′,6-diamidino-2-phenylindole (DAPI). Immunostaining of the negative control was performed (elimination of primary antibody), which did not show any antiserum immunolabeling. The percentage of PPAR-γ positive cells was expressed in relation to the total number of cells (by counting DAPI stained nucleus, 300–400 total cells per layer at 40× magnification). Immunoreactivity was visualized using a Nikon Eclipse 50i microscope equipped with a Nikon Digital Sight D5–U3 camera (Nikon Instruments Inc., Melville,

NY, USA) and NIS-Elements software (Nikon Instruments Inc., Melville, NY, USA). An image editing software program, Adobe Photoshop CS3 (Adobe Systems, San Jose, CA, USA) was used to adjust the contrast and brightness of microphotographs.

Table 1. Primers used for real-time polymerase chain reaction (PCR) analysis.

	Primers (5′-3′)	GBAN	bp
β-actin (ACTβ)	se, AGCCATGTACGTAGCCATCC as, ACCCTCATAGATGGGCACAG	NM_031144	115
Adiponectin (Adipoq)	se, AATCCTGCCCAGTCATGAAG as, TCTCCAGGAGTGCCATCTCT	NM_144744	159
CCAAT/enhancer binding protein alpha (C/EBPα)	se, CTGCGAGCACGAGACGTCTATAG as, TCCCGGGTAGTCAAAGTCACC	NM_012524	159
Glucocorticoid Receptor (GR)	se, TGCCCAGCATGCCGCTATCG as, GGGGTGAGCTGTGGTAATGCTGC	NW_047512	170
Mineralocorticoid Receptor (MR)	se, TCGCTCCGACCAAGGAGCCA as, TTCGCTGCCAGGCGGTTGAG	NM_013131	193
Leptin (Ob)	se, GAGACCTCCTCCATCTGCTG as, CTCAGCATTCAGGGCTAAGG	NM_013076	192
Peroxisome proliferator-activated receptor gamma 2 (PPAR-γ2)	se, AGGGGCCTGGACCTCTGCTG as, TCCGAAGTTGGTGGGCCAGA	NW_047696	185
Preadipocyte Factor 1 (Pref-1)	se, TGCTCCTGCTGGCTTTCGGC as, CCAGCCAGGCTCACACCTGC	NM_053744	113
Wingless-type MMTV integration site family member 10b (Wnt-10b)	se, AGGGGCTGCACATCGCCGTTC as, ACTGCGTGCATGACACCAGCAG	NW_047784	175
Zinc finger protein 423 (Zfp423)	se, CCGCGATCGGTGAAAGTTG as, CACGGCTGGATTTCCGATCA	NM_053583.2	121

Rat-specific primers for real-time PCR are listed in alphabetical order. se: sense; as: anti-sense; GBAN: GenBank Accession Number; amplicon length in bp.

2.8.3. Leptin Measurement

Medium LEP concentration was determined by specific RIA developed in our laboratory [32]. In this assay, the standard curve ranged between 0.05 and 25 ng/mL, with coefficients of intra- and inter-assay variation of 4%–7% and 9%–11%, respectively.

2.8.4. Cellular Lipid Content

Cell on Dd 10 were washed with PBS and fixed with 10% formalin (for 10–15 min) in PBS. Then, cells were quickly washed with PBS and stained for 1 h with Oil-Red O (ORO) solution (2:3 *vol/vol* H_2O:isopropanol, containing 0.5% ORO) [33]. After staining, cells were washed ($\times 3$ with PBS), and the dye from lipid droplets was extracted by adding 200 µL isopropanol (10 min). To quantify cell lipid content, sample OD was obtained at 510 nm in a spectrophotometer. Remaining cells were digested with 200 µL 0.25% trypsin solution in PBS-EDTA, at 37 °C for 24 h and centrifuged at $8000 \times g$ for 15 s. The OD of supernatants was read at 260 nm for DNA quantification, and cell lipid content (measured by ORO and expressed in OD units) was then expressed by the corresponding cell DNA content.

2.8.5. Cell Differentiation and Maturation

On Dd 10, differentiated cells were fixed with 10% formalin solution for 1 h at room temperature and then stained using the Papanicolaou technique. The percentage of differentiated cells was calculated by counting the total number of cells and that of cells containing lipid droplets, when visualized in a light microscope (after counting 200–250 total cells per layer, at $40\times$ magnification). Lipid-containing cells were assigned to 3 graded stages of maturation according to the nucleus position:

stage I (GI, central), stage II (GII, between central and peripheral) and stage III (GIII, completely peripheral) [34]. The percentage of cells corresponding to different maturation stages was expressed in relation to the total number of differentiated cells. Image analysis was assessed using a using a Nikon Eclipse 50i microscope equipped with a camera Nikon Digital Sight D5–U3 (Nikon Instruments Inc., Melville, NY, USA) and image analysis software (Image ProPlus 6.0, Rockville, MD, USA).

2.9. Statistical Analysis

Results are expressed as mean values $\pm$ SEM. Data were analyzed by ANOVA (one-way) followed by Fisher's test. To determine the differential effect of the treatment according to age, ANOVA (two-way) followed by the Bonferroni post-test were performed. For comparison of adipocyte size populations between groups, the non-parametric Mann–Whitney test was used. The normal or binomial distribution of adipocyte size data was determined by the Kruskal–Wallis test, followed by the Mann–Whitney test. In all cases, *p*-values lower than 0.05 were considered statistically significant. All statistical tests were performed using GraphPad Prism 6.0 (GraphPad Software Inc., San Diego, CA, USA).

3. Results

3.1. The MSG Rat Phenotype

Thirty-day-old MSG rats displayed lower BW (Table 2) and significantly higher LEP and CORT levels, as well as increased RPAT adipocyte diameter and RPAT/100 g of BW (Figure 1). Glu, INS and TG plasmatic levels remained similar to CTR litter-mate values (Table 2). As we have previously shown [28], 60-day-old MSG rats showed the same altered parameters as 30-day-old MSG rats (Table 2 and Figure 1), but when we compared all of these parameters in both ages, we found that the circulating levels of LEP and CORT, as well as RPAT/100 g of BW and RPAT adipocyte hypertrophy increased in MSG rats during development (Figure 1).

Table 2. Metabolic parameters of control (CTR) and Monosodium L-glutamate (MSG) treated rats.

	CTR 30-Day-Old	MSG 30-Day-Old	CTR 60-Day-Old	MSG 60-Day-Old
Body Weight (BW, g)	78.84 $\pm$ 1.78	71.23 $\pm$ 1.56 *	312.34 $\pm$ 9.32 [a,b,c]	242.50 $\pm$ 5.47 [*,a,b,c]
Insulin (INS, ng/mL)	0.25 $\pm$ 0.02	0.31 $\pm$ 0.04	2.01 $\pm$ 0.05 [a]	2.42 $\pm$ 0.35 [a]
Glucose (Glu, g/L)	1.26 $\pm$ 0.03	1.27 $\pm$ 0.03	1.17 $\pm$ 0.03	1.14 $\pm$ 0.06
Triglyceride (TG, g/L)	0.82 $\pm$ 0.06	1.19 $\pm$ 0.11	1.16 $\pm$ 0.14	1.24 $\pm$ 0.22

BW and plasma levels of INS, Glu and TG in CTR and MSG rats at 30 (*n* = 20 rats per group) and 60 days of age (*n* = 10 rats per group). Values are the means $\pm$ SEM. * *p* < 0.05 vs. CTR values of similar age. Two-way ANOVA: [a] those parameters significantly affected by age; [b] those parameters significantly affected by treatment; [c] a significant synergic effect of MSG treatment and age.

3.2. Proliferation Capacity of SVF Cells from MSG Rats at 30 Days of Age

After seeding, the proliferation capacity of RPAT SVF cells from both groups was assessed by counting the cell number every 24 h and recording those numbers throughout the proliferation period (Pd 1–Pd 9). Data indicated a significant (*p* < 0.05) decrease in the proliferation capacity of cells from the MSG group, which was noticed at the end of the proliferation period (158,083 $\pm$ 13,086 and 103,312 $\pm$ 17,028 cells/well on Pd 8 and 177,020 $\pm$ 11,097 and 115,688 $\pm$ 15,433 cells/well on Pd 9, in CTR and MSG groups, respectively). Moreover, the slopes of these curves were as follows: 21,722 $\pm$ 1457 and 16,628 $\pm$ 2055 cells per day, in CTR and MSG cell groups, respectively (*p* < 0.05).

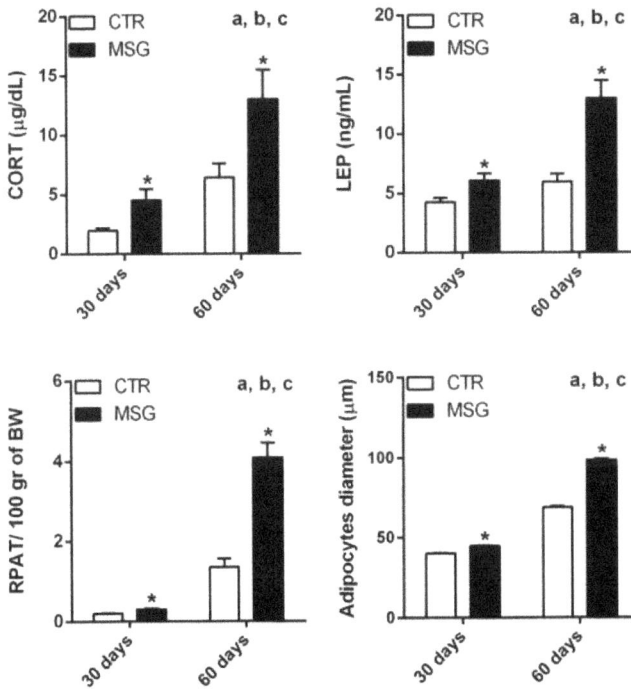

Figure 1. Comparison of hormone levels and retroperitoneal adipose tissue (RPAT) parameters from CTR and MSG rats. Corticosterone (CORT) and leptin (LEP) plasma levels; RPAT/100 g of BW and RPAT adipocyte size from rats at 30 and 60 days of age. Values are means $\pm$ SEM. * $p < 0.05$ vs. CTR values for similar ages. Two-way ANOVA: [a] those parameters significantly affected by age; [b] those significantly affected by treatment; [c] a significant synergic effect of MSG treatment and age.

3.3. Enhanced Terminal Differentiation of SVF Cells from MSG Rats at 30 Days of Age

On Dd 4, MSG cultured SVF cells showed a higher percentage of PPARγ positive cells (Figure 2A) in addition to enhanced PPARγ2 expression on the same culture day (Figure 2B). Intracellular lipid content and cell LEP release into the culture medium on Dd 10 were evaluated as parameters of adipocyte differentiation. As shown in Figure 3, MSG adipocytes displayed significantly ($p < 0.05$ vs. CTR values) higher lipid content (Figure 3A,B) and LEP release (Figure 3C). The expression of marker genes of fully-differentiated cells (on Dd 10), such as Ob, Adipoq, C/EBP-α and PPAR-γ2 mRNAs, were significantly ($p < 0.05$) higher in MSG than in CTR cells; conversely, no difference was noticed in Adipoq mRNA concentration (Figure 3D). Additionally, we determined the extent of adipogenesis in vitro by quantifying the percentage of differentiated cells at the end of the differentiation period (Dd 10). Our results showed no differences among groups for this parameter (53.99% $\pm$ 1.90% and 50.29% $\pm$ 2.8% of differentiated cells in the CTR and MSG groups, respectively; $n = 3$ independent experiments). However, differences in the percentage of cells at different maturation degrees were found. Indeed, MSG specimens showed a higher percentage of cells at an advanced maturation degree (GII and GIII; see Figure 3E,F), thus indicating that MSG cells mature faster than CTR cells.

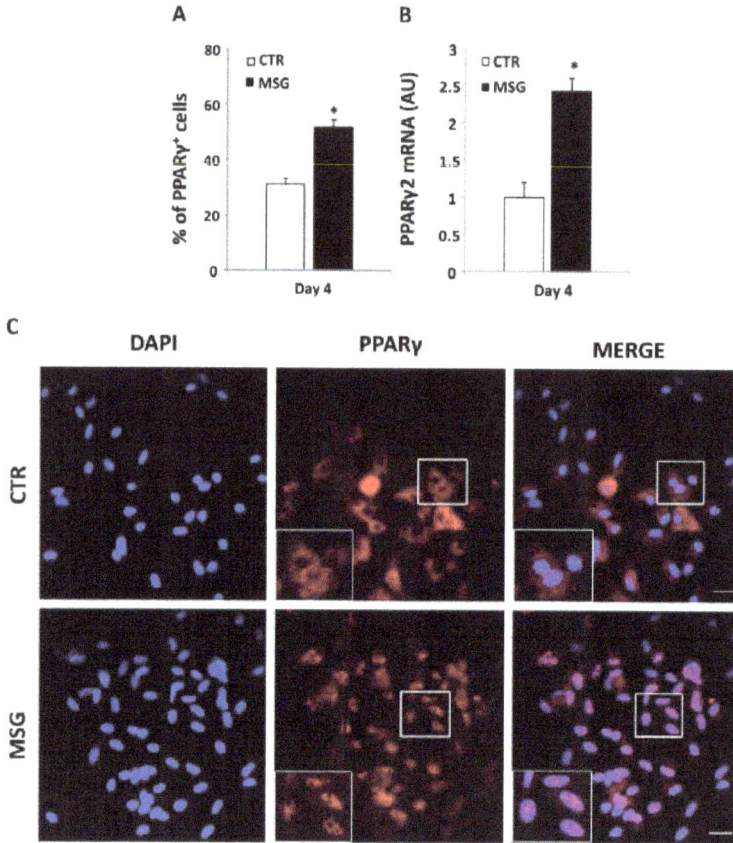

Figure 2. MSG cells display higher expression of Peroxisome proliferator-activated receptor (PPAR)γ2 during in vitro differentiation. (**A**) Percentage of PPARγ positive cells related to the total cell number counted by nucleus 4′,6-diamidino-2-phenylindole (DAPI) staining; (**B**) mRNA cell expression levels of PPARγ2 in CTR and MSG stromal vascular fraction (SVF) cells on Differentiation Day (Dd) 4 (AU: arbitrary units). Values are the means $\pm$ SEM (n = 5/6 different experiments). * $p < 0.05$ vs. CTR values; (**C**) Representative images of DAPI nucleus staining (blue), PPARγ positive cells (red) and merged image of CTR and MSG cells on Dd 4 (40× magnification, scale bar at 20 μm). The insert shows cytoplasmatic or nuclear PPARγ localization.

3.4. Age-Dependent Effect of GCs on APCs' Competency and Adipogenic Potential

Taking into account the differences found in the adipogenic capacity of MSG cells, the expression levels of several pro- and anti-adipogenic factors expressed by SVF cells were analyzed. MSG RPAT SVF cells expressed significantly ($p < 0.05$) lower levels of Pref-1 and Wnt-10b (Figure 4), whereas the expression of MR and GR genes remained the same. These results are different from those previously found for SVF cells from MSG rats at 60 days of age, where anti-adipogenic factors showed higher expression and the MR mRNA level was lower [28]. Similarly, the expression levels of Zfp423 and PPARγ2 were higher in SVF cells from MSG rats at 30 days of age (Figure 4), in contrast with the corresponding values previously found for SVF cells from MSG rats at 60 days of age [28]. Taken together, these data clearly indicate that high GC plasmatic levels induce a different effect on APCs' adipogenic competency, a fact probably dependent on the differential cell pattern of MR gene expression.

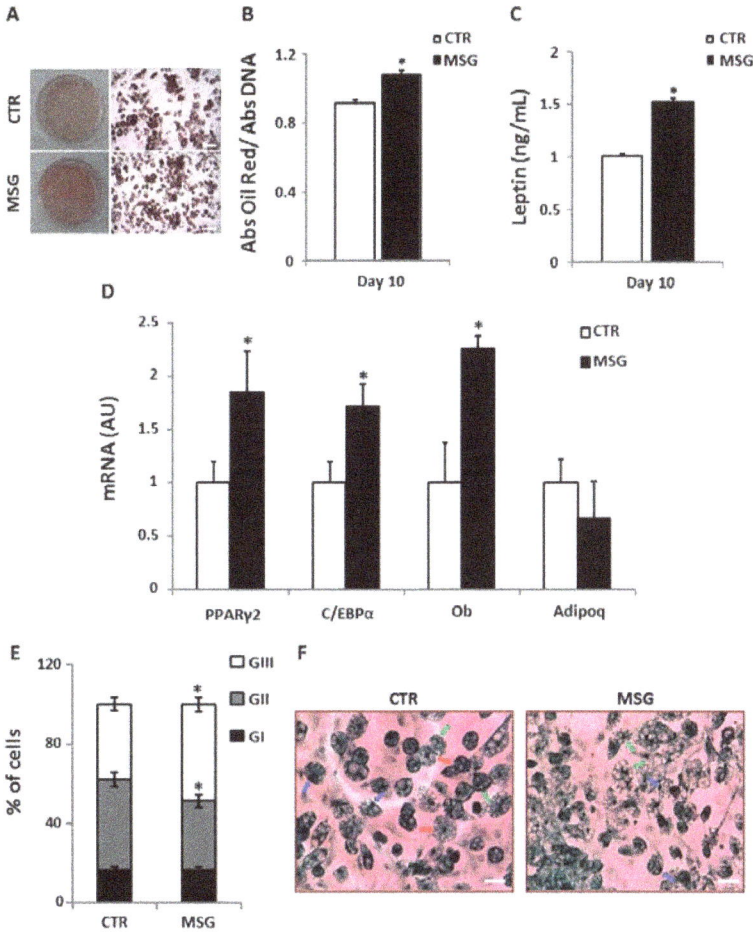

Figure 3. MSG cells exhibit increased in vitro adipocyte differentiation. (**A**) Macroscopic (left panel) and microscopic (right panel, magnification 10×, scale bars at 200 μm) views of the Oil Red O-stained dishes; (**B**) Quantification of intracellular lipid accumulation; (**C**) cell leptin secretion (*n* = 5/6 different experiments with 10/12 wells per day per experiment) and (**D**) cell mRNA expression levels of PPAR-γ2, CCAAT/enhancer binding protein (C/EBP)α, Leptin (Ob) and Adiponectin (Adipoq) on Differentiation day (Dd) 10 of SVF cells isolated from RPAT pads of 30 day-old CTR and MSG male rats (*n* = 5/6 different experiments) (AU: arbitrary units); (**E**) Percentages of cells according to their stages of maturation; (**F**) Representative fields containing in vitro differentiated CTR and MSG adipocytes (stained on Dd 10, magnification 40×, scale bars at 20 μm), displaying different degrees of maturation depending on the nucleus position: GI, central (red arrow); GII, displaced from the center (green arrow); and GIII: fully peripheral (blue arrow) (*n* = 4/5 different experiments; data from 200/250 cells were recorded in each experiment). Values are means ± SEM *, *p* < 0.05 vs. CTR values.

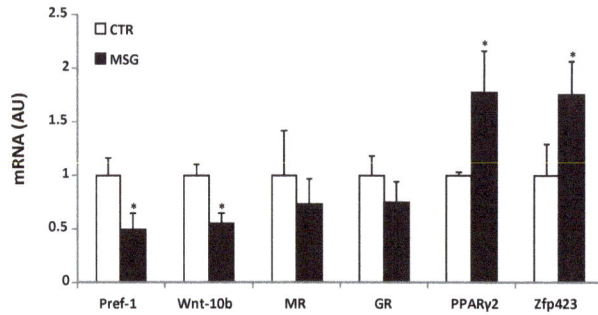

Figure 4. MSG SVF cells displayed higher competency, but lower anti-adipogenic factors expression. RPAT-SVF cell mRNA levels of anti-adipogenic (Pref-1 and Wnt-10b), glucocorticoid and mineralocorticoid receptors (GR and MR) and competency markers (PPAR-γ2 and Zfp423) from CTR and MSG male rats (AU: arbitrary units).Values are means ± SEM (*n* = 5/6 different experiments). * *p* < 0.05 vs. CTR values.

3.5. High Peripheral GC Levels Do Not Modify APC Number over Development

The adipogenic population ($CD34^+$/$CD31^-$/$CD45^-$) contained in the RPAT SVF from 30- and 60-day-old rats from both groups was evaluated in order to assess a possible GC effect on APC number. Interestingly, GCs exposure did not change the APC number at any age studied (Figure 5). These data strongly suggest that the main GC effect on SFV cells is on APCs' competency rather than on cell number.

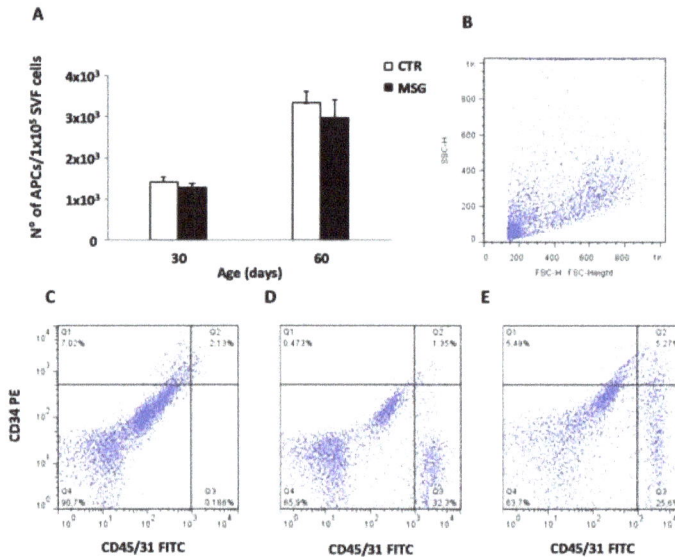

Figure 5. High GC exposure does not change adipocyte precursor cells (APCs) number. (**A**) Number of APCs in SVF from CTR and MSG animals at both ages. Adipocyte progenitors were identified by flow cytometry analysis using the $CD34^+$/$CD31^-$/$CD45^-$ profile; (**B**) Characteristic forward versus side scatter dot plot of freshly-isolated SVF cells from RPAT. Fluorescence profiles obtained for (**C**) IgG isotype control FITC conjugated combined with CD34 PE staining; (**D**) IgG1 isotype control PE conjugated combined with CD45/CD31 FITC staining and (**E**) APC subset (upper left quadrant). FITC: fluorescein isothiocyanate; PE: phycoerythrin. Values are means ± SEM (*n* = 3/4 different experiments).

3.6. Relationship between APCs' Competency and Adipogenic Capacity in MSG Rats

As described above, APCs from MSG rats at 30 days of age displayed an increased competency and differentiated rapidly when compared to CTR cells. Therefore, in order to establish any possible relationship between these data and the characteristic of in vivo RPAT mass expansion, the size distribution of mature adipocytes contained in RPAT pads from CTR and MSG rats of both age groups (Figure 6) was determined. Our data indicate that adipocytes from 30-day-old MSG animals were hypertrophic vs. age-matched CTR cells (Figure 6, upper panel). However, the smaller size of all adipocytes from 30-day-old rats compared to those from 60-day-old rats suggests that newly-generated adipocytes appeared at 30 days of age, regardless of the group examined. Interestingly, the profile of adipocyte size found in RPAT pads from 60-day-old MSG rats was conspicuous. In fact, while two adipocyte populations were found in the MSG group, one smaller and the other larger, a unique adipocyte size (intermediate) population characterizes CTR RPAT pads (Figure 6, lower panel). These data reveal that the in vivo activation of the adipogenic process could be dependent on a higher APCs competency in the 30-day-old MSG rat.

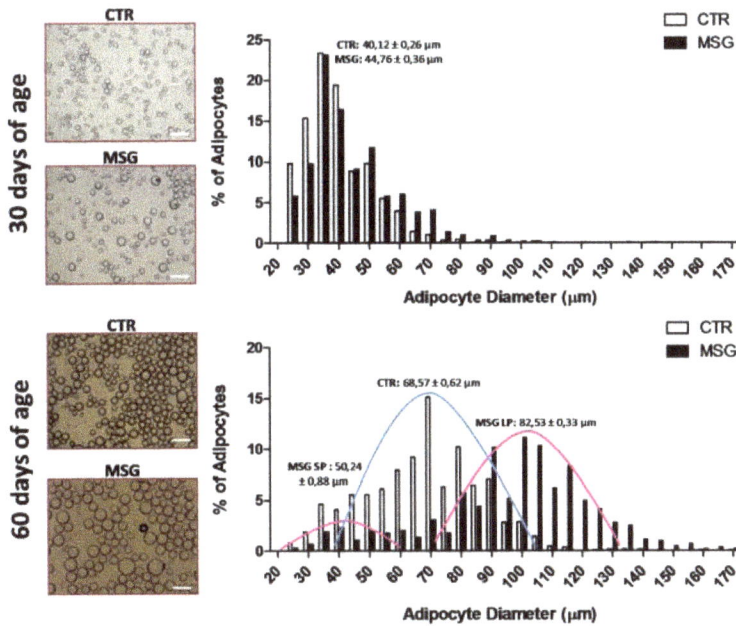

Figure 6. In vivo adipogenesis occurs in MSG animals. Adipocyte size distribution in RPAT depot from CTR and MSG rats at 30 (upper panel) and 60 days of age (lower panel). Purple and blue lines represent MSG (MSG SP: MSG small population; MSG LP: MSG large population) and CTR adipocyte populations, respectively. Representative images of mature adipocytes in cell suspension are shown for each group (magnification 10×, scale bars at 200 μm). Values are the means ± SEM (*n* = 3 animals per group).

4. Discussion

Enhanced VAT is associated with an increased risk of the development of several pathologies, such as diabetes mellitus type 2 and cardiovascular disease. Conversely, SCAT function is considered as protective against them [35,36]. This difference has been attributed, at least in part, to a higher adipogenic capacity of SCAT [37]. However, a system has been recently developed for the inducible and permanent labelling of mature adipocytes in vivo, which indicates that hyperplastic expansion of the AT occurs mainly at the epididymal, but not at the SCAT depot [38]. The present work showed that high chronic GC plasma levels are associated with early activation of adipogenesis (30-day-old MSG rats), supporting the concept that RPAT could expand through the generation of new adipocytes. In contrast, our previous studies revealed the inhibition of the RPAT adipogenic process at advanced age (60 day-old MSG rats) [28]. This age-/time-dependent shift in the adipogenic potential could be a consequence of changes in the expression levels of APCs' competency factors.

GCs have diverse effects on both AT functions [39,40] and distribution [41,42], favoring an increase in VAT, but not in SCAT mass. MSG rats share several features of the human CS phenotype, which is characterized by chronic high circulating levels of GC, enhanced AT mass and adipocyte size and an altered pattern of adipokine secretion, among others. In the MSG rat phenotype, restoring to normal the peripheral levels of GC reverses most of such dysfunctions [43]. Our present data indicate that the MSG animal phenotype is already established at 30 days of age, and some characteristic alterations get differentially worse over time.

Regarding the terminal stage of adipogenesis, an increase in all differentiation parameters was observed in MSG cells from 30-day-old rats. According to these findings, the expression of anti-adipogenic factors, such as Pref-1 and Wnt-10b decreased in undifferentiated MSG cells. In fact, the pro-adipogenic action of GCs is due to its inhibitory effect on Pref-1 and Wnt/b-catenin signaling pathway expression [21]. As mentioned above, these results show evidence of a dual behavior of the adipogenic process by itself in a GC-rich endogenous environment, characterized by adipogenesis activation at an initial step and the subsequent inhibition of the process, as shown before [28].

Cristancho et al. [15] distinguished between two functional terms: cell competency and cell commitment, where adipogenic competency refers to the cell's ability to differentiate into adipocyte upon the addition of defined stimuli, and adipogenic commitment indicates the multipotent cell type fate to undergo its conversion into adipocyte. Within this context, the adipogenic potential of an AT pad depends, besides any adipogenic stimulus environment, on the number and competency of APCs present in the local SVF. GCs are known to inhibit the proliferation capacity of APCs and to play an important role driving APCs to differentiate into adipocytes.

Over the last few years, great effort has been made to find cell surface markers that unequivocally identify APCs applying diverse criteria. Most of them agree that the CD34 antigen can distinguish between cells that are able or not to differentiate into mature adipocytes [44–46]. Interestingly, the expansion of different AT pads, both in mouse and human obese phenotypes, has been proposed to depend on changes in progenitor cell number [10,37,47]. To our knowledge, the effect of chronic exposure to high GC levels on APCs number in VAT pad has not been yet explored. In fact, our study is the first to show that APCs number in the SVF of RPAT from MSG rats is not altered at 30 or 60 days of age, and consequently, this parameter does not seem to be responsible for the changes observed in their adipogenic potential.

Zfp423 has been described as a marker of APCs competency, because it regulates PPARγ2 expression throughout the amplification of SMAD protein activity [17]. Thus, since PPARγ2 plays a key role within the overall adipogenic process, we are persuaded that PPARγ2 should be considered as a competency factor by itself. In SVF cells from 30 day-old MSG rats, the levels of PPARγ2 and Zfp423 mRNA were higher than in CTR SVF cells, which indicates high APC competency. These data are opposite to those found in 60 day-old MSG rat cells where both PPARγ2 and Zfp423 mRNA levels were low. Our results demonstrate that changes in APCs competency are responsible for the different adipogenic capacities of SVF cells from MSG rats of 30 and 60 days of age.

In obese phenotypes, a recruitment of immune cells occurs in VAT, including macrophages, lymphocytes and neutrophils, thus contributing to the development of a chronic inflammatory state [48–51]. Furthermore, there is a macrophage polarization toward the M1 type, which secretes pro-inflammatory cytokines (e.g., TNFα, IL1β and MCP-1) to the detriment of the anti-inflammatory M2 type (IL-10) [52,53]. These pro-inflammatory macrophage-secreted factors have been involved in an antiadipogenic activity, by decreasing the expression levels of adipogenic markers, such as aP2 and

PPARγ2 in human and 3T3-L1 preadipocytes [54,55]. The role of GCs mediating the inflammatory response in AT depends on the MR or GR activation, which will determine a pro- or anti-inflammatory response, respectively, due to the decrease or increase of pro-inflammatory cytokines' secretion [26]. Nevertheless, CS patients display increased adiposity, but the establishment of a chronic inflammatory state is controversial [56,57]. We have previously shown that RPAT expression of TNFα, IL-6, MCP-1 and F4/80 does not increase in 60-day-old MSG rats, probably due to the anti-inflammatory effect of GCs exerted through GR activation [28]. In this regard, further studies are needed to evaluate the AT inflammatory response in MSG rats at 30 days of age.

Pro-adipogenic activity of GCs has been clearly recognized; then, the co-existence of high GC levels and a reduced adipogenic cell capacity could be indicative of changes in the RPAT sensitivity to GCs. This could explain why high levels of a potent adipogenic factor do not stimulate the process continuously, preventing hypertrophy of VAT. It is known that aldosterone is able to promote differentiation of APCs in both 3T3-L1 [58] and human preadipocytes. Notably, expression silencing or activity blocking of MR in both cell types prevent adipogenesis, but this is not the same for GR inactivation [25,26]. We found that MR mRNA levels did not change in 30-day-old MSG rats, though they decreased in 60-day-old rats, coinciding with the low adipogenic capacity found in them [28]. This could suggest that MR is involved in the development of a GC-resistant state, although the participation of MR or GR in the biological actions of GCs upon the AT is still being debated [25–27]. However, the contribution of GR to the lack of GC effect cannot be ruled out, despite not finding any change in cell GR expression.

The distribution of adipocyte size has been previously used to determine the presence of AT hypertrophy and/or hyperplasia [10]. Analysis of the adipocyte size distribution in RPAT from MSG animals at both ages showed interesting data. Indeed, MSG rats at 30 days of age displayed one hypertrophic adipocyte population, while MSG rats at 60 days of age presented two adipocyte size populations, one smaller and another larger than the only adipocyte size population found in CTR pads. The additional presence of small adipocytes in 60-day-old MSG rats suggests that increased APC competency (seen in 30-day-old MSG rats) leads to adipogenesis stimulation between Days 30 and 60 of age.

5. Conclusions

The present study shows that changes in competency and/or number of APCs are two independent mechanisms that can modulate the adipogenic potential of an AT depot. In particular, long term in vivo cell exposure to high GC levels induces an early stimulation and subsequent inhibition of RPAT adipogenesis, a dual age-dependent process, mainly due to changes in APCs' competency, but not in number. Metabolic dysfunctions associated with obesity are dependent on the development of adipocyte hypertrophy; hence, the possibility of increased APC competency and/or number could result in the activation of the adipogenic process by activating hyperplastic VAT expansion, with consequent benefits for health.

Acknowledgments: This work was supported by grants from CONICET (PIP-2013-2015-0198), Fondo para la Investigación Científica y Tecnológica (FONCYT, PICT-2012-1415 and PICT-2013-0930) and Fondation pour la Recherche en Endocrinologie, Diabetologie et Metabolisme (FPREDM 062013). The authors are grateful to Rebecca Doyle for careful manuscript edition/correction. A.A., G.M., E.S. and A.G. are researchers from the National Research Council of Argentina (CONICET).

Author Contributions: A.G., M.G.Z. and E.S. conceived of and designed the experiments. M.G.Z. performed the research. A.A., D.C. and A.P. participated in the cell culture and qPCR assays and analyses. G.M. participated in the flow cytometry experiments and analyses. A.G. and M.G.Z. analyzed all of the data and wrote the manuscript. E.S. participated in the critical revision and correction of the final manuscript. All authors read and approved the final manuscript.

Conflicts of Interest: The authors declare no conflicts of interest.

References

1. Peckett, A.J.; Wright, D.C.; Riddell, M.C. The effects of glucocorticoids on adipose tissue lipid metabolism. *Metabolism* **2011**, *60*, 1500–1510. [CrossRef] [PubMed]
2. Lee, M.J.; Fried, S.K. Integration of hormonal and nutrient signals that regulate leptin synthesis and secretion. *Am. J. Physiol. Endocrinol. Metab.* **2009**, *296*, E1230–E1238. [CrossRef] [PubMed]
3. Lee, M.J.; Pramyothin, P.; Karastergiou, K.; Fried, S.K. Deconstructing the roles of glucocorticoids in adipose tissue biology and the development of central obesity. *Biochim. Biophys. Acta* **2014**, *1842*, 473–481. [CrossRef] [PubMed]
4. Rebuffé-Scrive, M.; Krotkiewski, M.; Elfverson, J.; Björntorp, P. Muscle and adipose tissue morphology and metabolism in Cushing's syndrome. *J. Clin. Endocrinol. Metab.* **1988**, *67*, 1122–1128. [CrossRef] [PubMed]
5. Mayo-Smith, W.; Hayes, C.W.; Biller, B.M.; Klibanski, A.; Rosenthal, H.; Rosenthal, D.I. Body fat distribution measured with CT: Correlations in healthy subjects, patients with anorexia nervosa, and patients with Cushing syndrome. *Radiology* **1989**, *170*, 515–518. [CrossRef] [PubMed]
6. Chanson, P.; Salenave, S. Metabolic syndrome in Cushing's syndrome. *Neuroendocrinology* **2010**, *92* (Suppl. 1), 96–101. [CrossRef] [PubMed]
7. Nemeroff, C.B.; Grant, L.D.; Bissette, G.; Ervin, G.N.; Harrell, L.E.; Prange, A.J. Growth, endocrinological and behavioral deficits after monosodium L-glutamate in the neonatal rat: Possible involvement of arcuate dopamine neuron damage. *Psychoneuroendocrinology* **1977**, *2*, 179–196. [CrossRef]
8. Perelló, M.; Gaillard, R.C.; Chisari, A.; Spinedi, E. Adrenal enucleation in MSG-damaged hyperleptinemic male rats transiently restores adrenal sensitivity to leptin. *Neuroendocrinology* **2003**, *78*, 176–184. [CrossRef] [PubMed]
9. Moreno, G.; Perelló, M.; Camihort, G.; Luna, G.; Console, G.; Gaillard, R.C.; Spinedi, E. Impact of transient correction of increased adrenocortical activity in hypothalamo-damaged, hyperadipose female rats. *Int. J. Obes.* **2006**, *30*, 73–82. [CrossRef] [PubMed]
10. Joe, A.W.B.; Yi, L.; Even, Y.; Vogl, A.W.; Rossi, F.M.V. Depot-specific differences in adipogenic progenitor abundance and proliferative response to high-fat diet. *Stem Cells* **2009**, *27*, 2563–2570. [CrossRef] [PubMed]
11. Wang, M.Y.; Grayburn, P.; Chen, S.; Ravazzola, M.; Orci, L.; Unger, R.H. Adipogenic capacity and the susceptibility to type 2 diabetes and metabolic syndrome. *Proc. Natl. Acad. Sci. USA* **2008**, *105*, 6139–6144. [CrossRef] [PubMed]
12. Franck, N.; Stenkula, K.G.; Ost, A.; Lindström, T.; Strålfors, P.; Nystrom, F.H. Insulin-induced GLUT4 translocation to the plasma membrane is blunted in large compared with small primary fat cells isolated from the same individual. *Diabetologia* **2007**, *50*, 1716–1722. [CrossRef] [PubMed]
13. Skurk, T.; Alberti-Huber, C.; Herder, C.; Hauner, H. Relationship between adipocyte size and adipokine expression and secretion. *J. Clin. Endocrinol. Metab.* **2007**, *92*, 1023–1033. [CrossRef] [PubMed]
14. Wåhlen, K.; Sjölin, E.; Löfgren, P. Role of fat cell size for plasma leptin in a large population based sample. *Exp. Clin. Endocrinol. Diabetes* **2011**, *119*, 291–294. [CrossRef] [PubMed]
15. Cristancho, A.G.; Lazar, M.A. Forming functional fat: a growing understanding of adipocyte differentiation. *Nat. Rev. Mol. Cell Biol.* **2011**, *12*, 722–734. [CrossRef] [PubMed]
16. Sengenès, C.; Lolmède, K.; Zakaroff-Girard, A.; Busse, R.; Bouloumié, A. Preadipocytes in the human subcutaneous adipose tissue display distinct features from the adult mesenchymal and hematopoietic stem cells. *J. Cell. Physiol.* **2005**, *205*, 114–122. [CrossRef] [PubMed]
17. Gupta, R.K.; Arany, Z.; Seale, P.; Mepani, R.J.; Ye, L.; Conroe, H.M.; Roby, Y.A.; Kulaga, H.; Reed, R.R.; Spiegelman, B.M. Transcriptional control of preadipocyte determination by Zfp423. *Nature* **2010**, *464*, 619–623. [CrossRef] [PubMed]
18. Tontonoz, P.; Spiegelman, B.M. Fat and beyond: the diverse biology of PPARgamma. *Annu. Rev. Biochem.* **2008**, *77*, 289–312. [CrossRef] [PubMed]
19. Smas, C.M.; Chen, L.; Zhao, L.; Latasa, M.J.; Sul, H.S. Transcriptional repression of pref-1 by glucocorticoids promotes 3T3-L1 adipocyte differentiation. *J. Biol. Chem.* **1999**, *274*, 12632–12641. [CrossRef] [PubMed]
20. Mulholland, D.J.; Dedhar, S.; Coetzee, G.A.; Nelson, C.C. Interaction of nuclear receptors with the Wnt/beta-catenin/Tcf signaling axis: Wnt you like to know? *Endocr. Rev.* **2005**, *26*, 898–915. [CrossRef] [PubMed]

21. Xiao, X.; Li, H.; Yang, J.; Qi, X.; Zu, X.; Yang, J.; Zhong, J.; Cao, R.; Liu, J.; Wen, G. Wnt/β-catenin signaling pathway and lipolysis enzymes participate in methylprednisolone induced fat differential distribution between subcutaneous and visceral adipose tissue. *Steroids* **2014**, *84*, 30–35. [CrossRef] [PubMed]

22. Christodoulides, C.; Lagathu, C.; Sethi, J.K.; Vidal-Puig, A. Adipogenesis and WNT signalling. *Trends Endocrinol. Metab. TEM* **2009**, *20*, 16–24. [CrossRef] [PubMed]

23. Wang, Y.; Hudak, C.; Sul, H.S. Role of preadipocyte factor 1 in adipocyte differentiation. *Clin. Lipidol.* **2010**, *5*, 109–115. [CrossRef] [PubMed]

24. Pantoja, C.; Huff, J.T.; Yamamoto, K.R. Glucocorticoid signaling defines a novel commitment state during adipogenesis in vitro. *Mol. Biol. Cell* **2008**, *19*, 4032–4041. [CrossRef] [PubMed]

25. Caprio, M.; Fève, B.; Claës, A.; Viengchareun, S.; Lombès, M.; Zennaro, M.C. Pivotal role of the mineralocorticoid receptor in corticosteroid-induced adipogenesis. *FASEB J.* **2007**, *21*, 2185–2194. [CrossRef] [PubMed]

26. Hoppmann, J.; Perwitz, N.; Meier, B.; Fasshauer, M.; Hadaschik, D.; Lehnert, H.; Klein, J. The balance between gluco- and mineralo-corticoid action critically determines inflammatory adipocyte responses. *J. Endocrinol.* **2010**, *204*, 153–164. [CrossRef] [PubMed]

27. Lee, M.J.; Fried, S.K. The glucocorticoid receptor, not the mineralocorticoid receptor, plays the dominant role in adipogenesis and adipokine production in human adipocytes. *Int. J. Obes.* **2014**, *38*, 1228–1233. [CrossRef] [PubMed]

28. Zubiría, M.G.; Vidal-Bravo, J.; Spinedi, E.; Giovambattista, A. Relationship between impaired adipogenesis of retroperitoneal adipose tissue and hypertrophic obesity: Role of endogenous glucocorticoid excess. *J. Cell. Mol. Med.* **2014**, *18*, 1549–1561. [CrossRef] [PubMed]

29. Giovambattista, A.; Gaillard, R.C.; Spinedi, E. Ghrelin gene-related peptides modulate rat white adiposity. *Vitam. Horm.* **2008**, *77*, 171–205. [PubMed]

30. Tchoukalova, Y.D.; Harteneck, D.A.; Karwoski, R.A.; Tarara, J.; Jensen, M.D. A quick, reliable, and automated method for fat cell sizing. *J. Lipid Res.* **2003**, *44*, 1795–1801. [CrossRef] [PubMed]

31. Maumus, M.; Sengenès, C.; Decaunes, P.; Zakaroff-Girard, A.; Bourlier, V.; Lafontan, M.; Galitzky, J.; Bouloumié, A. Evidence of in situ proliferation of adult adipose tissue-derived progenitor cells: Influence of fat mass microenvironment and growth. *J. Clin. Endocrinol. Metab.* **2008**, *93*, 4098–4106. [CrossRef] [PubMed]

32. Giovambattista, A.; Piermaría, J.; Suescun, M.O.; Calandra, R.S.; Gaillard, R.C.; Spinedi, E. Direct effect of ghrelin on leptin production by cultured rat white adipocytes. *Obesity (Silver Spring)* **2006**, *14*, 19–27. [CrossRef] [PubMed]

33. Chen, J.; Dodson, M.V.; Jiang, Z. Cellular and molecular comparison of redifferentiation of intramuscular- and visceral-adipocyte derived progeny cells. *Int. J. Biol. Sci.* **2010**, *6*, 80–88. [CrossRef] [PubMed]

34. Grégoire, F.; Todoroff, G.; Hauser, N.; Remacle, C. The stroma-vascular fraction of rat inguinal and epididymal adipose tissue and the adipoconversion of fat cell precursors in primary culture. *Biol. Cell* **1990**, *69*, 215–222. [CrossRef]

35. Wang, Y.; Rimm, E.B.; Stampfer, M.J.; Willett, W.C.; Hu, F.B. Comparison of abdominal adiposity and overall obesity in predicting risk of type 2 diabetes among men. *Am. J. Clin. Nutr.* **2005**, *81*, 555–563. [PubMed]

36. Tankó, L.B.; Bagger, Y.Z.; Alexandersen, P.; Larsen, P.J.; Christiansen, C. Peripheral adiposity exhibits an independent dominant antiatherogenic effect in elderly women. *Circulation* **2003**, *107*, 1626–1631. [CrossRef] [PubMed]

37. Macotela, Y.; Emanuelli, B.; Mori, M.A.; Gesta, S.; Schulz, T.J.; Tseng, Y.H.; Kahn, C.R. Intrinsic differences in adipocyte precursor cells from different white fat depots. *Diabetes* **2012**, *61*, 1691–1699. [CrossRef] [PubMed]

38. Wang, Q.A.; Tao, C.; Gupta, R.K.; Scherer, P.E. Tracking adipogenesis during white adipose tissue development, expansion and regeneration. *Nat. Med.* **2013**, *19*, 1338–1344. [CrossRef] [PubMed]

39. Hauner, H.; Schmid, P.; Pfeiffer, E.F. Glucocorticoids and insulin promote the differentiation of human adipocyte precursor cells into fat cells. *J. Clin. Endocrinol. Metab.* **1987**, *64*, 832–835. [CrossRef] [PubMed]

40. Lee, M.J.; Gong, D.W.; Burkey, B.F.; Fried, S.K. Pathways regulated by glucocorticoids in omental and subcutaneous human adipose tissues: A microarray study. *Am. J. Physiol. Endocrinol. Metab.* **2011**, *300*, E571–E580. [CrossRef] [PubMed]

41. Geer, E.B.; Shen, W.; Gallagher, D.; Punyanitya, M.; Looker, H.C.; Post, K.D.; Freda, P.U. MRI assessment of lean and adipose tissue distribution in female patients with Cushing's disease. *Clin. Endocrinol. (Oxf.)* **2010**, *73*, 469–475. [CrossRef] [PubMed]

42. Rockall, A.G.; Sohaib, S.A.; Evans, D.; Kaltsas, G.; Isidori, A.M.; Monson, J.P.; Besser, G.M.; Grossman, A.B.; Reznek, R.H. Computed tomography assessment of fat distribution in male and female patients with Cushing's syndrome. *Eur. J. Endocrinol.* **2003**, *149*, 561–567. [CrossRef] [PubMed]

43. Perelló, M.; Moreno, G.; Gaillard, R.C.; Spinedi, E. Glucocorticoid-dependency of increased adiposity in a model of hypothalamic obesity. *Neuro Endocrinol. Lett.* **2004**, *25*, 119–126. [PubMed]

44. Miranville, A.; Heeschen, C.; Sengenès, C.; Curat, C.A.; Busse, R.; Bouloumié, A. Improvement of postnatal neovascularization by human adipose tissue-derived stem cells. *Circulation* **2004**, *110*, 349–355. [CrossRef] [PubMed]

45. Rodeheffer, M.S.; Birsoy, K.; Friedman, J.M. Identification of white adipocyte progenitor cells in vivo. *Cell* **2008**, *135*, 240–249. [CrossRef] [PubMed]

46. Maumus, M.; Peyrafitte, J.; D'Angelo, R.; Fournier-Wirth, C.; Bouloumié, A.; Casteilla, L.; Sengenès, C.; Bourin, P. Native human adipose stromal cells: Localization, morphology and phenotype. *Int. J. Obes.* **2011**, *35*, 1141–1153. [CrossRef] [PubMed]

47. Tchoukalova, Y.; Koutsari, C.; Jensen, M. Committed subcutaneous preadipocytes are reduced in human obesity. *Diabetologia* **2007**, *50*, 151–157. [CrossRef] [PubMed]

48. Elgazar-Carmon, V.; Rudich, A.; Hadad, N.; Levy, R. Neutrophils transiently infiltrate intra-abdominal fat early in the course of high-fat feeding. *J. Lipid Res.* **2008**, *49*, 1894–1903. [CrossRef] [PubMed]

49. Talukdar, S.; Oh, D.Y.; Bandyopadhyay, G.; Li, D.; Xu, J.; McNelis, J.; Lu, M.; Li, P.; Yan, Q.; Zhu, Y.; et al. Neutrophils mediate insulin resistance in mice fed a high-fat diet through secreted elastase. *Nat. Med.* **2012**, *18*, 1407–1412. [CrossRef] [PubMed]

50. Nishimura, S.; Manabe, I.; Nagasaki, M.; Eto, K.; Yamashita, H.; Ohsugi, M.; Otsu, M.; Hara, K.; Ueki, K.; Sugiura, S.; et al. CD8+ effector T cells contribute to macrophage recruitment and adipose tissue inflammation in obesity. *Nat. Med.* **2009**, *15*, 914–920. [CrossRef] [PubMed]

51. Choe, S.S.; Huh, J.Y.; Hwang, I.J.; Kim, J.I.; Kim, J.B. Adipose tissue remodeling: Its role in energy metabolism and metabolic disorders. *Front. Endocrinol. (Lausanne)* **2016**, *7*, 30. [CrossRef] [PubMed]

52. Chawla, A.; Nguyen, K.D.; Goh, Y.P.S. Macrophage-mediated inflammation in metabolic disease. *Nat. Rev. Immunol.* **2011**, *11*, 738–749. [CrossRef] [PubMed]

53. Lumeng, C.N.; Bodzin, J.L.; Saltiel, A.R. Obesity induces a phenotypic switch in adipose tissue macrophage polarization. *J. Clin. Invest.* **2007**, *117*, 175–184. [CrossRef] [PubMed]

54. Lacasa, D.; Taleb, S.; Keophiphath, M.; Miranville, A.; Clement, K. Macrophage-secreted factors impair human adipogenesis: Involvement of proinflammatory state in preadipocytes. *Endocrinology* **2007**, *148*, 868–877. [CrossRef] [PubMed]

55. Lu, C.; Kumar, P.A.; Fan, Y.; Sperling, M.A.; Menon, R.K. A novel effect of growth hormone on macrophage modulates macrophage-dependent adipocyte differentiation. *Endocrinology* **2010**, *151*, 2189–2199. [CrossRef] [PubMed]

56. Barahona, M.J.; Sucunza, N.; Resmini, E.; Fernández-Real, J.M.; Ricart, W.; Moreno-Navarrete, J.M.; Puig, T.; Farrerons, J.; Webb, S.M. Persistent body fat mass and inflammatory marker increases after long-term cure of Cushing's syndrome. *J. Clin. Endocrinol. Metab.* **2009**, *94*, 3365–3371. [CrossRef] [PubMed]

57. Setola, E.; Losa, M.; Lanzi, R.; Lucotti, P.; Monti, L.D.; Castrignanò, T.; Galluccio, E.; Giovanelli, M.; Piatti, P. Increased insulin-stimulated endothelin-1 release is a distinct vascular phenotype distinguishing Cushing's disease from metabolic syndrome. *Clin. Endocrinol.* **2007**, *66*, 586–592. [CrossRef] [PubMed]

58. Rondinone, C.M.; Rodbard, D.; Baker, M.E. Aldosterone stimulated differentiation of mouse 3T3-L1 cells into adipocytes. *Endocrinology* **1993**, *132*, 2421–2426. [PubMed]

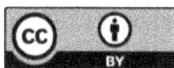

© 2016 by the authors. Licensee MDPI, Basel, Switzerland. This article is an open access article distributed under the terms and conditions of the Creative Commons Attribution (CC BY) license (http://creativecommons.org/licenses/by/4.0/).

nutrients

Article

Natural Course of Metabolically Healthy Overweight/Obese Subjects and the Impact of Weight Change

Ruizhi Zheng [1,†], Chengguo Liu [2,†], Chunmei Wang [3,†], Biao Zhou [4], Yi Liu [1], Feixia Pan [1], Ronghua Zhang [4,*] and Yimin Zhu [1,*]

[1] Department of Epidemiology & Biostatistics, School of Public Health, Zhejiang University, Hangzhou 310058, Zhejiang, China; canprezrz@126.com (R.Z.); lyzju_2012@163.com (Y.L.); pfx19911119@163.com (F.P.)

[2] Department of Endocrinology and Institute of Cardiovascular Diseases, Zhejiang Putuo Hospital, Zhoushan 316100, Zhejiang, China; Prylcg@mail.zsptt.zj.cn

[3] Tongxiang Center for Disease Control and Prevention, Tongxiang 314500, Zhejiang, China; chunmei328@sina.com

[4] Institute of Nutrition and Food Safety, Zhejiang Center for Disease Control and Prevention, Hangzhou 310000, Zhejiang, China; bzhou@cdc.zj.cn

* Correspondence: rhzhang@cdc.zj.cn (R.Z.); zhuym@zju.edu.cn (Y.Z.); Tel.: +86-571-8711-5111 (R.Z.); +86-571-8820-8138 (Y.Z.); Fax: +86-571-8711-5111 (R.Z.); +86-571-8820-8198 (Y.Z.)

† These authors contributed equally to this work.

Received: 19 May 2016; Accepted: 11 July 2016; Published: 15 July 2016

Abstract: Few studies have described the characteristics of metabolically healthy individuals with excess fat in the Chinese population. This study aimed to prospectively investigate the natural course of metabolically healthy overweight/obese (MH-OW/OB) adults, and to assess the impact of weight change on developing metabolic abnormalities. During 2009–2010, 525 subjects without any metabolic abnormalities or other obesity-related diseases were evaluated and reevaluated after 5 years. The subjects were categorized into two groups of overweight/obese and normal weight based on the criteria of BMI by 24.0 at baseline. At follow-up, the MH-OW/OB subjects had a significantly increased risk of developing metabolically abnormalities compared with metabolically healthy normal-weight (MH-NW) individuals (risk ratio: 1.35, 95% confidence interval: 1.17–1.49, *p* value < 0.001). In the groups of weight gain and weight maintenance, the MH-OW/OB subjects was associated with a larger increase in fasting glucose, triglycerides, systolic blood pressure, diastolic blood pressure and decrease in high-density lipoprotein cholesterol comparing with MH-NW subjects. In the weight loss group, no significant difference of changes of metabolic parameters was observed between MH-OW/OB and MH-NW adults. This study verifies that MH-OW/OB are different from MH-NW subjects. Weight management is needed for all individuals since weight change has a significant effect on metabolic health without considering the impact of weight change according to weight status.

Keywords: metabolically healthy; overweight and obese; weight change

1. Introduction

Obesity is a key risk factor for various diseases, including type 2 diabetes, cardiovascular disease (CVD), certain cancers, and musculoskeletal diseases [1]. However, it has been appreciated for many years that about 20% to 30% of obese adults exhibit fewer of these complications and do not meet all the criteria for metabolic syndrome [2]. Intense interest surrounds the "healthy" obese phenotype, which is defined as being obesity in the absence of metabolic syndrome (MetS), termed as metabolically healthy obesity (MHO) [3]. Despite the fact that there is no consensus on which criteria is preferable for defining MHO phenotype, longitudinal studies have suggested that this subtype of obesity are still at increased risk of diabetes and cardiovascular diseases [4–7]. Additionally, several studies have reported that MHO is not a permanent state and almost 30% to 50% of these individuals will convert to metabolically unhealthy status, with resultant increased cardiovascular risk [8,9]. Therefore, it has been speculated that the MHO subjects are not protected, but simply require additional time to develop adverse metabolic outcomes.

Weight change has a strong impact on metabolic status; however, several studies investigating the effects of weight loss by lifestyle intervention on metabolic status in the MHO subjects have yielded inconsistent results [10–12]. Most of these studies find that the MHO individuals obtain smaller improvements in MetS components from weight loss, compared with the metabolically abnormal obese (MAO) patients. Furthermore, it has been suggested that weight loss in postmenopausal MHO women may be unnecessary and paradoxically harmful given their favorable metabolic profiles [12]. Fabbrini et al. have evaluated the effect of a high-calorie diet on the metabolic status between the MHO and the MAO subjects [13]. The results demonstrate distinct differences in the response to weight gain. The MAO patients are predisposed to adverse metabolic effects of moderate weight gain, but not in the MHO subjects [13]. According to their conclusion, it can be speculated that the MHO subjects may maintain a healthy status in weight maintenance or even a little weight gain.

China has been experiencing an epidemic of obesity and metabolic disease in the last few decades; it has been estimated that almost 70% of Chinese adults are in the overweight and obesity category [14]. Furthermore, the Chinese population tend to accumulate fat intra-abdominally, and thus even lean subjects may have ectopic fat deposition and intra-abdominal obesity, accompanied with increasing cardiometabolic problems in overweight and obese subjects [15]. Our previous study found that 27.9% of obese participants are in metabolic health in the Chinese population [16]. However, little is known regarding the impact of weight changes on the metabolic profile for metabolically healthy overweight/obese subjects in Chinese population. Given this background, the aim of this study was to assess the metabolic response to 5-year weight change for metabolically healthy overweight/obese (MH-OW/OB) adults.

2. Materials and Methods

2.1. Subjects

During 2009–2010, the population aged over 30 and residing in the city of Tongxiang and Zhoushan in the Zhejiang province, China, were invited to participate in a health survey aimed at identifying risk factors for non-communicable diseases. A total of 3603 subjects participated in the prospective study, and data collected in 2009–2010 were used as the baseline for the present study. A clinical assessment was repeated 5 years later. This study was conducted according to the guidelines laid down in the Declaration of Helsinki and all procedures involving human subjects were approved by the Institutional Review Board of School of Medicine, Zhejiang University, Zhejiang, China (ethic approval code: ZGL201304-3). Written informed consents were obtained from all participants.

According to the objective for the current study, those with a history of chronic diseases were excluded (e.g., diabetes, cardiovascular disease, dyslipidemia, cancer, hypertension) ($n = 719$). After exclusion of those with body mass index (BMI) < 18.5 kg/m^2 ($n = 150$), and those who had missing anthropometric, metabolic detection data and questionnaire information ($n = 30$), 2704 participants were remained. Of these subjects, we selected those who had healthy metabolic status at baseline. Namely, all of the selected subjects had no metabolic abnormality of MetS definition of the International Diabetes Federation (IDF) criteria (waist circumference was not included in the definition of metabolic health because of collinearity with BMI), including elevated triglycerides (TG) ($\geq$1.7 mmol/L), low high-density lipoprotein cholesterol (HDL-C) (men < 1.03 mmol/L, women < 1.29 mmol/L), elevated systolic blood pressure (SBP) ($\geq$130 mm·Hg) or diastolic blood pressure (DBP) ($\geq$85 mm·Hg), elevated fasting plasma glucose (FPG) ($\geq$5.6 mmol/L) [17]. The selection yielded 630 subjects in metabolic health. After starting the study, 105 subjects (16.7%) were excluded for not attending a follow-up visit. Ultimately, 525 subjects were included in the analysis (Figure 1). General obesity was defined by BMI, which was recommended by the Working Group on Obesity in China (WGOC) [18]. There were 392 subjects in the normal weight category (BMI < 24.0 kg/m^2), 98 in the overweight category (BMI 24 textasciitilde 28 kg/m^2) and 35 in the obesity category (BMI $\geq$ 28 kg/m^2).

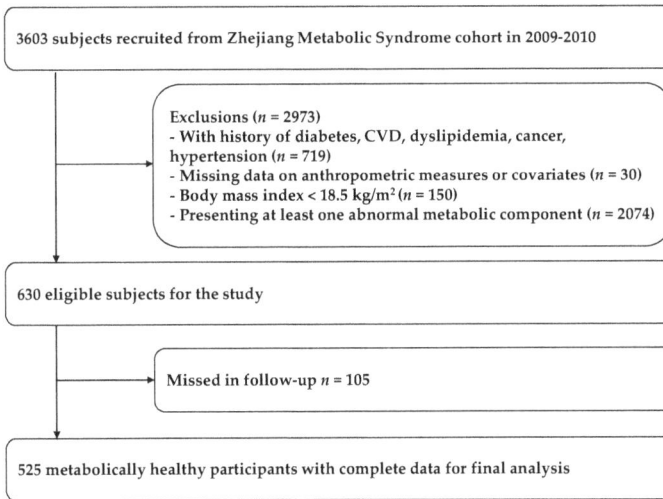

```
┌─────────────────────────────────────────────────────────────────────────┐
│ 3603 subjects recruited from Zhejiang Metabolic Syndrome cohort in 2009-2010 │
└─────────────────────────────────────────────────────────────────────────┘
        │
        │      ┌──────────────────────────────────────────────────────────┐
        │      │ Exclusions (n = 2973)                                       │
        │─────▶│ - With history of diabetes, CVD, dyslipidemia, cancer,      │
        │      │ hypertension (n = 719)                                      │
        │      │ - Missing data on anthropometric measures or covariates (n = 30) │
        │      │ - Body mass index < 18.5 kg/m² (n = 150)                    │
        │      │ - Presenting at least one abnormal metabolic component (n = 2074) │
        │      └──────────────────────────────────────────────────────────┘
        ▼
┌─────────────────────────────────────────────────────────────────────────┐
│ 630 eligible subjects for the study                                        │
└─────────────────────────────────────────────────────────────────────────┘
        │
        │─────▶ Missed in follow-up n = 105
        ▼
┌─────────────────────────────────────────────────────────────────────────┐
│ 525 metabolically healthy participants with complete data for final analysis │
└─────────────────────────────────────────────────────────────────────────┘
```

Figure 1. The flowchart of including subjects in the analysis.

2.2. Clinical Measurements at Baseline and Follow-up

Follow-up measurements took place 5 years after baseline examination. Both at baseline and follow-up investigation, the same measurements were conducted. Nurses collected anthropometric data (weight, height) and blood pressure using standard protocols. Height and weight were measured on a scale, with the subjects wearing light clothing and without shoes. Waist circumference was measured twice after a normal expiration halfway between the lowest rib and the top of the pelvis. The mean of the two measurements was calculated. Blood pressure was measured in a sitting position with a mercury sphygmomanometer. SBP and DBP were reported as the average of three repeat measurements with 30-s intervals.

After a 12-h overnight fast, whole blood and serum samples were collected for each subject. All of the laboratory tests were conducted on fresh samples in an ISO-9002 quality-assured, core facility laboratory. Glucose was analyzed with a glucose oxidase method with the Beckman Glucose Analyzer (Beckman Instruments, Irvine, CA, USA). Biochemical variables including, TG, total cholesterol (TC), HDL-C and low density lipoprotein cholesterol (LDL-C) were determined using biochemical auto-analyzers (Hitachi 7060, Tokyo, Japan).

2.3. Covariates

At baseline, each participant had completed a self-reported questionnaire to determine ethnicity and lifestyle factors such as smoking behavior, alcohol intake, history of disease and medication use. Smoking and alcohol consumption status were regarded as positive when the participant was currently smoking and drinking; in the case of former or never, it was regarded as negative. International Physical Activity Questionnaire (IPAQ) (short vision) was used for the assessment of the average amount of time per week engaged in exercise activities [19]. The energy expended for each activity in metabolic equivalent (MET) minutes per week (MET-m/week) was calculated and summed.

2.4. Outcome Measurement

Follow-up measurements were conducted 5 years later. To determine the incident of metabolic abnormalities, the same threshold levels previously mentioned according to MetS definition of IDF criteria was used, including elevated TG, low HDL-C, elevated FPG and elevated SBP or DBP. Participants who used medication for either high blood pressure or high fasting glucose or a reduced HDL cholesterol or elevated triglycerides were defined as having the corresponding metabolic abnormalities. The occurrence of metabolically abnormal status was defined as presenting one or more metabolic abnormalities. Changes in these components were calculated as the values at follow-up minus the values at baseline. For each observation, weight change was calculated as the percent change between follow-up relative to the baseline ((weight at follow-up—weight at baseline)/weight at baseline × 100%). Weight change groups included weight loss, weight maintenance and weight gain, which were defined as percent change of $<-3\%$, $\geqslant -3\%$ to $\leqslant 3\%$ and $>3\%$, respectively [20].

2.5. Statistical Analysis

We firstly classified the subjects into three groups by the BMI status at baseline (normal-weight, overweight and obesity). The software of Power Analysis and Sample Size (PASS) version 11 was used to calculate the statistical power for comparing the change of metabolic parameters (FPG, SBP, DBP, TG and HDL-C) among the groups of baseline BMI status. The results showed that statistical power ranged from 43% to 56%. Therefore, we combined the subjects in overweight and obesity. The subjects were classified as metabolically healthy normal weight (MH-NW) and metabolically healthy overweight/obese (MH-OW/OB). The statistical power increased to over 85%, which is enough to detect reasonable departures from the null hypothesis.

Continuous variables were checked for normality using the Kolmogorov-Smirnov test and the skewed variable (alanine aminotransferase) was log transformed. Categorical variables are presented as percentages. Chi-square tests were used for categorical variables. The comparisons of baseline clinical and anthropometry parameters between the groups were assessed using a 2-by-2 (body size-by-metabolic status at follow-up) ANCOVA, and Bonferroni correction was used to control for the inflation of type I error due to multiple comparisons.

Relationships between incident metabolic abnormalities were investigated with multivariable logistic regression analyses, and odds ratios (ORs) and 95% confidence intervals (95% CIs) were calculated with MH-NW subjects as the reference to assess the risk of developing metabolic abnormalities for MH-OW/OB. The OR and 95% CI were then used to compute risk ratio (RR) and 95% CI [21]. Models were adjusted for age, sex, smoking status, alcohol drinking status, physical activity, absolute weight change and the correspondingly metabolic parameters at baseline. Changes of metabolic parameters from baseline to follow-up were assessed by using mixed effects models with compound symmetry accounting for within-subjects correlation (multiple observation from a participant) with adjusting for the covariates previously mentioned.

We did not conduct sex-specific analyses because there were too few events in some subgroups to calculate stable risk estimates. A p-value < 0.05 was considered significant. All the statistical analysis was conducted using SAS software package (version 9.3; SAS institute, Cary, NC, USA).

3. Results

At baseline, the sample consisted of 630 individuals although loss to follow up resulted in a final analytic sample of 525 individuals. We checked for withdrawal bias by testing for differences in baseline variables between the participants who participated in follow-up measurements and those who did not participated in follow-up examinations. There were no differences in age, gender, metabolic parameters, BMI, smoking status, alcohol drinking status, and education level between the participated and non-participated individuals (Table S1).

At baseline, 392 participants were classified as MH-NW and 133 as MH-OW/OB. Baseline characteristics of the participants are presented in Table 1. The subjects in MH-OW/OB had larger values of baseline BMI and waist, and slightly higher DBP compared with MH-NW individuals.

Table 1. Characteristics of the metabolically healthy normal-weight (MH-NW) and metabolically healthy overweight/obese (MH-OW/OB) subjects at baseline and the incidences of the metabolic abnormalities at follow-up.

Variables	MH-NW (n = 392)	MH-OW/OB (n = 133)	p-Value
Female (n (%))	203 (51.8)	87 (65.4)	0.006
Age (years)	55.0 ± 9.0	55.6 ± 7.2	0.513
BMI (kg/m^2)	21.15 ± 1.77	25.95 ± 1.84	<0.001
Waist circumference (cm)	77.52 ± 5.60	87.58 ± 5.81	<0.001
SBP (mm·Hg)	115.0 ± 8.6	116.8 ± 8.1	0.066
DBP (mm·Hg)	73.5 ± 6.4	76.2 ± 6.3	<0.001
FPG (mmol/L)	4.85 ± 0.37	4.88 ± 0.38	0.555
TC (mmol/L)	4.95 ± 0.88	5.05 ± 0.91	0.121
TG (mmol/L)	0.93 ± 0.32	0.98 ± 0.34	0.059
HDL-C (mmol/L)	1.54 ± 0.33	1.50 ± 0.28	0.196
ALT (U/L) *	1.31 ± 0.17	1.33 ± 0.19	0.266
Current smoking (n (%))	135 (34.4)	37 (27.7)	0.121
Current drinking (n (%))	105 (26.8)	25 (18.8)	0.065
Percent in weight change (n (%))			
Weight loss	84 (21.4)	42 (31.6)	0.054
Weight maintenance	167 (42.6)	52 (39.1)	
Weight gain	141 (36.0)	39 (29.3)	
Changes in measurement			
Body weight (kg)	0.75 ± 3.93	−0.47 ± 6.07	0.007
BMI (kg/m^2)	0.24 ± 1.53	−0.24 ± 2.26	0.005
Waist circumference (cm)	2.48 ± 6.15	0.49 ± 5.42	0.026
FPG (mmol/L)	0.42 ± 0.59	0.55 ± 0.49	0.018
TG (mmol/L)	0.18 ± 0.55	0.29 ± 0.57	0.037
SBP (mm·Hg)	7.7 ± 13.6	12.1 ± 13.2	0.004
DBP (mm·Hg)	2.4 ± 8.3	4.1 ± 8.4	0.042
HDL-C (mmol/L)	−0.11 ± 0.32	−0.20 ± 0.31	0.016
Developing metabolic abnormalities at follow-up (n (%))			
Pre-diabetes	82 (20.9)	52 (39.1)	<0.001
Hypertriglyceridemia	51 (13.0)	28 (21.1)	0.026
High SBP	115 (29.3)	57 (42.9)	0.004
High DBP	51 (13.0)	31 (23.3)	0.005
Low HDL-C	77 (19.6)	49 (36.8)	<0.001
Developing one or more	218 (55.6)	100 (75.2)	<0.001

Abbreviations: MH-NW, metabolically healthy normal-weight; MH-OW/OB, metabolically healthy overweight/obese. BMI, body mass index; SBP, systolic blood pressure; DBP, diastolic blood pressure; FPG, fasting plasma glucose; TC, total cholesterol; TG, triglycerides; HDL-C, high-density lipoprotein cholesterol; LDL-C, low-density lipoprotein cholesterol; ALT, alanine aminotransferase. * Data were log transformed. Data are expressed as means ± standard deviation and number (percentage).

After 5 years, the proportion of individuals in each weight change category was not significantly different between MH-NW and MH-OW/OB participants. The MH-NW subjects had greater increase in body weight, BMI and waist circumference than that of MH-OW/OB subjects. However, the MH-OW/OB subjects had more detrimental changes in all the metabolic parameters compared with the MH-NW counterparts (Table 1). Correspondingly, higher incidents of metabolic abnormalities were observed in the MH-OW/OB than MH-NW subjects. Compared with the MH-NW subjects, MH-OW/OB group was at a significantly elevated risk for developing pre-diabetes (RR = 2.01, 95% CI = 1.42–2.57, $p < 0.001$), high SBP (RR = 1.50, 95% CI = 1.11–1.91, $p < 0.001$), low HDL-C (RR = 1.69, 95% CI = 1.18–2.29, $p < 0.001$) and one or more metabolic abnormalities (RR = 1.35,

95% CI = 1.17–1.49, $p < 0.001$) with adjusting for age, gender, smoking status, alcohol drinking status, physical activity, weight change and correspondingly baseline metabolic parameters.

Both baseline BMI status and weight change contributed to the changes of metabolic parameters over time (both $p < 0.01$). No interaction of baseline BMI status by weight change category ($p > 0.05$) was noted for the changes of metabolic parameters. Table 2 presents the comparison of the paired-difference of the metabolic parameters between the MH-NW and MH-OW/OB subjects within each weight change category. In the weight loss group, there was no significant difference in the changes of these metabolic parameters between the MH-NW and MH-OW/OB adults. In the weight maintenance category, the MH-OW/OB subjects had significantly larger increase in TG (0.34 vs. 0.16 mmol/L, $p = 0.040$), SBP (12.4 vs. 7.4 mm· Hg, $p = 0.020$), DBP (5.6 vs. 1.9 mm· Hg, $p = 0.001$) and decrease in HDL-C (−0.21 vs. −0.08 mmol/L, $p = 0.014$) compared with MH-NW peers. In weight gain category, significantly more deleterious changes in FPG, SBP, DBP and HDL-C were observed in the MH-OW/OB subjects.

The MH-NW subjects with weight maintenance and weight gain had larger increase in SBP compared with the subjects in weight loss. Among the MH-OW/OB adults, weight maintainers had larger increase in DBP (5.6 vs. 1.1 mm· Hg, $p = 0.003$) and decrease in HDL-C (−0.21 vs. −0.11 mmol/L, $p = 0.029$) than that of the subjects in weight loss. Both the MH-NW and the MH-OW/OB subjects in the weight gain group lead to worse changes in metabolic parameters compared with the subjects in the weight loss group.

Table 2. Comparison of 5-year change of the metabolic parameters between the subjects of MH-NW and MH-OW/OB and within weight change category.

Variables	Weight Loss (<−3%)		Weight Maintenance (≥−3% to ≤3%)		Weight Gain (>3%)	
	MH-NW (n = 84)	MH-OW/OB (n = 42)	MH-NW (n = 167)	MH-OW/OB (n = 52)	MH-NW (n = 141)	MH-OW/OB (n = 39)
ΔFPG (mmol/L)	0.40 ± 0.04	0.52 ± 0.06	0.39 ± 0.04	0.52 ± 0.08	0.52 ± 0.05 [b]	0.77 ± 0.09 [c,d]
ΔTG (mmol/L)	0.07 ± 0.05	0.17 ± 0.08	0.16 ± 0.05	0.34 ± 0.08 [d]	0.27 ± 0.05 [c]	0.35 ± 0.09
ΔSBP (mm·Hg)	4.7 ± 1.0	8.7 ± 1.9	7.4 ± 0.9 [a]	12.4 ± 1.8 [d]	10.0 ± 1.1 [c]	15.7 ± 2.18 [c,d]
ΔDBP (mm·Hg)	−0.1 ± 0.7	1.1 ± 1.0	1.9 ± 0.6	5.6 ± 1.1 [a,d]	3.9 ± 0.7 [c]	8.5 ± 1.4 [c,d]
ΔHDL-C (mmol/L)	−0.07 ± 0.03	−0.11 ± 0.05	−0.08 ± 0.02	−0.21 ± 0.04 [a,d]	−0.19 ± 0.02 [c]	−0.27 ± 0.04 [c,d]

Δ Absolute values between baseline and follow-up were expressed as mean ± standard error with adjustment for age, gender, smoking status, alcohol drinking status, and absolute weight change. Abbreviations: MH-NW, metabolically healthy normal-weight; MH-OW/OB, metabolically healthy overweight/obese; SBP, systolic blood pressure; DBP, diastolic blood pressure; FPG, fasting plasma glucose; TG, triglycerides; HDL-C, high-density lipoprotein cholesterol. [a] Significant difference between weight loss and weight maintenance within each baseline BMI category; [b] Significant difference between weight maintenance and weight gain within each baseline BMI category; [c] Significant difference between weight loss vs. weight gain within each baseline BMI category; [d] Significant difference between MH-NW and MH-OW/OB within each weight change category.

4. Discussion

This is, to the best of our knowledge, the first prospective study describing the characteristics of developing metabolic abnormalities in MH-OW/OB subjects in the Chinese population. In this prospective study, we found that the MH-OW/OB subjects had higher incidences of metabolic derangements compared with MH-NW counterparts as time passed. Our findings relating to stability in healthy individuals with excess fat over time were consistent with recently reported studies. Another prospective study in Spanish had shown that 30%–40% of healthy obese subjects had converted to the unhealthy status after 6 years of follow-up. Bobbioni et al. also examined the change of the metabolic status in the metabolically healthy overweight/obese individuals. At 3 years follow-up, the incidence of one or more cardiometabolic risk factors was 57.2% in the overweight/obese adults compared with 31.7% in the normal-weight subjects [22]. In the present study, the subjects in the overweight and obesity groups were positively correlated with higher incidences of metabolic abnormalities over time compared with the MH-NW subjects. This suggested that the MH-OW/OB individuals underwent more deterioration in metabolic change associated with excess fat. Our findings might explain the reason that the MH-OW/OB individuals had a higher risk for incident diabetes and cardiovascular events compared with that of MH-NW individuals [23]. Further longitudinal investigation of the sustainability and other predictors of the metabolic health subjects might better stratify the sub-type of obese individuals and provide potential intervention targets.

The beneficial effects of weight loss for the overweight and obese subjects have been well documented. However, intervention studies investigating the effect of weight loss on the metabolic status in MHO individuals had yielded contradictory results. Karelis et al. had carried out an intervention study in MHO subjects [12]. After 6-month energy-restricted diet, the MHO individuals exhibited significant reduction in body weight, accompanied with deterioration in insulin sensitivity [12]. Two similar studies observed no measureable effect of weight loss on inflammation levels in the MHO individuals [24,25]. Another two intervention studies also observed no significant improvements of the metabolic profiles in the MHO subjects [10,26]. However, a longer-term intensive lifestyle intervention including Mediterranean diet nutritional counselling and high-intensity interval training improved body composition and metabolic parameters in the MHO patients [27]. Similarly, three intervention studies found that energy-restricted diet and exercise intervention induced weight loss among the MHO subjects was associated with improvement in metabolic health status [28–30]. It was also suggested that the laparoscopic adjustable gastric banding was suitable for the morbidly obese individuals in metabolic health [31]. In the present study, under the natural conditions, the MH-NW and MH-OW/OB subjects in the weight loss group had similar changes in the metabolic parameters. They also presented better metabolic profiles than the subjects who gained weight.

Although weight maintenance literally implies no change in body weight, in free-living individuals, weight varies over time. The research by Forbes et al. showed that even with weight maintenance, adults lost about 1.5 kg of fat-free mass per decade [32]. In the present study, by using the definition of within ± 3.0 percent change of baseline weight as weight maintenance, it showed that fasting plasma glucose, triglycerides, systolic blood pressure and diastolic blood pressure were significantly increased, while HDL-cholesterol decreased in weight maintainers. Naturally, long-term trends were superimposed upon the effects of aging in the longitudinal study. Truesdale et al. and Cui et al. compared the changes of the metabolic profiles between normal weight and obese subjects who maintained their weight based on the data from the Atherosclerosis Risk in Communities (ARIC) study [33,34]. However, they obtained opposite conclusions. The research of Truesdale et al. observed more favorable changes of metabolic parameters in the obese maintainers compared with the normal weight individuals, while Cui et al. reported reverse results. In the present study, the overweight and obese weight maintainers had more deleterious changes in the metabolic profiles than that of the normal weight maintainers. It suggested that the notion of metabolically healthy overweight/obese subjects should be used in caution, since weight maintenance and weight gain was associated with much more deleterious changes of metabolic conditions in MH-OW/OB adults compared with MH-NW.

Theoretically, MHO subjects were protected from the adverse metabolic effects of weight gain and increased adiposity, which had been proved by Fabbrini et al. [13]. They compared the metabolic response to a high-calorie diet intervention between the MHO and metabolically unhealthy obese subjects. Their results suggested that MHO phenotypes were protected against the adverse metabolic effects of weight gain by increased adipose tissue capacity for lipogenesis. However, plenty of studies have challenged the existence of a healthy obese phenotype by demonstrating that such subjects had higher risk of incident hypertension, type 2 diabetes, cardiovascular diseases than that of MH-NW individuals [24]. In line with these studies, our findings indicated that both the MH-NW and MH-OW/OB subjects had higher risk of advancing to metabolic abnormal status as a result of weight gain. A recent Mendelian randomization study concluded that increased adiposity had causal adverse effects on numerous risk markers for cardiovascular disease and type 2 diabetes in non-obese young adults [35]. Therefore, guidelines advising health care professionals to treat, monitor and prevent weight gain covered the population in all BMI would benefit from interventions on developing cardiometabolic risk factors.

Since the MHO phenotype was first described, many investigators have explored the characteristics that might distinguish these individuals from those with unfavorable metabolic status [36]. However, there was still lack of consensus on the definition of metabolic health. One study summarized that, up to now, there were at least 30 different definitions had been used to define a metabolically healthy phenotype in the literature [2]. Without specific and precise definition of metabolic health, we might not obtain an accurate risk estimate of metabolic diseases for MHO subjects. However, even if there would be a gold standard to accurately differentiate healthy and unhealthy subjects, it might still be invalid in the research of metabolic diseases. Since it has been generally accepted that overweight-to-moderately-obese individuals can be either metabolically healthy or unhealthy, it is not clear to what degree an individual could switch "categories" [37]. It might be efficient and convenient to operationally dichotomizing a continuous metabolic parameter above or below a certain threshold of interest so as to target persons who were at risk, but it would ignore the variability of metabolic status and other influencing factors during the follow up. Data from the present study showed that weight change had a strong impact on the developing cardiometabolic risk factors. Dozens of longitudinal studies had assessed the risk of developing type 2 diabetes, fatty liver and cardiovascular disease for MHO subjects [38,39]. However, few of these studies had taken account of the effects of weight change after stratifying by body size and metabolic status category [40].

There were several limitations to this study. The relatively small sample size made it impossible to stratify the subjects into three categories by BMI categories (normal weight, overweight and obese). Secondly, it has been demonstrated that inflammation was secondary to obesity in humans. However, we did not have the information of inflammation markers, such as C-reactive protein. The inclusion of inflammation as a criterion might modify the identification of metabolically healthy and abnormal individuals at baseline. We were aware that the results from this study could be varied if we used a different definition of weight change. Yet owning to the relatively small sample size in the present study, when using the cut-off of 5.0% for weight change classification, the sample size became much less concentrated in weight loss and weight gain categories, but the results were similar to our primary analyses.

5. Conclusions

MH-OW/OB is a relatively unstable condition and a considerable portion of these individuals will transition into unhealthy status at follow-up. Therefore, the potential benefits of differentiating the MHO and metabolically unhealthy obese phenotypes in clinical practice in the Chinese population appear limited. Our results suggest that weight gain and weight maintenance are strong indicators for advancing to metabolic abnormalities. With regards to BMI, there is plentiful evidence that, for the same category of BMI, Chinese subjects have higher percentage of total body fat and higher risk of cardiometabolic disease compared with white subjects. Therefore, even though obesity management consumes considerable labor and expense, weight management is needed for all individuals since weight change has a significant effect on metabolic health without considering the effect of weight change according to weight status.

Supplementary Materials: The following are available online at http://www.mdpi.com/2072-6643/8/7/430/s1, Table S1: The comparison of the baseline characteristics of the people participated in follow-up examinations and lost to follow up.

Acknowledgments: This research was funded by National Key Technology R&D Program of China (2012BAI02B03); the National Natural Science Foundation of China (81172755 and 81102200). Fundamental Research Funds for the Central Universities and Program for Zhejiang Leading Team of Science and Technology Innovation (2010R50050); Zhejiang Provincial Program for the Cultivation of High-Level Innovative Health Talents. Acknowledgement included the contribution of the staff of Department of Endocrinology and Institute of Cardiovascular Diseases, Zhejiang Putuo Hospital, Tongxiang Center for Disease Control and Prevention, and Institute of Nutrition and Food Safety in Zhejiang Center for Disease Control and Prevention.

Author Contributions: Yimin Zhu, Ronghua Zhang and Ruizhi Zheng conceived the study. Chengguo Liu, Chunmei Wang, Biao Zhou, Yi Liu and Feixia Pan carried out the epidemiological investigation. Ruizhi Zheng were responsible for data cleaning and carried out the analyses, and drafted the manuscript. Yimin Zhu revised the manuscript. All authors read and approved the final manuscript.

Conflicts of Interest: The authors declare no conflict of interest.

References

1. Chatzigeorgiou, A.; Kandaraki, E.; Papavassiliou, A.G.; Koutsilieris, M. Peripheral targets in obesity treatment: A comprehensive update. *Obes. Rev.* **2014**, *15*, 487–503. [CrossRef] [PubMed]

2. Rey-Lopez, J.P.; de Rezende, L.F.; Pastor-Valero, M.; Tess, B.H. The prevalence of metabolically healthy obesity: A systematic review and critical evaluation of the definitions used. *Obes. Rev.* **2014**, *15*, 781–790. [CrossRef] [PubMed]

3. Primeau, V.; Coderre, L.; Karelis, A.D.; Brochu, M.; Lavoie, M.E.; Messier, V.; Sladek, R.; Rabasa-Lhoret, R. Characterizing the profile of obese patients who are metabolically healthy. *Int. J. Obes.* **2011**, *35*, 971–981. [CrossRef] [PubMed]

4. Kramer, C.K.; Zinman, B.; Retnakaran, R. Are metabolically healthy overweight and obesity benign conditions?: A systematic review and meta-analysis. *Ann. Int. Med.* **2013**, *159*, 758–769. [PubMed]

5. Bell, J.A.; Kivimaki, M.; Hamer, M. Metabolically healthy obesity and risk of incident type 2 diabetes: A meta-analysis of prospective cohort studies. *Obes. Rev.* **2014**, *15*, 504–515. [CrossRef] [PubMed]

6. Hinnouho, G.M.; Czernichow, S.; Dugravot, A.; Batty, G.D.; Kivimaki, M.; Singh-Manoux, A. Metabolically healthy obesity and risk of mortality: Does the definition of metabolic health matter? *Diabetes Care* **2013**, *36*, 2294–2300. [PubMed]

7. Aung, K.; Lorenzo, C.; Hinojosa, M.A.; Haffner, S.M. Risk of developing diabetes and cardiovascular disease in metabolically unhealthy normal-weight and metabolically healthy obese individuals. *J. Clin. Endocrinol. Metab.* **2014**, *99*, 462–468. [CrossRef] [PubMed]

8. Eshtiaghi, R.; Keihani, S.; Hosseinpanah, F.; Barzin, M.; Azizi, F. Natural course of metabolically healthy abdominal obese adults after 10 years of follow-up: The Tehran Lipid and Glucose Study. *Int. J. Obes.* **2015**, *39*, 514–519.

9. Hamer, M.; Bell, J.A.; Sabia, S.; Batty, G.D.; Kivimaki, M. Stability of metabolically healthy obesity over 8 years: The English Longitudinal Study of Ageing. *Eur. J. Endocrinol.* **2015**, *173*, 703–708. [PubMed]

10. Kantartzis, K.; Machann, J.; Schick, F.; Rittig, K.; Machicao, F.; Fritsche, A.; Haring, H.U.; Stefan, N. Effects of a lifestyle intervention in metabolically benign and malign obesity. *Diabetologia* **2011**, *54*, 864–868. [PubMed]

11. Perseghin, G. Is a nutritional therapeutic approach unsuitable for metabolically healthy but obese women? *Diabetologia* **2008**, *51*, 1567–1569. [PubMed]

12. Karelis, A.D.; Messier, V.; Brochu, M.; Rabasa-Lhoret, R. Metabolically healthy but obese women: Effect of an energy-restricted diet. *Diabetologia* **2008**, *51*, 1752–1754. [CrossRef] [PubMed]

13. Fabbrini, E.; Yoshino, J.; Yoshino, M.; Magkos, F.; Tiemann Luecking, C.; Samovski, D.; Fraterrigo, G.; Okunade, A.L.; Patterson, B.W.; Klein, S. Metabolically normal obese people are protected from adverse effects following weight gain. *J. Clin. Investig.* **2015**, *125*, 787–795. [CrossRef] [PubMed]

14. Xu, W.; Zhang, H.; Paillard-Borg, S.; Zhu, H.; Qi, X.; Rizzuto, D. Prevalence of Overweight and Obesity among Chinese Adults: Role of Adiposity Indicators and Age. *Obes. Facts* **2016**, *9*, 17–28. [CrossRef] [PubMed]
15. Mathew, H.; Farr, O.M.; Mantzoros, C.S. Metabolic health and weight: Understanding metabolically unhealthy normal weight or metabolically healthy obese patients. *Metabolism* **2016**, *65*, 73–80. [CrossRef] [PubMed]
16. Zheng, R.; Yang, M.; Bao, Y.; Li, H.; Shan, Z.; Zhang, B.; Liu, J.; Lv, Q.; Wu, O.; Zhu, Y.; et al. Prevalence and Determinants of Metabolic Health in Subjects with Obesity in Chinese Population. *Int. J. Environ. Res. Public Health* **2015**, *12*, 13662–13677. [CrossRef] [PubMed]
17. Alberti, K.G.; Zimmet, P.; Shaw, J.; Group IDFETFC. The metabolic syndrome—A new worldwide definition. *Lancet* **2005**, *366*, 1059–1062. [CrossRef]
18. Zhou, B.F.; Cooperative Meta-Analysis Group of the Working Group on Obesity in China. Predictive values of body mass index and waist circumference for risk factors of certain related diseases in Chinese adults—Study on optimal cut-off points of body mass index and waist circumference in Chinese adults. *Biomed. Environ. Sci.* **2002**, *15*, 83–96. [PubMed]
19. Craig, C.L.; Marshall, A.L.; Sjostrom, M.; Bauman, A.E.; Booth, M.L.; Ainsworth, B.E.; Pratt, M.; Ekelund, U.; Yngve, A.; Sallis, J.F.; et al. International physical activity questionnaire: 12-country reliability and validity. *Med. Sci. Sports Exerc.* **2003**, *35*, 1381–1395. [CrossRef] [PubMed]
20. Stevens, J.; Truesdale, K.P.; McClain, J.E.; Cai, J. The definition of weight maintenance. *Int. J. Obes.* **2006**, *30*, 391–399. [CrossRef] [PubMed]
21. Zhang, J.; Yu, K.F. What's the relative risk? A method of correcting the odds ratio in cohort studies of common outcomes. *JAMA* **1998**, *280*, 1690–1691. [CrossRef] [PubMed]
22. Bobbioni-Harsch, E.; Pataky, Z.; Makoundou, V.; Laville, M.; Disse, E.; Anderwald, C.; Konrad, T.; Golay, A.; Investigators, R. From metabolic normality to cardiometabolic risk factors in subjects with obesity. *Obesity* **2012**, *20*, 2063–2069. [CrossRef] [PubMed]
23. Zheng, R.; Zhou, D.; Zhu, Y. The long-term prognosis of cardiovascular disease and all-cause mortality for metabolically healthy obesity: A systematic review and meta-analysis. *J. Epidemiol. Commun. Health* **2016**. [CrossRef]
24. McLaughlin, T.; Abbasi, F.; Lamendola, C.; Liang, L.; Reaven, G.; Schaaf, P.; Reaven, P. Differentiation between obesity and insulin resistance in the association with C-reactive protein. *Circulation* **2002**, *106*, 2908–2912. [CrossRef] [PubMed]
25. Shin, M.J.; Hyun, Y.J.; Kim, O.Y.; Kim, J.Y.; Jang, Y.; Lee, J.H. Weight loss effect on inflammation and LDL oxidation in metabolically healthy but obese (MHO) individuals: Low inflammation and LDL oxidation in MHO women. *Int. J. Obes.* **2006**, *30*, 1529–1534. [CrossRef] [PubMed]
26. Arsenault, B.J.; Cote, M.; Cartier, A.; Lemieux, I.; Despres, J.P.; Ross, R.; Earnest, C.P.; Blair, S.N.; Church, T.S. Effect of exercise training on cardiometabolic risk markers among sedentary; but metabolically healthy overweight or obese post-menopausal women with elevated blood pressure. *Atherosclerosis* **2009**, *207*, 530–533. [CrossRef] [PubMed]
27. Dalzill, C.; Nigam, A.; Juneau, M.; Guilbeault, V.; Latour, E.; Mauriege, P.; Gayda, M. Intensive lifestyle intervention improves cardiometabolic and exercise parameters in metabolically healthy obese and metabolically unhealthy obese individuals. *Can. J. Cardiol.* **2014**, *30*, 434–440. [CrossRef] [PubMed]
28. Rondanelli, M.; Klersy, C.; Perna, S.; Faliva, M.A.; Montorfano, G.; Roderi, P.; Colombo, I.; Corsetto, P.A.; Fioravanti, M.; Solerte, S.B.; Rizzo, A.M. Effects of two-months balanced diet in metabolically healthy obesity: Lipid correlations with gender and BMI-related differences. *Lipids Health Dis.* **2015**, *14*, 139. [CrossRef] [PubMed]
29. Janiszewski, P.M.; Ross, R. Effects of weight loss among metabolically healthy obese men and women. *Diabetes Care* **2010**, *33*, 1957–1959. [CrossRef] [PubMed]
30. Liu, R.H.; Wharton, S.; Sharma, A.M.; Ardern, C.I.; Kuk, J.L. Influence of a clinical lifestyle-based weight loss program on the metabolic risk profile of metabolically normal and abnormal obese adults. *Obesity* **2013**, *21*, 1533–1539. [CrossRef] [PubMed]
31. Sesti, G.; Folli, F.; Perego, L.; Hribal, M.L.; Pontiroli, A.E. Effects of weight loss in metabolically healthy obese subjects after laparoscopic adjustable gastric banding and hypocaloric diet. *PLoS ONE* **2011**, *6*, e17737. [CrossRef] [PubMed]

32. Forbes, G.B. Longitudinal changes in adult fat-free mass: Influence of body weight. *Am. J. Clin. Nutr.* **1999**, *70*, 1025–1031. [PubMed]

33. Cui, Z.; Truesdale, K.P.; Bradshaw, P.T.; Cai, J.; Stevens, J. Three-year weight change and cardiometabolic risk factors in obese and normal weight adults who are metabolically healthy: The atherosclerosis risk in communities study. *Int. J. Obes.* **2015**, *39*, 1203–1208. [CrossRef] [PubMed]

34. Truesdale, K.P.; Stevens, J.; Cai, J. Nine-year changes in cardiovascular disease risk factors with weight maintenance in the atherosclerosis risk in communities cohort. *Am. J. Epidemiol.* **2007**, *165*, 890–900. [CrossRef] [PubMed]

35. Wurtz, P.; Wang, Q.; Kangas, A.J.; Richmond, R.C.; Skarp, J.; Tiainen, M.; Tynkkynen, T.; Soininen, P.; Havulinna, A.S.; Kaakinen, M.; et al. Metabolic signatures of adiposity in young adults: Mendelian randomization analysis and effects of weight change. *PLoS Med.* **2014**, *11*, e1001765. [CrossRef] [PubMed]

36. Samocha-Bonet, D.; Dixit, V.D.; Kahn, C.R.; Leibel, R.L.; Lin, X.; Nieuwdorp, M.; Pietilainen, K.H.; Rabasa-Lhoret, R.; Roden, M.; Scherer, P.E.; et al. Metabolically healthy and unhealthy obese—The 2013 Stock Conference report. *Obes. Rev.* **2014**, *15*, 697–708. [CrossRef] [PubMed]

37. Rey-Lopez, J.P.; de Rezende, L.F.; de Sa, T.H.; Stamatakis, E. Is the metabolically healthy obesity phenotype an irrelevant artifact for public health? *Am. J. Epidemiol.* **2015**, *182*, 737–741. [CrossRef] [PubMed]

38. Heianza, Y.; Arase, Y.; Tsuji, H.; Fujihara, K.; Saito, K.; Hsieh, S.D.; Tanaka, S.; Kodama, S.; Hara, S.; Sone, H. Metabolically healthy obesity; presence or absence of fatty liver; and risk of type 2 diabetes in Japanese individuals: Toranomon Hospital Health Management Center Study 20 (TOPICS 20). *J. Clin. Endocrinol. Metab.* **2014**, *99*, 2952–2960. [CrossRef] [PubMed]

39. Jung, C.H.; Lee, M.J.; Kang, Y.M.; Jang, J.E.; Leem, J.; Hwang, J.Y.; Kim, E.H.; Park, J.Y.; Kim, H.K.; Lee, W.J. The risk of incident type 2 diabetes in a Korean metabolically healthy obese population: The role of systemic inflammation. *J. Clin. Endocrinol. Metab.* **2015**, *100*, 934–941. [CrossRef] [PubMed]

40. Soriguer, F.; Gutierrez-Repiso, C.; Rubio-Martin, E.; Garcia-Fuentes, E.; Almaraz, M.C.; Colomo, N.; Esteva de Antonio, I.; de Adana, M.S.; Chaves, F.J.; Morcillo, S.; et al. Metabolically healthy but obese; a matter of time? Findings from the prospective Pizarra study. *J. Clin. Endocrinol. Metab.* **2013**, *98*, 2318–2325. [CrossRef] [PubMed]

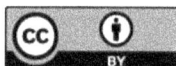

© 2016 by the authors. Licensee MDPI, Basel, Switzerland. This article is an open access article distributed under the terms and conditions of the Creative Commons Attribution (CC BY) license (http://creativecommons.org/licenses/by/4.0/).

nutrients

MDPI

Article

Metabolically Healthy Overweight and Obesity Is Associated with Higher Adherence to a Traditional Dietary Pattern: A Cross-Sectional Study among Adults in Lebanon

Joane Matta [1,†], Lara Nasreddine [2,†], Lamis Jomaa [2], Nahla Hwalla [2], Abla Mehio Sibai [3], Sebastien Czernichow [4,5,6], Leila Itani [7] and Farah Naja [2,*]

[1] Department of Nutrition, Faculty of Agricultural and Food Sciences, Holy Spirit University, P.O. Box 446, Jounieh, Lebanon; joanematta@usek.edu.lb

[2] Department of Nutrition and Food Science, Faculty of Agricultural and Food Sciences and Nutrition for Health Program (NHP), Office of Strategic Health Initiatives American University of Beirut, Beirut 1107-2020, Lebanon; ln10@aub.edu.lb (L.N.); lj18@aub.edu.lb (L.J.); Nahla@aub.edu.lb (N.H.)

[3] Department of Epidemiology and Population Health, American University of Beirut, Beirut 1107-2020, Lebanon; am00@aub.edu.lb

[4] INSERM, UMS 011, Villejuif UMS 011, France; sebastien.czernichow@aphp.fr

[5] Department of Nutrition, Hopital Europeen Georges Pompidou, Paris 75015, France

[6] School of Medicine, Paris Descartes University, Paris 75006, France

[7] Department of Nutrition & Dietetics, Faculty of Health Sciences, Beirut Arab University, P.O. Box 11-5020 Riad El Solh, Beirut 11072809, Lebanon; itani.leila@gmail.com

* Correspondence: fn14@aub.edu.lb; Tel.: +961-1-350-000 (ext. 4504)

† These authors contributed equally to this work.

Received: 18 May 2016; Accepted: 13 July 2016; Published: 20 July 2016

Abstract: This study aimed to examine the proportion and socio-demographic correlates of Metabolically Healthy Overweight and Obesity (MHOv/O) among Lebanese adults and to investigate the independent effect of previously identified dietary patterns on odds of MHOv/O. Data were drawn from the National Nutrition and Non-Communicable Disease Risk Factor Survey (Lebanon 2008–2009). Out of the 337 adult participants who had complete socio-demographic, lifestyle, dietary as well as anthropometric and biochemical data, 196 had a BMI ≥ 25 kg/m^2 and their data were included in this study. MHOv/O was identified using the Adult Treatment Panel criteria. Dietary patterns previously derived in this study population were: Fast Food/Dessert, Traditional-Lebanese and High-Protein. The proportion of MHOv/O in the study sample was 37.2%. Females, higher education and high level of physical activity were positively associated with odds of MHOv/O. Subjects with higher adherence to the Traditional-Lebanese pattern had higher odds of MHOv/O (OR: 1.83, 95% CI: 1.09–3.91). No significant associations were observed between the Fast Food/Dessert and the high-protein patterns with MHOv/O. Follow-up studies are needed to confirm those findings and understand the mechanisms by which the Traditional-Lebanese pattern may exert a protective effect in this subgroup of overweight and obese adults.

Keywords: metabolically healthy obesity; Lebanese dietary pattern; traditional dietary pattern

1. Introduction

Obesity is generally associated with numerous metabolic disorders such as insulin resistance (IR) and type 2 diabetes [1], hypertension [2–4], dyslipidemia, and some forms of cancer [5–7]. However, studies have shown that a subset of overweight and obese individuals does not display such cardio-metabolic abnormalities and were identified under a phenotype termed 'Metabolically

Healthy Obese: MHO'. Those individuals present with favorable metabolic profiles such as insulin sensitivity, normal blood pressure and lipids profiles [8]. Additional protective factors identified among individuals with MHO include lower levels of circulating C-reactive protein (CRP) [9] and a possible elevation of adiponectin [10]. It has been suggested that this subset of overweight and obese subjects may also have a lower risk of mortality and a better prognosis than their non-metabolically healthy obese counterparts [11,12].

The prevalence of MHO varies according to the definitions used to characterize this phenotype and could reach up to 40% among obese adults [13,14]. Given the possible protective effects of MHO on morbidity and its considerable prevalence, the identification of underlying characteristics that may be associated with it may help provide a better understanding of the factors that may protect overweight and obese individuals from developing metabolic disturbances [12,15]. Some studies have shown that the prevalence of MHO is higher among younger vs. older individuals and among women vs. men [16,17]. Physical activity has been suggested as one of the lifestyle factors that may be associated with a metabolically healthy profile among overweight and obese subjects [16,17]. Similarly, it was suggested that specific dietary factors may be associated with the MHO phenotype, even though the number of studies in this field is still limited [18]. For instance, a study conducted among adult overweight and obese women showed that the MHO phenotype was positively associated with higher daily intakes of fiber and a higher number of daily servings of vegetables [18]. However, subsequent studies failed to confirm similar associations [19,20]. Results from a recent investigation of food groups, macro- and micronutrients' intakes in a multi-ethnic group of 775 obese Americans did not support the hypothesis that dietary intake is associated with MHO [21]. This controversy may partly result from the use of traditional methods in nutritional epidemiology which focuses on the intake of individual nutrients, foods or food groups when investigating the association between diet and MHO. Such a conventional approach has several limitations mainly the interaction between nutrients, confounding by foods/nutrients not eaten and the problem of collinearity [22]. In this context, and to overcome the limitations of the traditional methods of examining single foods or nutrients, dietary pattern analysis was proposed as an approach that allows the examination of the holistic effect of diet on disease [23]. In fact, the dietary pattern approach looks beyond single nutrients or foods and attempts to capture the broader picture of diet that is hypothesized to be linked to health. In addition, results stemming from dietary patterns analyses are more helpful in disseminating diet-related messages to consumers who seem more likely to adhere to these messages rather than those stemming related to single foods or nutrients [22].

In Lebanon, similarly to other Eastern Mediterranean countries, the rate of overweight and obesity among adults is reported to follow an escalating secular trend, with its prevalence estimates increasing from 54.4% to 65.0% over the past decade [24]. Such an alarming trend coupled with the potential protective effect of MHO on disease risk, underscores the need to examine the proportions of overweight and obese individuals who are metabolically healthy and to investigate associated dietary and lifestyle factors. This study aims to (1) examine the proportion of Metabolically Healthy Overweight and Obesity (MHOv/O) among Lebanese adults (2) evaluate the socio-demographic and lifestyle correlates of MHOv/O; and (3) investigate the independent effect of previously identified dietary patterns on odds of MHOv/O in the study population.

2. Materials and Methods

2.1. Study Design and Participants

Data for this study were drawn from the cross-sectional National Nutrition and Non-Communicable Disease Risk Factor Survey (2008–2009) described elsewhere [25]. In brief, households, the primary sampling units, were drawn using a stratified cluster random sampling frame. The strata were the six administrative Lebanese governorates, while the clusters were further selected at the level of districts. Using the household roster, one adult from each household was selected. The distribution of the study sample by sex and 5-year age group was similar to that of the Lebanese population as estimated by the Central Administration for Statistics in Lebanon (2004) [26]. Out of 2202 visited households, 1982 accepted to participate in the study (response rate 90%) [27]. Of those, participants who had no chronic diseases and were not taking blood pressure, sugar or lipid lowering medications were contacted to give blood samples (n = 1331). From these participants, 337 subjects provided written consent and gave a blood sample. Comparison of subjects who gave blood and those who did not showed that both groups were comparable across the sociodemographic characteristics except for marital status (62% of respondents vs. 50% of non-respondents are married). In addition, significantly higher proportions of overweight and obesity were found among those who gave blood as compared to those who did not (Overweight 36%, Obesity: 22% vs. Overweight 33%, Obesity 16% respectively, $p < 0.05$). (Unpublished data). Of these 337 subjects, 196 were overweight and obese individuals (BMI $\geqslant$ 25 kg/m^2), and their data are included in this study (overweight: n = 119; obese: n = 77).

2.2. Data Collection

At the participants' homes, data collection was conducted by trained field workers, phlebotomists and dietitians. Data collection procedures followed the WHO STEP wise approach to Surveillance (STEPS) [26] and included socio-demographic and lifestyle questionnaires, anthropometric measurements, biochemical assessment, as well as a food frequency questionnaire (FFQ) for the evaluation of dietary intake. The study protocol was reviewed and approved by the Institutional Review Board of the American University of Beirut, and informed consent was obtained from all participants in the study.

Socio-demographic characteristics were age, sex, marital status, education level, crowding index, and family history of obesity. Crowding index was defined as the average number of people per room, excluding the kitchen and bathroom. Previous studies have shown that a higher crowding index was correlated with a lower socioeconomic status [28–30]. This finding was further validated in the Lebanese context [31]. A positive family history of obesity was defined as either one of the two parents (mother or father) identified as obese. Lifestyle factors included smoking, physical activity, weekly frequency of breakfast, snack consumption as well as frequency of eating at TV and eating out. Snacking was defined as an intake occasion that was not considered a main meal, light meal/breakfast or drink-only [32]. 'Eating out' and 'Eating at TV' were examined in terms of number of occasions per week. Physical activity was assessed using the short version of the International Physical Activity Questionnaire, and three levels of physical activity were determined based on metabolic equivalents-min per week (low, moderate, high) [33].

Anthropometric measurements obtained included weight, height and waist circumference, all of which were obtained using standardized protocols. The percent body fat was computed using skinfold thickness measurements according to the Durnin and Womersley formula [34]. Blood pressure was measured using a standard mercury sphygmomanometer. Two readings were obtained for both systolic and diastolic blood pressure, at 5-min intervals, and their average was used in this study.

Metabolic and biochemical assessments were measured after an overnight fast and included serum triglycerides, HDL and LDL-cholesterol, fasting blood glucose, fasting blood insulin, and CRP. Details regarding blood collection and analysis were described elsewhere [25].

Dietary patterns in the study population: Previous work by our research group derived dietary patterns among survey participants who had complete socio-demographic, lifestyle, dietary as well as anthropometric and biochemical data [25]. The FFQ used to assess dietary intake had 61 items and measured food intake over the past year. For each food item listed in the FFQ, a standard portion size was indicated and five frequency choices were given. This FFQ was designed by a panel of nutritionists and included culture specific dishes and recipes. It was tested on a convenient sample to check for clarity and cultural sensitivity. For the derivation of the dietary patterns, food items were grouped into 25 food groups based on similarities in ingredients, nutrient profile, and/or culinary usage [25]. Food items having a unique composition (e.g., eggs, olives, and mayonnaise) were classified individually. The total consumption for each group was determined by summing the daily gram intake of each item within the group. Using the dietary intake of these 25 food groups, dietary patterns were identified by factor analysis. The latter is a data-driven technique which identifies foods that are frequently consumed together by grouping food items based on the degree to which the amounts eaten are correlated together [35]. The number of factors/patterns to be retained was based on three criteria: (1) the Kaiser criterion (eigenvalues > 1); (2) inflection point of the scree plot; and (3) the interpretability of factors. The rotated factor loadings matrix was extracted (Varimax rotation). The derived dietary patterns were labeled based on food groups having a rotated factor loading greater than 0.4. Factor scores were calculated by multiple regressions; a higher factor score indicated a greater adherence to the respective factor or pattern [36].

Accordingly, three dietary patterns were identified: Fast Food/Dessert, Traditional-Lebanese, and High Protein. The Fast Food/Dessert pattern consisted mainly of hamburger, shawarma, pizza and pies, falafel sandwiches, desserts, as well as carbonated beverages and juices. The Traditional-Lebanese pattern was identified as a variant of the Mediterranean diet [37] and included foods such as dairy products, olives, fruits, legumes, grains, eggs, vegetable oil, dried fruits, and traditional sweets. The High Protein pattern was characterized by high intakes of fish, chicken, meat, and low fat dairy products. Further details about the patterns and the loadings of each food items are presented in Appendix. The patterns' scores for Fast Food/Dessert, Traditional-Lebanese, and High Protein of overweight and obese participants (BMI $\geq 25\text{kg/m}^2$) were included in the analyses of this study.

2.3. MHOv/O Classification

To date, there is no consensus on the MHO phenotype's definition. A commonly used definition is The Adult Treatment Panel criteria for the metabolic syndrome (ATP-III) criterion, which was used in this study. Accordingly, an overweight or obese subject was classified as MHOv/O if he/she had one or none of the following: triglycerides $\geq$1.7 mmol/L; systolic blood pressure (BP) $\geq$130 mm·Hg; diastolic blood pressure $\geq$85 mm·Hg; fasting blood glucose $\geq$5.6 mmol/L; and HDL- cholesterol <1.04 mmol/L for men and <1.29 mmol/L for women. Overweight and obese subjects with more than one of these conditions were classified as Metabolically Unhealthy Overweight and Obese (MUHOv/O).

2.4. Statistical Analyses

Descriptive statistics for socio-demographic, lifestyle, anthropometric, and biochemical characteristics of study participants were presented as means $\pm$ SD and proportions for continuous and categorical variables, respectively. Chi-square and independent t-tests were used to compare MHO and MUHOv/O groups. The association of each of the characteristics of study participants with MHOv/O was assessed using simple logistic regression analysis. In order to evaluate the determinants of MHOv/O, a multiple logistic regression model was used. In this model, variables were included if they were significantly associated with the outcome in the univariate analysis. Simple and multiple logistic regression models were also used to evaluate the associations between the dietary patterns of the study population and the odds of the MHOv/O phenotype. In these models, scores of the dietary pattern were the independent variable (grouped as low adherence-1st tertile- and high adherence-2nd and 3rd tertile), and MHOv/O phenotype as dependent variable (MHOv/O vs. MUHOv/O). These models were adjusted for variables found to be significantly associated with MHOv/O. Tests for linearity (Tolerance > 0.4) of the covariates included in the regression models were performed. Normality of the residuals was assessed by the histogram of standardized residuals and normal probability plot in all regression models. All analyses were undertaken using SPPS software version 22 (IBM Corp. Released 2013. IBM SPSS Statistics for Windows, Version 22.0. IBM Corp: Armonk, NY, USA).

3. Results

The proportion of MHOv/O in the study population was 37.24%, 95% CI (30.78–44.19). Descriptive characteristics of the study population and their association with MHOv/O, as derived by simple logistic regression, are shown in Table 1. Of socio-demographic characteristics, sex, and education level were associated with MHOv/O status. Females and participants with a higher education level had higher odds of MHOv/O. Belonging to the 'High Physical Activity' category was also associated with a higher odd of MHOv/O. While BMI and percent body fat were not associated with MHOv/O, a one unit increase in waist circumference led to significantly lower odds of MHOv/O in the study population.

Table 1. Descriptive characteristics of the study population and their association with Metabolically Healthy Overweight and Obesity (MHOv/O), as derived by simple logistic regression ($n = 196$).

	MUHOv/O ($n = 123$)	MHOv/O ($n = 73$)	p-Value [†]	OR (95% CI)
Age (years)	42.7 ± 15.7	39.2 ± 13.0	0.12	0.98 (0.96–1.00)
Sex			0.00	
Males	81 (66)	29 (40)		Ref
Females	42 (34)	44 (60)		2.93 (1.61–5.33)
Marital status			0.93	
Single	38 (31)	23 (32)		Ref
Married	85 (69)	50 (68)		0.97 (0.52–1.81)
Education			0.06	
Middle school	60 (49)	23 (31)		Ref
High school	32 (26)	27 (37)		1.93 (0.94–3.99)
University & Higher education	31 (25)	23 (32)		2.20 (1.09–4.44)
Family history of obesity			0.84	
No	69 (56)	42 (57)		Ref
Yes	54 (44)	31 (43)		0.94 (0.523–1.69)
Crowding index	1.0 ± 0.5	1.2 ± 0.5	0.10	1.56 (0.91–2.66)
<1person per room	52 (43)	22 (31)		Ref
≥1 person per room	70 (57)	50 (69)		1.69 (0.91–3.13)
Breakfast per week	5.0 ± 2.8	5.3 ± 2.5	0.40	1.05 (0.94–1.17)
Breakfast Skippers (≤5 times/week)	44 (36)	24 (33)		Ref
Breakfast consumers (>5 times/week)	79 (64)	49 (67)		1.14 (0.62–2.10)
Smoking			0.24	
No	83 (67)	55 (75)		Ref
Yes	40 (33)	18 (25)		0.68 (0.35–1.30)
Physical activity level			0.00	
Low	49 (40)	18 (25)		Ref
Moderate	29 (24)	9 (12)		0.85 (0.34–2.13)
High	45 (36)	46 (63)		2.78 (1.41–5.49)
Snack per day	1.5 ± 1.2	1.5 ± 0.9	0.60	0.93 (0.71–1.23)
Eating at TV per week	2.6 ± 3.1	2.4 ± 3.2	0.57	0.97 (0.89–1.07)
Eating out per week	1.5 ± 2.2	0.8 ± 1.4	0.03	0.84 (0.70–1.01)
BMI (Kg/m^2)	30.2 ± 4.1	29.3 ± 3.7	0.13	0.94 (0.87–1.02)
Waist circumference (cm)	97.4 ± 11.1	92.6 ± 10.4	<0.01	0.95 (0.93–0.98)
Insulin (μU/mL)	29.5 ± 22.6	21.2 ± 8.3	<0.01	0.95 (0.91–0.98)
CRP (mg/dl)	6.9 ± 9.2	5.6 ± 5.6	0.29	0.985 (0.93–1.02)
Percent body fat	32.0 ± 7.6	32.7 ± 6.9	0.56	1.01 (0.97–1.06)

Numbers in this table represent mean $\pm$ SD for continuous variables and n (%) for categorical variables.
[†] p-values were derived from chi square test for categorical variables and from independent samples t-test for continuous variables.

Correlates of the MHOv/O status were examined by multiple logistic regression, and the resulting OR and their corresponding 95% CI are presented in Table 2. After adjustment, female sex, higher education, and physical activity levels were associated with a higher odd of MHOv/O among study participants.

The OR and 95% CI for the association of adherence to these dietary patterns with the odds of MHOv/O are presented in Table 3. These odds were derived from multiple logistic regression adjusted for sex, education, and physical activity. Results indicated that a high adherence to the Traditional-Lebanese pattern was associated with 83% increase in the odds of MHOv/O (OR: 1.83, 95% CI: 1.09–3.91). No significant association was noted between the Fast Food/Dessert and the High Protein patterns and the odds of MHOv/O in the study population.

Table 2. Multiple logistic regression for the association between socio-demographic and lifestyle characteristics with MHOv/O in the study population (n = 196).

Demographic and Lifestyle Variables	OR (95% CI)
Age (years)	0.99 (0.97–1.02)
Sex	
Males	Ref
Females	3.81 (1.95–7.40) **
Education	
Middle school	Ref
High school	2.66 (1.19–5.96) *
University & Higher education	2.49 (1.10–5.70)
Physical activity level	
Low	Ref
Moderate	0.59 (0.22–1.60)
High	2.35 (1.13–4.92) *

* p-value ⩽ 0.05. ** p-value ⩽ 0.001.

Table 3. Crude and adjusted logistic regression models describing the association between the various dietary patterns and MHOv/O in the study population, as derived by logistic regression (n = 196) *,†.

	Crude Model OR; 95% CI	Adjusted Model OR; 95% CI
Fast Food/Dessert		
Low adherence	Ref	Ref
High adherence	0.79 (0.43–1.45)	1.38 (0.66–2.92)
Traditional-Lebanese Pattern		
Low adherence	Ref	Ref
High adherence	1.29 (0.69–2.40)	1.83 (1.09–3.91)
High Protein Pattern		
Low adherence	Ref	Ref
High adherence	1.17(0.63–2.17)	1.36 (0.69–2.70)

* Low adherence was defined as belonging to the 1st tertile of the pattern score, while high adherence was defined as belonging to the 2nd and 3rd tertiles. † The adjusted model included sex, education, and physical activity.

4. Discussion

This study is the first in Lebanon and the region to assess the proportion and correlates of MHOv/O and investigate its association with dietary patterns among overweight and obese adults. The results showed that the proportion of MHOv/O in the current study sample is 38.2%, implying that approximately one out of three overweight/obese individuals is considered metabolically healthy. This proportion is higher than a recent estimate from a prospective cohort of 4397 adults in Spain, where prevalence of MHOv/O was found to be 28.7% [38]. Such a difference could be attributed to the fact that overweight and obese participants with medical complications were not included in the denominator for calculating the proportion of MHOv/O in the study sample, given that subjects were excluded if they had a known history of chronic diseases and/or were taking blood pressure, sugar, or lipid lowering medications. Such an exclusion criterion was chosen to avoid reverse causality in the association between MHOv/O and dietary patterns.

The findings of this study showed that, even though BMI and percent body fat were not associated with MHOv/O, a negative association between waist circumference and MHOv/O was observed. Recognizing waist circumference as a proxy measure of visceral adiposity [39], these findings implicate a possible role for visceral fat in modulating the metabolic profile in overweight and obese subjects. In fact, it has been proposed that metabolically healthy individuals have lower amounts of visceral fats [40,41]. Abdominal obesity, with its characteristic increase in visceral fat, is associated with an increase in the levels of free fatty acids (FFA) and abnormal adipokine profiles, which can result in the development of insulin resistance and other metabolic abnormalities including dyslipidemia, hyperglycemia, and elevated blood pressure.

In this study, investigation of the correlates of MHOv/O showed that female gender, higher education levels, and higher physical activity are significantly associated with higher odds of this phenotype. The fact that MHOv/O status was positively associated with female gender is in line with what has been reported in other investigations on MHO [40] and may be a reflection of the lower visceral fat deposition in women compared to men, when matched for BMI [42,43]. The positive association between female gender and MHOv/O is also in agreement with studies reporting women as being more health-conscious and followers of dietary recommendations than men [44,45]. Higher education may also be a driving factor towards healthier diets and lifestyles, and therefore higher odds of being metabolically healthy [46]. Our findings regarding the positive association between physical activity and MHOv/O are in accordance with what has been previously reported [13] and may be explained by several mechanisms including stimulation of fatty acid uptake and oxidation and increasing insulin sensitivity [47].

In the present study, we have opted to use the dietary pattern approach in investigating the association between diet and the MHOv/O phenotype. Previous studies conducted by our group on a national sample of Lebanese adults, which included normal weight, overweight and obese subjects, documented a positive association between metabolic syndrome and adherence to the Fast Food/Dessert pattern, a pattern that contains most of the food groups characteristic of the "Western Pattern" [25,48] and which was found to be associated with higher intakes of fat, saturated fat, sugar, and sodium coupled with lower intakes of dietary fiber and calcium, when compared to traditional Lebanese dietary pattern [25]. However, in the present study, which focuses on overweight and obese subjects only, we did not observe an association between the MHOv/O status and adherence to the Fast Food/Desert pattern. These results suggest that the negative effects of the Fast Food/Desert pattern on cardio-metabolic risk and the metabolic syndrome could be mediated mainly by its effects on increasing adiposity and obesity itself. In addition, even though previous studies conducted by our group did not document an association between the Traditional-Lebanese pattern and obesity risk [48], the results of this study showed that higher adherence to the Lebanese pattern was associated with higher odds of MHOv/O in overweight and obese adults. Taken together, these findings suggest that, although the Traditional-Lebanese dietary pattern may not be protective against obesity, it may offset or buffer adiposity-related metabolic abnormalities in overweight and obese subjects. The Traditional-Lebanese dietary pattern, a variant of the Mediterranean diet [37], is in fact a pattern that is rich in fruits, vegetables, legumes, olives, olive oil, and dairy products. This dietary pattern was also found to be associated with higher intakes of monounsaturated fats, polyunsaturated fats, fiber, and calcium while being characterized by lower intakes of protein, cholesterol, saturated fat, and sugars [25]. Dietary fiber, through its colonic, intrinsic and hormonal effects, and mono- and polyunsaturated fats, through their ability to buffer lipid and insulin fluctuations and peaks, may work in concert to increase insulin sensitivity, enhance fat oxidation, and decrease cardio-metabolic risk [49–52]. In addition, the beneficial combinations of phytochemicals, antioxidants, and fiber brought by a diet rich in legumes, fruits, and vegetables may decrease oxidative stress, temper the inflammatory response, and therefore enhance insulin sensitivity [53]. Dairy products, which also characterize the Lebanese dietary pattern, have been associated with decreased visceral fat, an effect that is likely to be mediated by independent or synergistic effects of calcium and dairy protein, on lipolysis, lipogenesis, and thermogenesis [54,55]. Our findings related to the positive association between the Lebanese dietary pattern and the MHOv/O phenotype are similar to those reported by Phillips et al. [20], whereby in a cross-sectional study among adults aged 45–74 years, greater compliance with the food pyramid recommendations and higher dietary quality were positively associated with metabolic health in obese subjects.

The findings of this study ought to be considered within the context of its limitations. First, we have included in our sample both overweight and obese individuals and not only obese. Descriptive statistics, however, have demonstrated that there was no significant difference in BMI between MHOv/O and MUHOv/O, indicating that overweight individuals did not have higher odds of belonging to the MHOv/O phenotype over obese participants. Second, the MHOv/O state may not be a stable phenotype, and there remain open questions related to whether MHOv/O represents a transient phenotype changing with aging and behavioral and environmental factors [56]. Third, the percentage of survey participants who agreed to give blood (respondents) was low (24.3%). Comparison of respondents and non-respondents showed that both groups were comparable across the sociodemographic characteristics except for marital status and proportions of overweight and obesity (as indicated in the Methods section). Lastly, the cross-sectional design of this study does not allow for causality inference. Longitudinal studies are needed to further confirm the role of dietary patterns in modulating metabolic profiles in high risk individuals.

5. Conclusions

In conclusion, the study showed that overweight and obese subjects with higher adherence to the Traditional-Lebanese dietary pattern had higher odds of belonging to the MHOv/O phenotype, independent of other socio-demographic, lifestyle characteristics. These findings suggest that the Traditional-Lebanese dietary pattern, a variant of the Mediterranean diet, may be associated with offset or delayed development of adiposity-related metabolic abnormalities. In this context, interventions and strategies aiming at preserving and promoting the traditional diet could be proposed in Lebanon. It is important to note that, even though this study has identified factors that modulate the odds of MHOv/O, maintaining a healthy body weight remains the most impactful public health recommendation to decrease metabolic abnormalities and associated diseases.

Acknowledgments: The authors thank all participants of National Nutrition and Non-Communicable Disease Risk Factor Survey. This work was funded by the Training Programs in Epidemiology and Public Health Interventions Network (TEPHINET). Additional funds were contributed by the World Health organization (WHO-Lebanon) and the Lebanese National Council for Scientific Research (LNCSR).

Author Contributions: J.M. and L.N. equally contributed to the conception and study design, interpretation of the data, and drafting the manuscript. L.J. contributed to the statistical analysis and interpretations of the data. N.H. and A.M.S. contributed to the conception and study design, obtaining funding and to the critical revision of the manuscript. S.C. contributed to the critical revision of the manuscript. F.N. contributed to the conception and study design, analysis and interpretation of the data, drafting of the manuscript as well as the critical revision of the manuscript. All authors read and approved the final version of the manuscript.

Conflicts of Interest: The authors declare no conflict of interest.

Appendix A

Table A1. Food items/groups constituting the dietary patterns prevalent in the study population [*,†].

Dietary Patterns		
Fast Food/Dessert	Traditional-Lebanese	High protein
Hamburger (0.76)	Dairy products-full fat (0.58)	Fish (0.70)

Table A1. *Cont*

Dietary Patterns		
Shawarma (0.72)	Olives (0.56)	Chicken (0.69)
Pizza and pies (0.70)	Fruits and vegetables (0.49)	Meat (0.60)
Falafel Sandwiches (0.61)	Legumes (0.47)	Dairy products-low fat (0.54)
Desserts (0.41)	Grains (0.47)	Breakfast cereals (0.23)
Carbonated beverages and juices (0.4)	Eggs (0.45)	-
Mayonnaise (0.35)	Vegetable oil (0.43)	-
Butter (0.22)	Nuts and dried fruits (0.40)	-
Alcoholic beverages (0.2)	Traditional sweets (0.37)	-

* Factor loading of the various food groups/items are presented in (). † The dietary patterns and the food items-and their factor loading-making up these patterns were taken from Naja et al. (2013) [29].

References

1. Eckel, R.H.; Kahn, R.; Robertson, R.M.; Rizza, R.A. Preventing cardiovascular disease and diabetes a call to action from the american diabetes association and the american heart association. *Circulation* **2006**, *113*, 2943–2946. [CrossRef] [PubMed]

2. Rahmouni, K.; Correia, M.L.; Haynes, W.G.; Mark, A.L. Obesity-associated hypertension new insights into mechanisms. *Hypertension* **2005**, *45*, 9–14. [CrossRef] [PubMed]

3. Ying, A.; Arima, H.; Czernichow, S.; Woodward, M.; Huxley, R.; Turnbull, F.; Perkovic, V.; Neal, B. Effects of blood pressure lowering on cardiovascular risk according to baseline body-mass index: A meta-analysis of randomised trials. *Lancet* **2015**, *385*, 867–874. [PubMed]

4. Czernichow, S.; Castetbon, K.; Salanave, B.; Vernay, M.; Barry, Y.; Batty, G.D.; Hercberg, S.; Blacher, J. Determinants of blood pressure treatment and control in obese people: Evidence from the general population. *J. Hypertens.* **2012**, *30*, 2338–2344. [CrossRef] [PubMed]

5. Lau, D.C.; Douketis, J.D.; Morrison, K.M.; Hramiak, I.M.; Sharma, A.M.; Ur, E.; Members of the Obesity Canada Clinical Practice Guidelines Expert Panel. 2006 Canadian clinical practice guidelines on the management and prevention of obesity in adults and children (summary). *Can. Med. Assoc. J.* **2007**, *176*, S1–S13. [CrossRef] [PubMed]

6. Adams, K.F.; Schatzkin, A.; Harris, T.B.; Kipnis, V.; Mouw, T.; Ballard-Barbash, R.; Hollenbeck, A.; Leitzmann, M.F. Overweight, obesity, and mortality in a large prospective cohort of persons 50 to 71 years old. *N. Engl. J. Med.* **2006**, *355*, 763–778. [CrossRef] [PubMed]

7. Hossain, P.; Kawar, B.; el Nahas, M. Obesity and diabetes in the developing world—A growing challenge. *N. Engl. J. Med.* **2007**, *356*, 213–215. [CrossRef] [PubMed]

8. Karelis, A.D.; Faraj, M.; Bastard, J.-P.; St-Pierre, D.H.; Brochu, M.; Prud'homme, D.; Rabasa-Lhoret, R. The metabolically healthy but obese individual presents a favorable inflammation profile. *J. Clin. Endocrinol. Metab.* **2005**, *90*, 4145–4150. [CrossRef] [PubMed]

9. Semple, R.K.; Savage, D.B.; Cochran, E.K.; Gorden, P.; O'Rahilly, S. Genetic syndromes of severe insulin resistance. *Endocr. Rev.* **2011**, *32*, 498–514. [CrossRef] [PubMed]

10. Fagerberg, B.; Hultén, L.M.; Hulthe, J. Plasma ghrelin, body fat, insulin resistance, and smoking in clinically healthy men: The atherosclerosis and insulin resistance study. *Metabolism* **2003**, *52*, 1460–1463. [CrossRef]

11. Calori, G.; Lattuada, G.; Piemonti, L.; Garancini, M.P.; Ragogna, F.; Villa, M.; Mannino, S.; Crosignani, P.; Bosi, E.; Luzi, L. Prevalence, metabolic features, and prognosis of metabolically healthy obese italian individuals the cremona study. *Diabetes Care* **2011**, *34*, 210–215. [CrossRef] [PubMed]

12. Hamer, M.; Stamatakis, E. Metabolically healthy obesity and risk of all-cause and cardiovascular disease mortality. *J. Clin. Endocrinol. Metab.* **2012**, *97*, 2482–2488. [CrossRef] [PubMed]

13. Wildman, R.P.; Muntner, P.; Reynolds, K.; McGinn, A.P.; Rajpathak, S.; Wylie-Rosett, J.; Sowers, M.R. The obese without cardiometabolic risk factor clustering and the normal weight with cardiometabolic risk factor clustering: Prevalence and correlates of 2 phenotypes among the us population (nhanes 1999–2004). *Arch. Intern. Med.* **2008**, *168*, 1617–1624. [CrossRef] [PubMed]

14. Hinnouho, G.-M.; Czernichow, S.; Dugravot, A.; Batty, G.D.; Kivimaki, M.; Singh-Manoux, A. Metabolically healthy obesity and risk of mortality does the definition of metabolic health matter? *Diabetes Care* **2013**, *36*, 2294–2300. [CrossRef] [PubMed]

15. Primeau, V.; Coderre, L.; Karelis, A.D.; Brochu, M.; Lavoie, M.E.; Messier, V.; Sladek, R.; Rabasa-Lhoret, R. Characterizing the profile of obese patients who are metabolically healthy. *Int. J. Obes.* **2011**, *35*, 971–981. [CrossRef] [PubMed]
16. Bell, J.A.; Hamer, M.; van Hees, V.T.; Singh-Manoux, A.; Kivimaki, M.; Sabia, S. Healthy obesity and objective physical activity. *Am. J. Clin. Nutr.* **2015**, *102*, 268–275. [CrossRef] [PubMed]
17. Fung, M.D.; Canning, K.L.; Mirdamadi, P.; Ardern, C.I.; Kuk, J.L. Lifestyle and weight predictors of a healthy overweight profile over a 20-year follow-up. *Obesity* **2015**, *23*, 1320–1325. [CrossRef] [PubMed]
18. Camhi, S.M.; Crouter, S.E.; Hayman, L.L.; Must, A.; Lichtenstein, A.H. Lifestyle behaviors in metabolically healthy and unhealthy overweight and obese women: A preliminary study. *PLoS ONE* **2015**, *10*, e0138548. [CrossRef] [PubMed]
19. Hankinson, A.L.; Daviglus, M.L.; van Horn, L.; Chan, Q.; Brown, I.; Holmes, E.; Elliott, P.; Stamler, J. Diet composition and activity level of at risk and metabolically healthy obese american adults. *Obesity* **2013**, *21*, 637–643. [CrossRef] [PubMed]
20. Phillips, C.M.; Dillon, C.; Harrington, J.M.; McCarthy, V.J.; Kearney, P.M.; Fitzgerald, A.P.; Perry, I.J. Defining metabolically healthy obesity: Role of dietary and lifestyle factors. *PLoS ONE* **2013**, *8*, e76188. [CrossRef] [PubMed]
21. Kimokoti, R.W.; Judd, S.E.; Shikany, J.M.; Newby, P.K. Metabolically healthy obesity is not associated with food intake in white or black men. *J. Nutr.* **2015**, *145*, 2551–2561. [CrossRef] [PubMed]
22. Jacques, P.F.; Tucker, K.L. Are dietary patterns useful for understanding the role of diet in chronic disease? *Am. J. Clin. Nutr.* **2001**, *73*, 1–2. [PubMed]
23. Hu, F.B. Dietary pattern analysis: A new direction in nutritional epidemiology. *Curr. Opin. Lipidol.* **2002**, *13*, 3–9. [CrossRef] [PubMed]
24. Nasreddine, L.; Naja, F.; Chamieh, M.C.; Adra, N.; Sibai, A.-M.; Hwalla, N. Trends in overweight and obesity in lebanon: Evidence from two national cross-sectional surveys (1997 and 2009). *BMC Public Health* **2012**. [CrossRef] [PubMed]
25. Naja, F.; Nasreddine, L.; Itani, L.; Adra, N.; Sibai, A.; Hwalla, N. Association between dietary patterns and the risk of metabolic syndrome among lebanese adults. *Eur. J. Nutr.* **2013**, *52*, 97–105. [CrossRef] [PubMed]
26. Central Administration for Statistics (Lebanon). *Living Conditions of Households: The National Survey of Household Living Condition 2004*; Presidency of the Council of Ministers: Beiut, Lebanon, 2006.
27. Sibai, A.; Hwalla, N. *Who Steps Chronic Disease Risk Factor Surveillance: Data Book for Lebanon, 2009*; American University of Beirut; World Health Organization: Beirut, Lebanon, 2010.
28. Freedman, J.L. What is crowding? In *Crowding and Behavior*; Freedman, J., Ed.; WH Freedman: San francisco, CA, USA, 1975; pp. 1–11.
29. Baum, A.; Epstein, Y. Crowding: Historical and contemporary trends in crowding research. In *Human Response to Crowding*; Baum, A., Epstein, Y., Eds.; L Earlbaum: Hillsdale, NJ, USA, 1978; pp. 3–22.
30. Uday, J. Introduction. In *The Psychological Consequences of Crowding*; Sage: New Delhi, India, 1978; pp. 15–46.
31. Melki, I.; Beydoun, H.; Khogali, M.; Tamim, H.; Yunis, K. Household crowding index: A correlate of socioeconomic status and inter-pregnancy spacing in an urban setting. *J. Epidemiol. Community Health* **2004**, *58*, 476–480. [CrossRef] [PubMed]
32. Forslund, H.B.; Torgerson, J.S.; Sjöström, L.; Lindroos, A.-K. Snacking frequency in relation to energy intake and food choices in obese men and women compared to a reference population. *Int. J. Obes.* **2005**, *29*, 711–719. [CrossRef] [PubMed]
33. IPAQ Group. Guidelines for Data Processing and Analysis of the International Physical Activity Questionnaire (ipaq)—Short and Long Forms, 2005. Available online: https://f0362602-a-62cb3a1a-s-sites.googlegroups.com/site/theipaq/scoring-protocol/scoring_protocol.pdf?attachauth=ANoY7co5OoW4Eu7VLGVZ1PVOxLBkNNMvcHYE7MZPCWYhQGe044Qyk7CWS-5o0qNLRJ04batH-A4f3Sx9GLg-QNQ2ICwKBliWJYZPLSCfCnXGdi1l7Ru1_ihH_ALirUwbqpmQIAWvxbe_tK3Wn5XGRGm7ij1jREYqi80x4KPX2A5H3UwI9EGHejJRewxbOQmbo5WUwQqnNVa78fMiUVyPcE90l-pfqIsBZtNx-uRTMI-6dciYNdzDGB4%3D&attredirects=0 (accessed on 14 July 2016).
34. Durnin, J.; Wormsley, J. Determination of percent body fat from the sum of biceps, triceps, subscapular and suprailiac skinfolds of male and female subjects. *Br. J. Nutr.* **1974**, *12*, 95–99.
35. Michels, K.B.; Schulze, M.B. Can dietary patterns help us detect diet–disease associations? *Nutr. Res. Rev.* **2005**, *18*, 241–248. [CrossRef] [PubMed]

36. Field, A.P. *Discovering Statistics Using SPSS for Windows*, 2nd ed.; Sage Publications: London, UK, 2005.
37. Naja, F.; Hwalla, N.; Itani, L.; Baalbaki, S.; Sibai, A.; Nasreddine, L. A novel mediterranean diet index from lebanon: Comparison with Europe. *Eur. J. Nutr.* **2014**, *54*, 1229–1254. [CrossRef] [PubMed]
38. Lopez-Garcia, E.; Guallar-Castillón, P.; Garcia-Esquinas, E.; Rodríguez-Artalejo, F. Metabolically healthy obesity and health-related quality of life: A prospective cohort study. *Clin. Nutr.* **2016**. in press. [CrossRef] [PubMed]
39. Lee, K.; Lee, S.; Kim, Y.J.; Kim, Y.J. Waist circumference, dual-energy X-ray absortiometrically measured abdominal adiposity, and computed tomographically derived intra-abdominal fat area on detecting metabolic risk factors in obese women. *Nutrition* **2008**, *24*, 625–631. [CrossRef] [PubMed]
40. Gonçalves, C.G.; Glade, M.J.; Meguid, M.M. Metabolically healthy obese individuals: Key protective factors. *Nutrition* **2015**, *32*, 14–20. [CrossRef] [PubMed]
41. Brochu, M.; Tchernof, A.; Dionne, I.J.; Sites, C.K.; Eltabbakh, G.H.; Sims, E.A.; Poehlman, E.T. What are the physical characteristics associated with a normal metabolic profile despite a high level of obesity in postmenopausal women? *J. Clin. Endocrinol. Metab.* **2001**, *86*, 1020–1025. [PubMed]
42. Heitmann, B.L. Obesity and gender. In *Clinical Obesity in Adults and Children*, 3rd ed.; Kopelman, P.G., Caterson, I.D., William, H.D., Eds.; John Wiley & Sons: West Sussex, UK, 2010; pp. 58–64.
43. Brunzell, J.D. Dyslipidemia of the metabolic syndrome. In *Obesity: Mechanisms and Clinical Management*; Eckel Robert, H., Ed.; Lippincott Williams & Wilkins: Philadelphia, PA, USA, 2003; pp. 378–396.
44. Nasreddine, L.; Hwalla, N.; Sibai, A.; Hamze, M.; Parent-Massin, D. Food consumption patterns in an adult urban population in beirut, lebanon. *Public Health Nutr.* **2006**, *9*, 194–203. [CrossRef] [PubMed]
45. Fagerli, R.A.; Wandel, M. Gender differences in opinions and practices with regard to a "healthy diet". *Appetite* **1999**, *32*, 171–190. [CrossRef] [PubMed]
46. Darmon, N.; Drewnowski, A. Does social class predict diet quality? *Am. J. Clin. Nutr.* **2008**, *87*, 1107–1117. [PubMed]
47. Van der Heijden, G.J.; Toffolo, G.; Manesso, E.; Sauer, P.J.; Sunehag, A.L. Aerobic exercise increases peripheral and hepatic insulin sensitivity in sedentary adolescents. *J. Clin. Endocrinol. Metab.* **2009**, *94*, 4292–4299. [CrossRef] [PubMed]
48. Naja, F.; Nasreddine, L.; Itani, L.; Chamieh, M.C.; Adra, N.; Sibai, A.M.; Hwalla, N. Dietary patterns and their association with obesity and sociodemographic factors in a national sample of lebanese adults. *Public Health Nutr.* **2011**, *14*, 1570–1578. [CrossRef] [PubMed]
49. Sleeth, M.L.; Thompson, E.L.; Ford, H.E.; Zac-Varghese, S.E.; Frost, G. Free fatty acid receptor 2 and nutrient sensing: A proposed role for fibre, fermentable carbohydrates and short-chain fatty acids in appetite regulation. *Nutr. Res. Rev.* **2010**, *23*, 135–145. [CrossRef] [PubMed]
50. Anderson, J.W.; Baird, P.; Davis, R.H., Jr.; Ferreri, S.; Knudtson, M.; Koraym, A.; Waters, V.; Williams, C.L. Health benefits of dietary fiber. *Nutr. Rev.* **2009**, *67*, 188–205. [CrossRef] [PubMed]
51. Fernandez, M.L.; West, K.L. Mechanisms by which dietary fatty acids modulate plasma lipids. *J. Nutr.* **2005**, *135*, 2075–2078. [PubMed]
52. Lopez, S.; Bermudez, B.; Ortega, A.; Varela, L.M.; Pacheco, Y.M.; Villar, J.; Abia, R.; Muriana, F.J. Effects of meals rich in either monounsaturated or saturated fat on lipid concentrations and on insulin secretion and action in subjects with high fasting triglyceride concentrations. *Am. J. Clin. Nutr.* **2011**, *93*, 494–499. [CrossRef] [PubMed]
53. Esmaillzadeh, A.; Kimiagar, M.; Mehrabi, Y.; Azadbakht, L.; Hu, F.B.; Willett, W.C. Fruit and vegetable intakes, c-reactive protein, and the metabolic syndrome. *Am. J. Clin. Nutr.* **2006**, *84*, 1489–1497. [PubMed]
54. Zemel, M.B. Mechanisms of dairy modulation of adiposity. *J. Nutr.* **2003**, *133*, 252s–256s. [PubMed]
55. Zemel, M.B. Role of dietary calcium and dairy products in modulating adiposity. *Lipids* **2003**, *38*, 139–146. [CrossRef] [PubMed]
56. Blüher, M. Mechanisms in endocrinology: Are metabolically healthy obese individuals really healthy? *Eur. J. Endocrinol.* **2014**, *171*, R209–R219. [CrossRef] [PubMed]

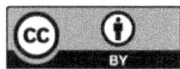

© 2016 by the authors. Licensee MDPI, Basel, Switzerland. This article is an open access article distributed under the terms and conditions of the Creative Commons Attribution (CC BY) license (http://creativecommons.org/licenses/by/4.0/).

nutrients

MDPI

Review

Dietary Interventions and Changes in Cardio-Metabolic Parameters in Metabolically Healthy Obese Subjects: A Systematic Review with Meta-Analysis

Marta Stelmach-Mardas [1,2,*] and Jarosław Walkowiak [2]

[1] Department of Epidemiology, German Institute of Human Nutrition, Potsdam-Rehbruecke, Arthur-Scheunert-Allee 114-116, Nuthetal 14558, Germany
[2] Department of Pediatric Gastroenterology and Metabolic Diseases, Poznan University of Medical Sciences, Szpitalna Str 27/33, Poznan 60-572, Poland; jarwalk@ump.edu.pl
* Correspondence: stelmach@dife.de; Tel.: +49-3200-88-2723; Fax: +49-33200-88-2721

Received: 8 May 2016; Accepted: 25 July 2016; Published: 28 July 2016

Abstract: The aim of this systematic review was to assess the effect of diet on changes in parameters describing the body size phenotype of metabolically healthy obese subjects. The databases Medline, Scopus, Web of Knowledge and Embase were searched for clinical studies carried out between 1958 and June 2016 that reported the effect of dietary intervention on BMI, blood pressure, concentration of fasting triglyceride (TG), high density lipoprotein cholesterol (HDL-C), fasting glucose level, the homoeostatic model assessment of insulin resistance (HOMA-IR) and high sensitivity C-Reactive Protein (hsCRP) in metabolically healthy, obese subjects. Twelve clinical studies met inclusion criteria. The combined analyzed population consists of 1827 subjects aged 34.4 to 61.1 with a BMI > 30 kg/m^2. Time of intervention ranged from eight to 104 weeks. The baseline characteristics related to lipid profile were more favorable for metabolically healthy obese than for metabolically unhealthy obese. The meta-analyses revealed a significant associations between restricted energy diet and BMI (95% confidence interval (CI): −0.88, −0.19), blood pressure (systolic blood pressure (SBP): −4.73 mmHg; 95% CI: −7.12, −2.33; and diastolic blood pressure (DBP): −2.75 mmHg; 95% CI: −4.30, −1.21) and TG (−0.11 mmol/l; 95% CI: −0.16, −0.06). Changes in fasting glucose, HOMA-IR and hsCRP did not show significant changes. Sufficient evidence was not found to support the use of specific diets in metabolically healthy obese subjects. This analysis suggests that the effect of caloric restriction exerts its effects through a reduction in BMI, blood pressure and triglycerides in metabolically healthy obese (MHO) patients.

Keywords: metabolically healthy obese; diet; biomarkers

1. Introduction

The prevalence of obesity is increasing worldwide with prognoses expected to affect more than one billion people by 2030 [1]. An association between obesity and increased risk of co-morbidities, i.e., metabolic syndrome (MetS) and cardiovascular disease (CVD) leading to significantly higher all-causes of mortality, has been observed [2]. However, the metabolically healthy obese (MHO) phenotype was described in the early 1980s [3], and, to date, there is no single consistent definition that covers "the metabolic health" approach in relation to differentiated dietary habits in obese subjects [4–6].

So far, the direct mechanism, which contributes to the different effects of weight loss in MHO and metabolically unhealthy obese (MUHO) subjects is not known, though it seems that it may vary as a function of different baseline metabolic profiles in MHO and MUHO groups. Only limited data are available with regards to dietary behaviors in MHO [7]. The prevalence of MHO is predicted to be 30%–40% of the obese population, with higher rates in younger subjects and in females [4,8]. Nevertheless, it should be taken under consideration that MHO subjects can shift to the metabolically unhealthy phenotype, a change confirmed by Schröder et al. [9] in a 10 years follow-up study.

Due to the fact that the effectiveness of dietary interventions in MHO is not very well known, we aimed to describe the influence of applied diet from intervention studies on changes in parameters describing the body size phenotype (body mass index—BMI, blood pressure—BP and concentration of selected biomarkers) of MHO.

2. Experimental Section

2.1. Search Strategy

The databases Medline, Scopus, Web of Knowledge and Embase were searched for clinical studies carried out between 1958 and June 2016 that reported the effect of dietary intervention on BMI and selected cardio-metabolic parameters (blood pressure and concentration of selected biomarkers) as primary or secondary outcomes in MHO. Search strategy was restricted to humans, English language and full length, original articles. The search based upon the listed below following index terms and title: #1 "Benign Obesity, Metabolically" OR "Metabolically Healthy Obesity" OR "Healthy Obesity, Metabolically" OR "Obesity, Metabolically Healthy" OR "Metabolically Benign Obesity" OR "Metabolically normal" OR "Metabolic syndrome" AND #2 "Diet" OR "Diet, carbohydrate-restricted" OR "Diet, fat-restricted" OR "Diet, protein-restricted" OR "Ketogenic diet" OR "Diet, high-fat" OR "Diet, reducing" OR "Weight reduction programs" OR "Caloric restriction" OR "Lifestyle intervention" NOT "Animals". The Preferred Reporting Items for Systematic Reviews and Meta-Analyses (PRISMA) Statement was followed [10].

2.2. Metabolically Healthy Obese—Definition

The criteria for MHO used in the studies include: absence of abdominal obesity on the basis of waist circumference, absence of metabolic syndrome components, e.g., normal blood pressure, normal lipid values, normal fasting glucose concentrations (at times also including normal C-reactive protein concentrations), insulin sensitivity determined on the basis of the homoeostatic model assessment of insulin resistance (HOMA-IR) and a high level of cardiorespiratory fitness [11]. All features were also used in the long-term prognosis of cardiovascular disease and all-cause mortality for MHO by Bo et al. [12], Calori et al., [13] and Hammer et al. [14].

Specifically, the criteria for the body size phenotype of MHO subjects include: a BMI $\geqslant 30$ kg/m^2 and <2 cardio-metabolic abnormalities (systolic/diastolic blood pressure (SBP/DBP) $\geqslant 130/85$ mmHg or antihypertensive medication use; fasting triglyceride (TG) level $\geqslant 150$ mg/dL (1.693 mmol/L)); decreased high density lipoprotein cholesterol (HDL-C) level < 40 mg/dL (1.0344 mmol/L) in men and <50 mg/dL (1.293 mmol/L) in women or lipid-lowering medication use; fasting glucose (Glc) level $\geqslant 100$ mg/dL (5.55 mmol/L) or antidiabetic medication use; insulin resistance: HOMA-IR > 5.13, i.e., the 90th percentile; systemic inflammation: high sensitivity C-Reactive Protein (hsCRP) level > 0.1 mg/L, i.e., the 90th percentile) [6]. Similar criteria were proposed by Meigs et al. [5] including the addition of waist circumference (WC) (>102 cm in men and >88 cm in women) and expanding the definition to include up to <3 cardio-metabolic abnormalities.

2.3. Inclusion and Exclusion Criteria

Only studies conducted with subjects described as metabolically healthy obese subjects, indicating the changes in BMI, blood pressure and selected blood parameters after various dietary interventions, were included. The intervention studies (randomized controlled trial and non-randomized trial) were taken into consideration. The articles that did not meet inclusion criteria (animal studies, other than the type of documents mentioned above, articles in any other language than English) were excluded.

2.4. Data Extraction and Analysis

Relevant articles were identified by screening the abstracts, titles and full-texts. The study selection process was performed by two independent researchers (M.S.-M. and J.W.) in parallel for each database. In every step of assessment, all disagreements between researchers were resolved after consultation. In the case of disagreement during the title assessment process, the paper was included in the next step. The process outline and workflow is presented in Figure 1.

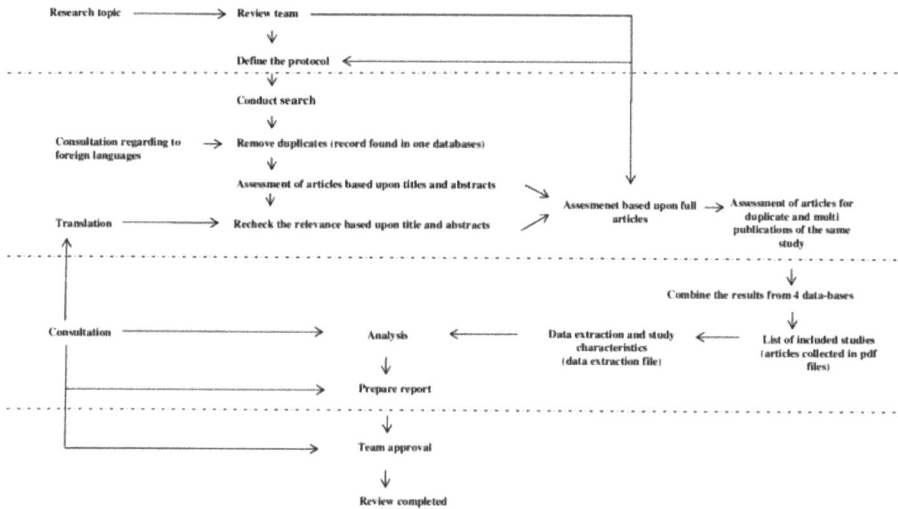

Figure 1. Process flow sheet.

Eligible studies were evaluated according to: the number of participants, study design, type of dietary intervention, changes in BMI (defined as body mass divided by the square of the height), and criteria for body size phenotype of MHO defined according to Third Report of the National Cholesterol Education Program Adult Treatment Panel (NCEP ATP III) [6]. To assess the study quality, a nine-point scoring system according to the Newcastle-Ottawa Scale was used. The maximum score was nine, with a high-quality study defined by a threshold of $\geqslant 7$ points [15].

The recorded biomarkers concentrations were converted to mmol/L (fasting glucose, Triglycerides, HDL-Cholesterol) and mg/L (hsCRP) in order to standardize results. A meta-analysis was performed to combine the results of individual studies. Data were analyzed using a random-effects model. The effect size of a study was investigated by calculating the standardized mean difference with a 95% confidence interval (CI). The heterogeneity of the sum of studies was tested for significance. As a measure for quantifying inconsistency, I^2 was selected [16]. Although included studies in our analysis were heterogeneous, careful inclusion of the suited arms (MHO group) in different interventions allowed us to combine the collected papers and run our analyses. The results of the meta-analysis were visualized using a forest plot which illustrates the results of the individual studies and the summary effect. The analysis was performed with Review Manager (RevMan, V5.3, The Nordic Cochrane Centre, the Cochrane Collaboration, Copenhagen, Denmark, 2014).

3. Results

3.1. Search Results

Using wide terms to describe the metabolically healthy obese patients, we end up with more than 14,000 articles that were screened. After initial exclusion criteria, 135 papers were assigned for full-text review with 12 articles included for data extraction and analysis [17–28] (Figure 2).

PRISMA 2009 Flow Diagram

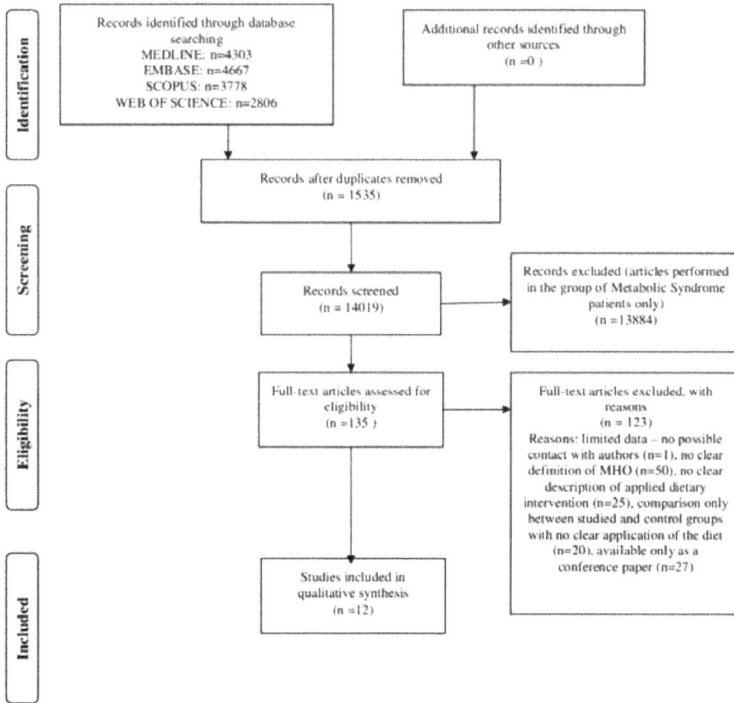

Figure 2. Process of literature search on the association between diet and selected cardio-metabolic parameters in metabolically healthy obese.

3.2. Studies and Populations Characteristics

The characteristics of clinical studies (randomized and non-randomized) and populations are presented in Table 1. The population consists of 1827 subjects and was characterized by a baseline BMI > 30 kg/m^2, a mean age from 34.4 [18] to 61.1 [20], and representing Caucasian and Asian ethnicities. Time of interventions ranged from 12 to 104 weeks and were based on diet only [18,21–27] or diet with combination of light to moderate physical activity (PA) [19,20,28] that supported the daily energy deficit.

Table 1. Characteristics of the included studies and study populations.

Study	Country	Total Number (Number of MHO)	Age (Years) Mean ± SD	Study Design	Intervention	Time of Intervention	Study Quality (Newcastle-Ottawa Scale)
Rondanelli et al., 2015 [17]	Italy	MHO: 103	MHO: 42.2 ± 9.2	Clinical study: non-RCT	Low-energy mix, well-balanced (55% carbohydrates, 30% lipids and 15% proteins) diet providing 600 kcal less than individually estimated energy requirements based on the measured Resting Energy Expenditure	8-week	7
Ruiz et al., 2013 [18]	Spain	78 (MHO: 25)	MHO: 34.4 ± 6.8 MUHO: 37.8 ± 6.9	Clinical study: non-RCT	Low-energy mixed diet (55% carbohydrates, 30% lipids and 15% proteins) providing 600 kcal less than individually estimated energy requirements based on measured resting metabolic rate (RMR) and multiplied by a factor of 1.3, corresponding to a low physical activity level	12-week	8
Kantartzis et al., 2011 [19]	Germany	262 (MHO: 26)	MHO: 46.8 ± 2.2 MUHO: 47.1 ± 1.3	Clinical study: non-RCT	Lifestyle intervention program with aim to reduce body weight by $\geq 5\%$, to reduce the intake of energy from fat to $<30\%$ and particularly the intake of saturated fat to $\leq 10\%$ of energy consumed and to increase the intake of dietary fiber to at least 15 g/4184 kJ (1000 kcal). Moderate sports per week: at least 3 h	36-week	7
Janiszewski & Ross, 2010 [20]	Canada	106 (MHO: 63)	MHO a. women: 61.1 ± 12.0 b. men: 61.4 ± 11.8 MUHO a. women: 46.5 ± 10.7 b. men: 53.1 ± 14.8	Clinical study: RCT	Men: program (diet or exercise) designed to induce a daily 700-kcal energy deficit Women: program (diet or exercise) designed to induce a daily 500-kcal energy deficit	Men: 12-week Women: 14-week	7
Shin et al., 2006 [21]	Korea	129 (MHO: 23)	MHO: 36.4 ± 11.2 MUHO: 39.8 ± 13.3	Clinical study: non-RCT	Weight loss program consisting of a 300 kcal/day reduction of usual caloric intakes to achieve the goal of losing a minimum of 3% of initial body weight	12-week	7
Liu et al., 2012 [22]	Canada	392 (MHO: 83)	53.6 ± 12.3	Clinical study: non-RCT	Calorie restricted meal plan of approximately 500–1000 calories below the patient's baseline daily caloric requirement to achieve the goal of losing a 5% of initial body weight	>12-week	8
Sesti et al., 2011 [23]	Italy	190	MHO: 38 ± 10 MUHO: 40 ± 10	Clinical study: non-RCT	Diet applied after Laparoscopic Adjustable Gastric Banding First month: a semiliquid diet of 800 and 950 kcal/day in women and men, respectively (33% proteins, 19% lipids, 48% carbohydrates). Second month: a solid diet was reintroduced. Third month: the suggested diet was 970 and 1090 kcal/day in women and men, respectively (diet included 48% carbohydrates (starch or bread), 33% proteins (fat-free parts of different animals and fish), and 19% lipids (olive oil)	>12-week	7

Table 1. *Cont.*

Study	Country	Total Number (Number of MHO)	Age (Years) Mean ± SD	Study Design	Intervention	Time of Intervention	Study Quality (Newcastle-Ottawa Scale)
Haro et al., 2015 [24]	Spain	MHO: 20	The LFHCC diet (a low-fat, high-complex carbohydrate diet) 61.4 ± 2.6 The Med diet (Mediterranean diet) 65.2 ± 3.2	Clinical study: RCT	The LFHCC diet contained 28% fat (12% monounsaturated; 8% polyunsaturated and 8% saturated) The Med diet contained 35% fat (22% monounsaturated; 6% polyunsaturated and 7% saturated)	52-week	8
Madero et al., 2011 [25]	Mexico	MHO: 131	The low-fructose diet 37.56 ± 1.14 The moderate natural fructose diet 40.15 ± 1.01	Clinical study: RCT	Energy-restricted diets: I. The low-fructose diet: first 2-week period of less than 10 g of fructose per day followed by a 4-week period of less than 20 g of fructose per day. II. The moderate natural fructose diet: consisted of 50 to 70 g of fructose consisting of mostly natural fructose from fruits.	6-week	7
Foster et al., 2010 [26]	US	MHO: 307	A low-carbohydrate diet 46.2 ± 9.2 A low-fat diet 44.9 ± 10.2	Clinical study: RCT	A low-carbohydrate diet which consisted of limited carbohydrate intake (20 g/day for 3 months) in the form of low-glycemic index vegetables with unrestricted consumption of fat and protein. After 3 months, participants in the low-carbohydrate diet group increased their carbohydrate intake (5 g per week) until a stable and desired weight was achieved A low-fat diet consisted of limited energy intake (1200 to 1800 kcal/day; ≤30% calories from fat)	104-week	8
Hermsdorff et al., 2011 [27]	Spain	MHO: 30	36.0 ± 8.0	Clinical study: RCT	The macronutrient-balanced diets (control and legume-based dietary approaches) were designed to provide a similar macronutrients distribution: 53% of energy as carbohydrates, 17% as proteins and 30% as fat	4-week	6
Christiansen et al., 2011 [28]	Denmark	MHO: 79	DIO group: 35.6 ± 7.0 DEX group: 37.5 ± 8.0	Clinical study: RCT	A liquid, very low energy diet of 600 and 800 kcal/day, respectively (proteins 41 g, carbohydrates 29 g, fat 5.6 g per 100 g), for 8 week followed by a weight maintenance diet for 4 week. In Diet-induced weight loss using a very low energy diet (DIO) and exercise and diet-induced weight-loss combined (DEX) groups the subjects should obtain similar weight losses to observe the possible specific, weight-independent effect of exercise. Thus, the subjects in the DEX group were allowed to consume 150–200 kcal more per day than the DIO group, reflecting the estimated extra energy expenditure of 1500 kcal/week during exercise activity. The supervised aerobic exercise three times per week with duration of 60–75 min per training session, with an estimated energy expenditure of 500–600 kcal per session	8-week	7

MHO: metabolically healthy obese; MUHO: metabolically unhealthy obese; non-RCT: non randomized control trial; LFHCC diet: a low-fat, high-complex carbohydrate diet; the Med diet: Mediterranean diet; DIO: a very low energy diet; DEX: exercise and diet-induced weight-loss combined.

3.3. Changes in Body Mass Index and Selected Cardio-Metabolic Outcomes during Dietary Interventions

The changes in BMI and selected cardio-metabolic outcomes during dietary interventions are presented in Table 2. Reduction in BMI, from baseline to the final day of intervention, ranged from 1.1 to 2.9 kg/m^2 in MHO, and were statistically significant in seven of twelve studies [18,20,22,23,25,27,28] within the study group. Kantartzis et al. [19], Haro et al. [24], and Foster et al. [26] failed to report exact values of baseline BMIs. The quantitative meta-analysis revealed a significant association between the restricted energy diets ($p < 0.0001$, $I^2 = 99\%$) and change in BMI (-2.70 kg/m^2; 95% CI: -4.01, -1.39) (Figure 3). The changes in systolic and diastolic blood pressure during the dietary interventions were measured only in six studies [20,22,25–28]. However, the meta-analysis showed statistically significant reduction in SBP (-4.73 mmHg; 95% CI: -7.12, -2.33; $p = 0.0001$, $I^2 = 87\%$) and DBP (-2.75 mmHg; 95% CI: -4.30, -1.21; $p = 0.0005$, $I^2 = 86\%$) within MHO group after applied dietary interventions, clinical relevance cannot be considered (Figure 4). The concentrations of TG and HDL-C were reported in all selected studies, where the baseline characteristic with regards to blood lipids was mostly more favorable for MHO than for metabolically unhealthy obese (MUHO) [19,21,23]. Nevertheless, the statistically significant association was observed only between energy restricted diets and the reduction in TG concentration (-0.11 mmol/L; 95% CI: -0.16, -0.06; $p < 0.0001$, $I^2 = 59\%$) (Figure 5). Fasting glucose was assessed in ten studies [15–18,20–23,25,26] with no significant decrease (-0.05 mmol/L; 95% CI: -0.14, 0.03; $p = 0.21$, $I^2 = 81\%$). Additionally, in the meta-analysis of studies reporting changes in HOMA-IR [17–19,21,25,27,28] in relation to dietary intervention, no significant reduction was observed within MHO group (-0.08; 95% CI: -0.31, 0.14; $p = 0.47$, $I^2 = 85\%$) (Figure 6). The reduction in hsCRP concentration were reported in only four studies [17,18,21,27] with no significant association with dietary intervention found (-0.19 mg/L; 95% CI: -1.35, 0.97; $p = 0.75$, $I^2 = 98\%$) (Figure 7). The funnel plot did not reveal asymmetry despite selected studies being outliers, suggesting no real evidence of a publication bias (Figure S1).

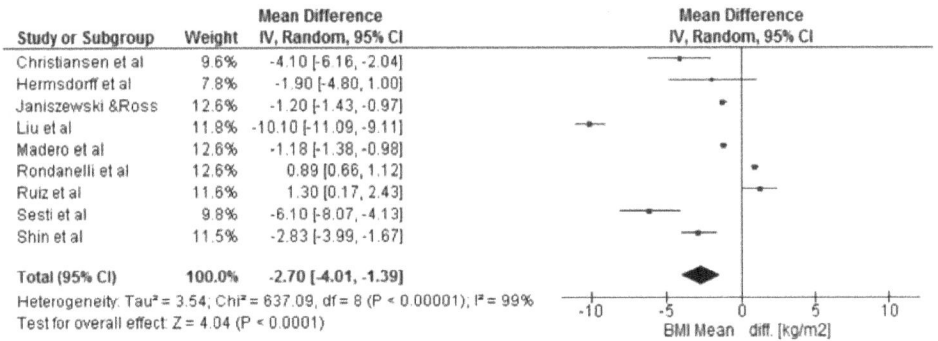

Study or Subgroup	Weight	Mean Difference IV, Random, 95% CI
Christiansen et al	9.6%	-4.10 [-6.16, -2.04]
Hermsdorff et al	7.8%	-1.90 [-4.80, 1.00]
Janiszewski &Ross	12.6%	-1.20 [-1.43, -0.97]
Liu et al	11.8%	-10.10 [-11.09, -9.11]
Madero et al	12.6%	-1.18 [-1.38, -0.98]
Rondanelli et al	12.6%	0.89 [0.66, 1.12]
Ruiz et al	11.6%	1.30 [0.17, 2.43]
Sesti et al	9.8%	-6.10 [-8.07, -4.13]
Shin et al	11.5%	-2.83 [-3.99, -1.67]
Total (95% CI)	100.0%	-2.70 [-4.01, -1.39]

Heterogeneity: Tau^2 = 3.54; Chi^2 = 637.09, df = 8 (P < 0.00001); I^2 = 99%
Test for overall effect: Z = 4.04 (P < 0.0001)

Figure 3. Forest plot of the random-effects meta-analysis of changes in BMI according to reduction in energy intake shown as polled standard differences in the means with 95% Cis and in randomized and non-randomized trials. * For each study, the square represents the point estimate of the intervention effect. Horizontal lines join the lower and upper limits of the 95% CI of this effect. The area of shaded squares reflects the relative weight of the study in the meta-analysis. Diamonds represent the subgroup mean difference and pooled mean differences. CI indicates confidence interval.

Nutrients 2016, 8, 455

Table 2. Changes in Body Mass Index and parameters describing cardio-metabolic outcomes in metabolically healthy obese.

Study	Intervention	Groups	BMI (kg/m²) Mean ± SD		Systolic/Diastolic Blood Pressure (mmHg) Mean ± SD		TG (mmol/L) Mean ± SD		HDL-C (mmol/L) Mean ± SD		Fasting Glucose (mmol/L) Mean ± SD		HOMA-IR Mean ± SD		hsCRP (mg/L) Mean ± SD	
			B'	I''	B'	I''	B'	I''	B'	I''	B'	I''	B'	I''	B'	I''
Rondanelli et al., 2015 [17]	Diet ONLY	MHO	0.89 (0.66 to 1.12)	-		-	0.03 (−0.21 to 0.27)*		−0.06 (−0.10 to 0.02)*		−0.06 (−0.17 to 0.05)*		−0.18 (−0.33 to 0.52)*		−4.00 (−6.00 to −1.00)*	
Ruiz et al., 2013 [18]	Diet ONLY	MHO:	+2.88 ± 1.3*		-		−0.03 ± 0.9*		+0.14 ± 0.3*		+1.2 ± 5.6*		+0.56 ± 0.7*		+1.51 ± 0.15*	
		MUHO:	+3.08 ± 1.1*				+0.31 ± 0.79*		+0.20 ± 0.28*		+2.1 ± 6.4*		+0.59 ± 0.66*		+0.38 ± 1.88	
Kantartzis et al., 2011 [19]	Diet AND exercise	MHO:	>30		-		1.71 ± 0.41	1.62 ± 0.44	1.37 ± 0.08	1.30 ± 0.05	5.07 ± 0.08	5.17 ± 0.10	1.16 ± 0.06	1.23 ± 0.08		
		MUHO:					1.56 ± 0.12	1.49 ± 0.08	1.27 ± 0.03	1.22 ± 0.03	5.42 ± 0.06	5.26 ± 0.06	2.98 ± 0.13	2.44 ± 0.14		
Janiszewski & Ross, 2010 [20]		MHO:											-			
		Men	−1.3 ± 1.0*		−3.0 ± 11.0*/−2.1 ± 6.4*		−0.2 ± 0.4*		+0.1 ± 0.1*		−0.1 ± 0.4*					
		Women	−1.1 ± 0.8*		−0.1 ± 11.3*/−1.5 ± 7.1*		0.0 ± 0.3*		0.0 ± 0.2*		0.0 ± 0.4					
	Diet OR exercise	MUHO:														
		Men	−1.9 ± 0.9*		−2.1 ± 11.9*/−2.9 ± 10.4*		−0.5 ± 0.7*		+0.1 ± 0.1*		−0.6 ± 0.7*					
		Women	−1.8 ± 1.0*		−1.9 ± 18.0*/0.3 ± 9.9*		−0.3 ± 0.5*		−0.0 ± 0.1*		−0.3 ± 0.8*					
Shin et al., 2006 [21]	Diet ONLY	MHO:	−2.83 ± 2.74**		-		1.09 ± 0.37	1.25 ± 0.54	1.33 ± 0.24	1.32 ± 0.25	-		1.80 ± 1.27	1.68 ± 0.76	0.74 ± 0.41	0.82 ± 0.45
		MUHO:	−3.16 ± 4.08**				1.72 ± 0.73	1.54 ± 0.78	1.09 ± 0.26	1.16 ± 0.26			2.60 ± 1.61	2.40 ± 2.3	1.9 ± 1.98	1.50 ± 1.3
Liu et al., 2012 [22]	Diet AND Supporting education	MHO:														
		<5% BW loss	−0.2 ± 3.4		−8.0 ± 1.0		−0.03 ± 0.07		0.08 ± 0.03		0.1 ± 0.15					
		>5% BW loss	−10.1 ± 4.6		−4.0 ± 1.0		−0.14 ± 0.07		−0.015 ± 0.03		0.0 ± 0.15					
		MUHO:														
		<5% BW loss	−1.1 ± 3.1		−4.0 ± 1.0		−0.19 ± 0.05		0.05 ± 0.01		−0.16 ± 0.09					
		>5% BW loss	−11.4 ± 5.6		−2.0 ± 1.0		−0.02 ± 0.05		0.02 ± 0.01		−0.07 ± 0.09					
Sesti et al., 2011 [23]	Diet Applied after LAGB'''	MHO:	41.1 ± 5.5	35.0 ± 5.3			1.34 ± 0.60	1.13 ± 0.52	1.24 ± 0.31	1.34 ± 0.31	5.2 ± 0.7	4.9 ± 0.7	-			
		MUHO:	44.0 ± 6.4	38.2 ± 5.6			1.58 ± 0.78	1.30 ± 0.55	1.27 ± 0.31	1.32 ± 0.34	5.7 ± 0.8	5.3 ± 0.7				
Haro et al., 2015 [24]	Diet ONLY	MHO:											-		-	
		LFHCC diet #	31.6 ± 0.8	-	129 ± 9.4	-	1.16 ± 0.09	1.11 ± 0.09	1.04 ± 0.06	1.03 ± 0.05	5.2 ± 0.2	5.1 ± 0.2				
		Med diet §	32.8 ± 0.5		136 ± 3.7		1.18 ± 0.13	0.97 ± 0.13	1.09 ± 0.06	1.16 ± 0.05	5.1 ± 0.2	5.4 ± 0.2				

Table 2. *Cont.*

Study	Intervention	Groups	BMI (kg/m²) Mean ± SD		Systolic/Diastolic Blood Pressure (mmHg) Mean ± SD		TG (mmol/L) Mean ± SD		HDL-C (mmol/L) Mean ± SD		Fasting Glucose (mmol/L) Mean ± SD		HOMA-IR Mean ± SD		hsCRP (mg/L) Mean ± SD	
			B'	I''	B'	I''	B'	I''	B'	I''	B'	I''	B'	I''	B'	I''
Madero et al., 2011 [25]	Diet ONLY	MHO: A low-fructose diet		−1.18 + 0.82		−9.46 + 7.77/ −5.17 + 4.69		−0.26 ± 0.78		0.0 ± 0.49		−0.30 ± 1.70		−0.29 ± 0.93		-
		A moderate natural fructose diet		−1.57 ± 1.08		−7.85 ± 8.73/ −6.04 ± 5.40		−0.35 ± 0.62		0.0 ± 0.31		−0.4 ± 0.5		−0.37 ± 0.57		-
Foster et al., 2010 [26]	Diet AND Supporting education	MHO: A low-carbohydrate diet		-		−2.68 (−5.08 to −0.27/ −3.19 (−4.66 to −1.73)		−0.13 (−0.25 to −0.01)		0.20 (0.15 to 0.25)		-		-		
		A low-fat diet				−2.59 (−5.07 to −0.12/ −0.50 (−2.13 to 1.13)		−0.16 (−0.28 to −0.03)		0.10 (0.08 to 0.16)						
Hermsdorff et al., 2011 [27]	Diet ONLY	MHO: Calorie-restricted legume-free diet	31.3 ± 4.0	29.4 ± 4.1	115 ± 9/ 76 ± 9	111 ± 12/ 72 ± 10	1.17 ± 0.32	1.17 ± 0.57	1.50 ± 0.26	1.27 ± 0.31	5.1 ± 0.5	5.0 ± 0.4	2.1 ± 1.7	1.6 ± 1.0	2.0 ± 1.0	1.9 ± 0.8
		Calorie-restricted legume-based diet	33.7 ± 4.7	31.7 ± 3.9	115 ± 13/ 76 ± 6	106 ± 10/ 70 ± 6	1.11 ± 0.43	1.09 ± 0.42	1.27 ± 0.26	1.14 ± 0.18	5.2 ± 0.3	5.1 ± 0.3	1.8 ± 0.9	1.6 ± 0.9	2.7 ± 2.4	1.6 ± 0.9
Christiansen et al., 2011 [28]	Diet OR Exercise OR Diet with Exercise	Exercise only (EXO)	33.3 ± 4	32.2 ± 4	126 ± 15/ 76 ± 12	118 ± 8/ 68 ± 9	1.6 ± 0.7	1.5 ± 0.4	1.3 ± 0.4	1.3 ± 0.5	5.6 ± 0.4	5.6 ± 5	2.3 ± 1.0	1.8 ± 1.0		
		Diet-induced weight loss using a very low energy diet (DIO)	35.3 ± 4	31.2 ± 4	129 ± 10/ 78 ± 12	122 ± 12/ 82 ± 12	1.5 ± 0.5	1.1 ± 0.3	1.2 ± 0.3	1.2 ± 0.3	5.5 ± 0.6	5.1 ± 0.5	3.1 ± 2.0	2.1 ± 1.0		-
		Exercise and diet-induced weight-loss combined (DEX)	34.2 ± 3	30.3 ± 3	140 ± 17/ 82 ± 12	129 ± 18/ 72 ± 13	1.8 ± 0.6	1.2 ± 0.5	1.2 ± 0.3	1.3 ± 0.3	5.6 ± 0.4	5.4 ± 0.5	3.2 ± 2.0	2.0 ± 1.0		

' B—Baseline; '' I—Intervention; * absolute changes; ** percent changes; statistically significant $p < 0.05$; MHO: metabolically healthy obese; MUHO: metabolically unhealthy obese; BMI: Body Mass Index; TG: triglycerides; HDL-C: high density lipoprotein cholesterol; HOMA-IR: homeostatic model assessment of insulin resistance; hsCRP: high-sensitivity C-reactive protein; BW—body weight changes; ''' LAGB: Laparoscopic Adjustable Gastric Banding; # LFHCC diet (a low-fat, high-complex carbohydrate diet); § The Med diet (Mediterranean diet) 65.2 ± 3.2.

Study or Subgroup	Weight	Mean Difference IV, Random, 95% CI
Christiansen et al	10.0%	-7.00 [-12.69, -1.31]
Foster et al	18.7%	-2.68 [-5.08, -0.28]
Hermsdorff et al	10.7%	-4.00 [-9.37, 1.37]
Janiszewski &Ross	17.7%	-1.60 [-4.34, 1.14]
Liu et al	22.9%	-4.00 [-4.22, -3.78]
Madero et al	20.1%	-9.46 [-11.35, -7.57]
Total (95% CI)	100.0%	-4.73 [-7.12, -2.33]

Heterogeneity: Tau² = 6.52; Chi² = 37.14, df = 5 (P < 0.00001); I² = 87%
Test for overall effect Z = 3.86 (P = 0.0001)

SBP Mean diff [mmHg]

Study or Subgroup	Weight	Mean Difference IV, Random, 95% CI
Christiansen et al	5.0%	4.00 [-2.18, 10.18]
Foster et al	20.6%	-3.19 [-4.66, -1.72]
Hermsdorff et al	7.3%	-4.00 [-8.81, 0.81]
Janiszewski &Ross	19.7%	-1.80 [-3.44, -0.16]
Liu et al	25.1%	-2.00 [-2.21, -1.79]
Madero et al	22.2%	-5.17 [-6.31, -4.03]
Total (95% CI)	100.0%	-2.75 [-4.30, -1.21]

Heterogeneity: Tau² = 2.47; Chi² = 35.21, df = 5 (P < 0.00001), I² = 86%
Test for overall effect Z = 3.49 (P = 0.0005)

DBP Mean diff [mmHg]

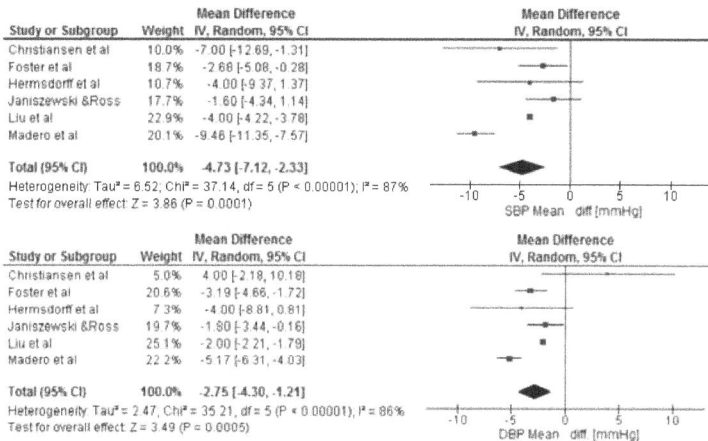

Figure 4. Forest plot of the random-effects meta-analysis of changes in Systolic and Diastolic Blood Pressure according to reduction in energy intake shown as polled standard differences in the means with 95% Cis and in randomized and non-randomized trials. * For each study, the square represents the point estimate of the intervention effect. Horizontal lines join the lower and upper limits of the 95% CI of this effect. The area of shaded squares reflects the relative weight of the study in the meta-analysis. Diamonds represent the subgroup mean difference and pooled mean differences. CI indicates confidence interval.

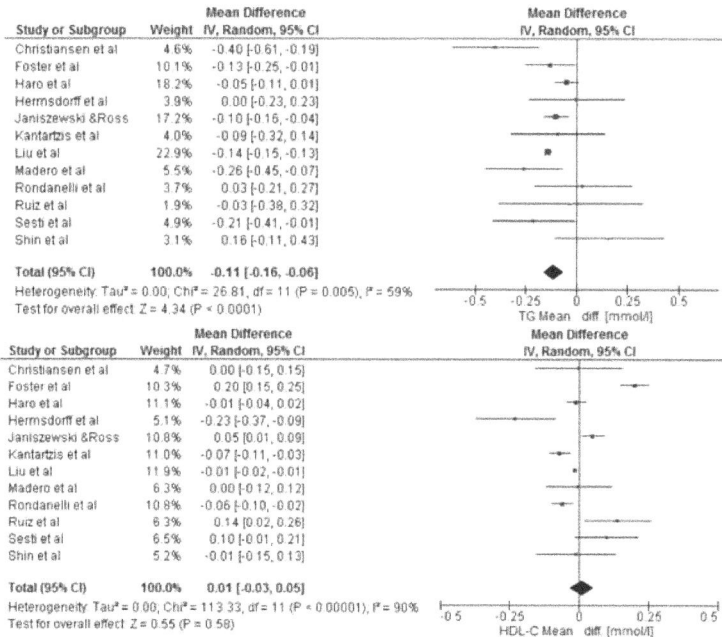

Study or Subgroup	Weight	Mean Difference IV, Random, 95% CI
Christiansen et al	4.6%	-0.40 [-0.61, -0.19]
Foster et al	10.1%	-0.13 [-0.25, -0.01]
Haro et al	18.2%	-0.05 [-0.11, 0.01]
Hermsdorff et al	3.9%	0.00 [-0.23, 0.23]
Janiszewski &Ross	17.2%	-0.10 [-0.16, -0.04]
Kantartzis et al	4.0%	-0.09 [-0.32, 0.14]
Liu et al	22.9%	-0.14 [-0.15, -0.13]
Madero et al	5.5%	-0.26 [-0.45, -0.07]
Rondanelli et al	3.7%	0.03 [-0.21, 0.27]
Ruiz et al	1.9%	-0.03 [-0.38, 0.32]
Sesti et al	4.9%	-0.21 [-0.41, -0.01]
Shin et al	3.1%	0.16 [-0.11, 0.43]
Total (95% CI)	100.0%	-0.11 [-0.16, -0.06]

Heterogeneity: Tau² = 0.00; Chi² = 26.81, df = 11 (P = 0.005), I² = 59%
Test for overall effect Z = 4.34 (P < 0.0001)

TG Mean diff [mmol/l]

Study or Subgroup	Weight	Mean Difference IV, Random, 95% CI
Christiansen et al	4.7%	0.00 [-0.15, 0.15]
Foster et al	10.3%	0.20 [0.15, 0.25]
Haro et al	11.1%	-0.01 [-0.04, 0.02]
Hermsdorff et al	5.1%	-0.23 [-0.37, -0.09]
Janiszewski &Ross	10.8%	0.05 [0.01, 0.09]
Kantartzis et al	11.0%	-0.07 [-0.11, -0.03]
Liu et al	11.9%	-0.01 [-0.02, -0.01]
Madero et al	6.3%	0.00 [-0.12, 0.12]
Rondanelli et al	10.8%	-0.06 [-0.10, -0.02]
Ruiz et al	6.3%	0.14 [0.02, 0.26]
Sesti et al	6.5%	0.10 [-0.01, 0.21]
Shin et al	5.2%	-0.01 [-0.15, 0.13]
Total (95% CI)	100.0%	0.01 [-0.03, 0.05]

Heterogeneity: Tau² = 0.00; Chi² = 113.33, df = 11 (P < 0.00001), I² = 90%
Test for overall effect Z = 0.55 (P = 0.58)

HDL-C Mean diff [mmol/l]

Figure 5. Forest plot of the random-effects meta-analysis of changes in Triglycerides and HDL-cholesterol according to reduction in energy intake shown as polled standard differences in the means with 95% Cis and in randomized and non-randomized trials. * For each study, the square represents the point estimate of the intervention effect. Horizontal lines join the lower and upper limits of the 95% CI of this effect. The area of shaded squares reflects the relative weight of the study in the meta-analysis. Diamonds represent the subgroup mean difference and pooled mean differences. CI indicates confidence interval.

Study or Subgroup	Weight	Mean Difference IV, Random, 95% CI
Christiansen et al	5.8%	-0.40 [-0.68, -0.12]
Haro et al	13.0%	-0.10 [-0.22, 0.02]
Hermsdorff et al	7.7%	-0.10 [-0.33, 0.13]
Janiszewski &Ross	14.6%	-0.05 [-0.15, 0.05]
Kantartzis et al	17.1%	0.10 [0.05, 0.15]
Liu et al	17.7%	0.10 [0.07, 0.13]
Madero et al	3.3%	-0.30 [-0.71, 0.11]
Rondanelli et al	13.8%	-0.06 [-0.17, 0.05]
Ruiz et al	0.1%	1.20 [-1.00, 3.40]
Sesti et al	6.7%	-0.30 [-0.55, -0.05]
Total (95% CI)	100.0%	-0.05 [-0.14, 0.03]

Heterogeneity: Tau² = 0.01; Chi² = 47.77, df = 9 (P < 0.00001); I² = 81%
Test for overall effect: Z = 1.25 (P = 0.21)

Fasting Glc Mean diff. [mmol/l]

Study or Subgroup	Weight	Mean Difference IV, Random, 95% CI
Christiansen et al	5.8%	-1.00 [-1.81, -0.19]
Hermsdorff et al	7.1%	-0.50 [-1.21, 0.21]
Kantartzis et al	22.5%	0.07 [0.03, 0.11]
Madero et al	18.5%	-0.29 [-0.52, -0.06]
Rondanelli et al	20.6%	-0.18 [-0.33, -0.03]
Ruiz et al	17.0%	0.56 [0.29, 0.83]
Shin et al	8.7%	-0.12 [-0.72, 0.48]
Total (95% CI)	100.0%	-0.08 [-0.31, 0.14]

Heterogeneity: Tau² = 0.06, Chi² = 41.12, df = 6 (P < 0.00001); I² = 85%
Test for overall effect: Z = 0.72 (P = 0.47)

HOMA Mean diff.

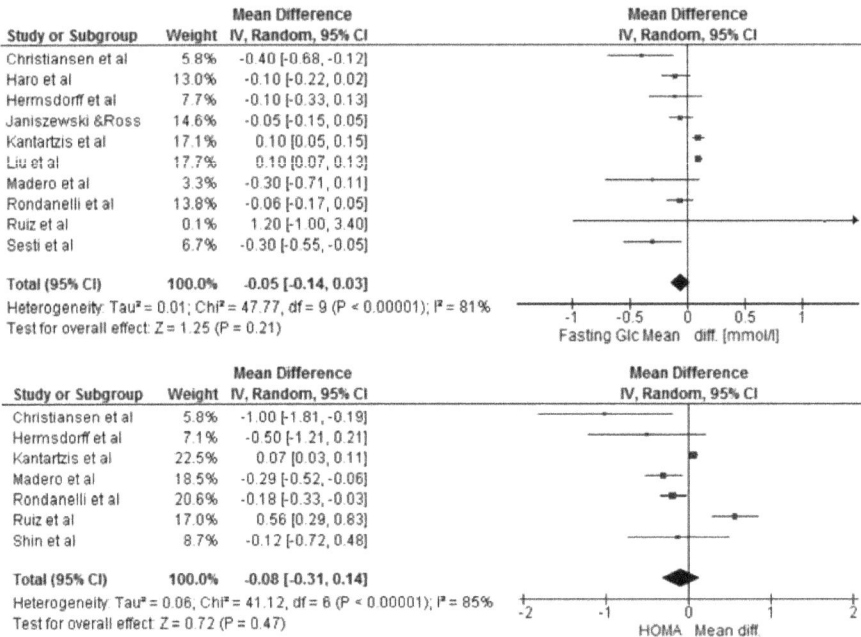

Figure 6. Forest plot of the random-effects meta-analysis of changes in Fasting Glucose and HOMA-IR according to reduction in energy intake shown as polled standard differences in the means with 95% Cis and in randomized and non-randomized trials. * For each study, the square represents the point estimate of the intervention effect. Horizontal lines join the lower and upper limits of the 95% CI of this effect. The area of shaded squares reflects the relative weight of the study in the meta-analysis. Diamonds represent the subgroup mean difference and pooled mean differences. CI indicates confidence interval.

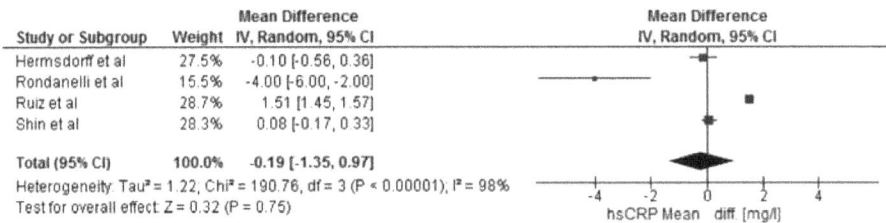

Study or Subgroup	Weight	Mean Difference IV, Random, 95% CI
Hermsdorff et al	27.5%	-0.10 [-0.56, 0.36]
Rondanelli et al	15.5%	-4.00 [-6.00, -2.00]
Ruiz et al	28.7%	1.51 [1.45, 1.57]
Shin et al	28.3%	0.08 [-0.17, 0.33]
Total (95% CI)	100.0%	-0.19 [-1.35, 0.97]

Heterogeneity: Tau² = 1.22, Chi² = 190.76, df = 3 (P < 0.00001); I² = 98%
Test for overall effect: Z = 0.32 (P = 0.75)

hsCRP Mean diff. [mg/l]

Figure 7. Forest plot of the random-effects meta-analysis of changes in high sensitivity C-Reactive Protein according to reduction in energy intake shown as polled standard differences in the means with 95% Cis and in randomized and non-randomized trials. * For each study, the square represents the point estimate of the intervention effect. Horizontal lines join the lower and upper limits of the 95% CI of this effect. The area of shaded squares reflects the relative weight of the study in the meta-analysis. Diamonds represent the subgroup mean difference and pooled mean differences. CI indicates confidence interval.

4. Discussion

Here, we present the first review summarizing the results from clinical studies performed in MHO with a primary interest in changes in BMI and selected cardio-metabolic outcomes. The findings of the conducted systematic review with meta-analysis did not find sufficient evidence to support the use of some specific diet in metabolically healthy obese subjects. However, it seems that effect of caloric restriction is related to reduction in BMI, blood pressure and triglycerides in the group of MHO patients.

It was imperative for the conducted review to show that the MHO subjects should be recognized as the core group with a primary interest in a changing lifestyle being the determinant of "metabolic health". Other longitudinal studies [29,30] with shorter follow-up (6–8.2 years) have indicated that only approximately half of MHO subjects maintained their "metabolic health" status. It was also suggested that initially MHO subjects undergo adverse metabolic changes associated with obesity over time [31]. Nevertheless, there is no clear data regarding the most beneficial dietary interventions, nor the effectiveness, of energy restricted diets in MHO patients taking into account clinical significance.

As previously demonstrated [32,33], obesity can be associated with a higher relative risk for CVD and cancer mortality compared to non-obese subjects. Therefore, the decrease in BMI can reflect the improvement in body composition, and consequently, reduce the mortality [34]. We have observed a significant association between the applications of energy restricted diets and BMI reduction in MHO individuals. Recently, Phillips and Perry [35] has also indicated that greater low density lipoprotein cholesterol (LDL-C) and HDL-C and less very low density lipoprotein cholesterol (VLDL-C) particles increase the likelihood of MHO. However, the results of our meta-analysis, through the applied dietary interventions, indicated only significantly beneficial association with the TG concentration within the MHO group. However, the inflammatory status in MHO can be reduced [36], partially stemming from more favorable fatty acid profiles [37] compared to MUHO, a significant decrease in hsCRP concentration was not observed in our analysis. As has been highlighted by Karelis et al. [38] health status may strongly influence the response to diet. For example, it was indicated in the MHO sedentary obese postmenopausal women without type 2 diabetes that the response to an energy-restricted diet may be different compared to at-risk individuals who achieve a similar weight loss, in that insulin sensitivity significantly improved in at-risk participants, but significantly deteriorated in MHO individuals in response to long-term diet. In our study, we did not find significant relation between energy restricted diets and biomarkers related to carbohydrates metabolism, i.e., fasting glucose and HOMA-IR within the MHO group of individuals. As shown in previously published studies [31,33], the baseline characteristic of metabolic profile can be more favorable in MHO compared to MUHO, which stay in line with some data selected for this systematic review [19,21]. As reported in Karelis et al. [39], MHO may have higher insulin sensitivity and a more favorable lipid profile. It has also been confirmed by Badoud et al. [40] that MHO individuals may show preserved insulin sensitivity and a greater ability to adapt to a caloric challenge compared to MUHO individuals. The postprandial response (i.e., area under the curve, AUC) for serum glucose and insulin were similar between MHO and lean healthy individuals and significantly lower than MUHO individuals ($p < 0.05$) [32]. However, a healthy metabolic profile and the absence of diabetic risk factors did not protect young adults from incident diabetes associated with overweight and obesity [40]. The intake of contraceptive pills by premenopausal women studied by Ruiz et al. [18] suggested that obtained results might be applied only for this sex and age group. Interestingly, the potential differences in body composition between MHO and MUHO were assessed in adults from the Pennington Center Longitudinal Study showing differences consistent between genders in both analyzed groups [34]. In clinical practice, as a goal for reducing CVD risk, the importance of body weight loss contributing to the maintenance of body weight loss is highlighted [4,41,42]. Camhi et al. [43] indicated that MHO young women demonstrate healthier lifestyle habits with less sedentary behavior, more time doing light physical activity, and healthier dietary quality for fat type and fiber in comparison to MUHO. Therefore, MUHO subjects are characterized by a higher risk of diabetes compared to MHO, which has been previously observed in Korean populations [44]. Indeed, metabolic health status, obesity and weight change were all independently associated with increased incidences of diabetes over five years of follow-up [44]. Nevertheless, we focused in our analysis on the MHO group of individuals only looking at the consequence of the applied dietary interventions. The data from the

International Population Study on Macro/Micronutrients and Blood Pressure (INTERMAP) cohort study did not support the hypothesis that diet composition accounts for the absence of cardio-metabolic abnormalities in MHO [45]. Furthermore, it has also been confirmed by Kimokoti et al. [46] in the cross-sectional analysis from the REasons for Geographic And Racial Differences in Stroke (REGARDS) study. Although HOMA-IR index can be slightly higher in MHO subjects than in subjects characterized by normal weight, it may also be lower compared to MUHO [21]. It has been also shown that a long-term intensive lifestyle program, including Mediterranean diet nutritional counselling and high-intensity interval training, may be an appropriate intervention in MHO and MUHO subjects with similar potential clinical health benefits including an improved body composition, blood pressure, fasting glucose levels, insulin sensitivity, peak oxygen uptake, and muscle endurance [47]. Therefore, it could be beneficial that the results obtained in intervention studies with regards to analyzed cardio-metabolic outcomes may have yielded stronger and more consistent support from the results of observational studies. More broadened interventional studies are needed to assess different dietary approaches in MHO subjects.

5. Limitations

The present findings are based on limited ethnicity (Caucasian, Asian), and, therefore, results could vary as a function of ethnic background. Although the duration of interventions in analyzed studies was relatively long, we could not analyze long-term follow-up changes of analyzed cardio-metabolic parameters (no data available in the literature). Although the applied dietary interventions were very different and heterogeneous in nature, all of them were based on energy restriction.

6. Conclusions

Based on the limited body of extracted data, we did not find sufficient evidence to support the use of some specific diet in metabolically healthy obese subjects. In general, it seems that the effect of caloric restriction is related to reduction in BMI, blood pressure and triglycerides in MHO individuals.

Supplementary Materials: The following are available online at http://www.mdpi.com/2072-6643/8/8/455/s1, Figure S1: Funnel plot of standard error by standard differences in means of (a) Body Mass Index; (b) Systolic Blood Pressure; (c) Diastolic Blood Pressure; (d) Trygliceride; (e) HDL-cholesterol; (f) Fasting Glucose; (g) HOMA-OR; (h) hsCRP.

Acknowledgments: The authors are grateful to Robert J. Tower for English correction of the manuscript and Marcin Mardas for help in the updated search process.

Author Contributions: M.S.M. and J.W. designed the research and conducted the search. M.S.M. wrote the manuscript and analyzed data. J.W. critically reviewed manuscript content.

Conflicts of Interest: The authors declare no conflict of interest.

References

1. Kelly, T.; Yang, W.; Chen, C.S.; Reynolds, K.; He, J. Global burden of obesity in 2005 and projections to 2030. *Int. J. Obes.* **2008**, *32*, 1431–1437. [CrossRef] [PubMed]
2. Flegal, K.M.; Kit, B.K.; Orpana, H.; Graubard, B.I. Association of all-cause mortality with overweight and obesity using standard body mass index categories: A systematic review and meta-analysis. *JAMA* **2013**, *309*, 71–82. [CrossRef] [PubMed]
3. Ruderman, N.B.; Schneider, S.H.; Berchtold, P. The "metabolically obese", normal-weight individual. *Am. J. Clin. Nutr.* **1981**, *34*, 1617–1621. [CrossRef] [PubMed]
4. Wildman, R.P.; Muntner, P.; Reynolds, K.; McGinn, A.P.; Rajpathak, S.; Wylie-Rosett, J.; Sowers, M.R. The obese without cardiometabolic risk factor clustering and the normal weight with cardiometabolic risk factor clustering: Prevalence and correlates of 2 phenotypes among the US population (NHANES 1999–2004). *Arch. Intern. Med.* **2008**, *168*, 1617–1624. [CrossRef] [PubMed]

5. Meigs, J.B.; Wilson, P.W.; Fox, C.S.; Vasan, R.S.; Nathan, D.M.; Sullivan, L.M.; D'Agostino, R.B. Body mass index, metabolic syndrome, and risk of type 2 diabetes or cardiovascular disease. *J. Clin. Endocrinol. Metab.* **2006**, *91*, 2906–2912. [CrossRef] [PubMed]

6. Executive summary of the third report of the National Cholesterol Education Program (NCEP) expert panel on detection, evaluation, and treatment of high blood cholesterol in adults (adult treatment panel III). *JAMA* **2001**, *285*, 2486–2497.

7. Van Vliet-Ostaptchouk, J.V.; Nuotio, M.L.; Slagter, S.N.; Doiron, D.; Fischer, K.; Foco, L.; Gaye, A.; Gögele, M.; Heier, M.; Hiekkalinna, T.; et al. The prevalence of metabolic syndrome and metabolically healthy obesity in Europe: A collaborative analysis of ten large cohort studies. *BMC Endocr. Disord.* **2014**, *14*, 9. [CrossRef] [PubMed]

8. Soriguer, F.; Gutiérrez-Repiso, C.; Rubio-Martín, E.; García-Fuentes, E.; Almaraz, M.C.; Colomo, N.; de Antonio, I.E.; de Adana, M.S.R.; Chaves, F.J.; Morcillo, S.; et al. Metabolically healthy but obese, a matter of time? Findings from the prospective Pizarra study. *J. Clin. Endocrinol. Metab.* **2013**, *98*, 2318–2325. [CrossRef] [PubMed]

9. Schröder, H.; Ramos, R.; Baena-Díez, J.M.; Mendez, M.A.; Canal, D.J.; Fito, M.; Sala, J.; Elosua, R. Determinants of the transition from a cardiometabolic normal to abnormal overweight/obese phenotype in a Spanish population. *Eur. J. Nutr.* **2013**, *53*, 1345–1353. [CrossRef] [PubMed]

10. Moher, D.; Liberati, A.; Tetzlaff, J.; Altman, D.G.; PRISMA Group. Preferred reporting items for systematic reviews and meta-analyses: The PRISMA statement. *PLoS Med.* **2009**, *6*, e1000097. [CrossRef] [PubMed]

11. Stefan, N.; Häring, H.U.; Hu, F.B.; Schulze, M.B. Metabolically healthy obesity: Epidemiology, mechanisms, and clinical implications. *Lancet Diabetes Endocrinol.* **2013**, *1*, 152–162. [CrossRef]

12. Bo, S.; Musso, G.; Gambino, R.; Villois, P.; Gentile, L.; Durazzo, M.; Cavallo-Perin, P.; Cassader, M. Prognostic implications for insulin-sensitive and insulin-resistant normal-weight and obese individuals from a population-based cohort. *Am. J. Clin. Nutr.* **2012**, *96*, 962–969. [CrossRef] [PubMed]

13. Calori, G.; Lattuada, G.; Piemonti, L.; Garancini, M.P.; Ragogna, F.; Villa, M.; Mannino, S.; Crosignani, P.; Bosi, S.; Luzi, L.; et al. Prevalence, metabolic features, and prognosis of metabolically healthy obese Italian Individuals: The Cremona Study. *Diabetes Care* **2011**, *34*, 210–215. [CrossRef] [PubMed]

14. Hamer, M.; Stamatakis, E. Metabolically healthy obesity and risk of all-cause and cardiovascular disease mortality. *J. Clin. Endocrinol. Metab.* **2012**, *97*, 2482–2488. [CrossRef] [PubMed]

15. Wells, G.; Shea, B.; O'Connell, D.; Peterson, J.; Welch, V.; Losos, M.; Tugwell, P. The Newcastle-Ottawa Scale (NOS) for Assessing the Quality of Nonrandomized Studies in Meta–Analyses. Available online: http://www.ohri.ca/programs/clinical_epidemiology/oxford.htm (accessed on 17 June 2016).

16. Borenstein, M.; Hedges, L.V.; Higgins, J.P.T.; Rothstein, H.R. *Introduction to Meta-Analysis*; John Wiley & Sons Ltd.: Chichester, UK, 2009.

17. Rondanelli, M.; Klersy, C.; Perna, S.; Faliva, M.A.; Montorfano, G.; Roderi, P.; Colombo, I.; Corsetto, P.A.; Fioravanti, M.; Solerte, S.B.; et al. Effects of two-months balanced diet in metabolically healthy obesity: Lipid correlations with gender and BMI-related differences. *Lipids Health Dis.* **2015**, *14*, 139. [CrossRef] [PubMed]

18. Ruiz, J.R.; Ortega, F.B.; Labayen, I. A weight loss diet intervention has a similar beneficial effect on both metabolically abnormal obese and metabolically healthy but obese premenopausal women. *Ann. Nutr. Metab.* **2013**, *62*, 223–230. [CrossRef] [PubMed]

19. Kantartzis, K.; Machann, J.; Schick, F.; Rittig, K.; Machicao, F.; Fritsche, A.; Häring, H.-U.; Stefan, N. Effects of a lifestyle intervention in metabolically benign and malign obesity. *Diabetologia* **2011**, *54*, 864–868. [CrossRef] [PubMed]

20. Janiszewski, P.M.; Ross, R. Effects of weight loss among metabolically healthy obese men and women. *Diabetes Care* **2010**, *33*, 1957–1959. [CrossRef] [PubMed]

21. Shin, M.J.; Hyun, Y.J.; Kim, O.Y.; Kim, J.Y.; Jang, Y.; Lee, J.H. Weight loss effect on inflammation and LDL oxidation in metabolically healthy but obese (MHO) individuals: Low inflammation and LDL oxidation in MHO women. *Int. J. Obes.* **2006**, *30*, 1529–1534. [CrossRef] [PubMed]

22. Phillips, C.M. Metabolically healthy obesity: Definitions, determinants and clinical implications. *Rev. Endocr. Metab. Disord.* **2013**, *14*, 219–227. [CrossRef] [PubMed]

23. Liu, R.H.; Wharton, S.; Sharma, A.M.; Ardern, C.I.; Kuk, J.L. Influence of a clinical lifestyle-based weight loss program on the metabolic risk profile of metabolically normal and abnormal obese adults. *Obesity* **2013**, *21*, 1533–1539. [CrossRef] [PubMed]

24. Sesti, G.; Folli, F.; Perego, L.; Hribal, M.L.; Pontiroli, A.E. Effects of weight loss in metabolically healthy obese subjects after laparoscopic adjustable gastric banding and hypocaloric diet. *PLoS ONE* **2011**, *6*, e17737. [CrossRef] [PubMed]

25. Haro, C.; Montes-Borrego, M.; Rangel-Zúñiga, O.A.; Alcalá-Díaz, J.F.; Gómez-Delgado, F.; Pérez-Martínez, P.; Delgado-Lista, J.; Quintana-Navarro, G.M.; Tinahones, F.J.; Landa, B.B.; et al. Two Healthy Diets Modulate Gut Microbial Community Improving Insulin Sensitivity in a Human Obese Population. *J. Clin. Endocrinol. Metab.* **2016**, *101*, 233–242. [CrossRef] [PubMed]

26. Madero, M.; Arriaga, J.C.; Jalal, D.; Rivard, C.; McFann, K.; Pérez-Méndez, O.; Vázquez, A.; Ruiz, A.; Lanaspa, M.A.; Jimenez, C.R.; et al. The effect of two energy-restricted diets, a low-fructose diet versus a moderate natural fructose diet, on weight loss and metabolic syndrome parameters: A randomized controlled trial. *Metabolism* **2011**, *60*, 1551–1559. [CrossRef] [PubMed]

27. Foster, G.D.; Wyatt, H.R.; Hill, J.O.; Makris, A.P.; Rosenbaum, D.L.; Brill, C.; Stein, R.I.; Mohammed, B.S.; Miller, B.; Rader, D.J.; et al. Weight and metabolic outcomes after 2 years on a low-carbohydrate versus low-fat diet: A randomized trial. *Ann. Intern. Med.* **2010**, *153*, 147–157. [CrossRef] [PubMed]

28. Hermsdorff, H.H.M.; Zulet, M.Á.; Abete, I.; Martínez, J.A. A legume-based hypocaloric diet reduces proinflammatory status and improves metabolic features in overweight/obese subjects. *Eur. J. Nutr.* **2011**, *50*, 61–69. [CrossRef] [PubMed]

29. Christiansen, T.; Paulsen, S.K.; Bruun, J.M.; Pedersen, S.B.; Richelsen, B. Exercise training versus diet-induced weight-loss on metabolic risk factors and inflammatory markers in obese subjects: A 12-week randomized intervention study. *Am. J. Physiol. Endocrinol. Metab.* **2010**, *298*, E824–E831. [CrossRef] [PubMed]

30. Chang, Y.; Ryu, S.; Suh, B.S.; Yun, K.E.; Kim, C.-W.; Cho, S.-I. Impact of BMI on the incidence of metabolic abnormalities in metabolically healthy men. *Int. J. Obes.* **2012**, *36*, 1187–1194. [CrossRef] [PubMed]

31. Ortega, F.B.; Lee, D.C.; Katzmarzyk, P.T.; Ruiz, J.R.; Sui, X.; Church, T.S.; Blair, S.N. The intriguing metabolically healthy but obese phenotype: Cardiovascular prognosis and role of fitness. *Eur. Heart J.* **2013**, *34*, 389–397. [CrossRef] [PubMed]

32. Arnlov, J.; Ingelsson, E.; Sundstrom, J.; Lind, L. Impact of body mass index and the metabolic syndrome on the risk of cardiovascular disease and death in middle-aged men. *Circulation* **2010**, *121*, 230–236. [CrossRef] [PubMed]

33. Berentzen, T.L.; Jakobsen, M.U.; Halkjaer, J.; Tjønneland, A.; Overvad, K.; Sørensen, T.I.A. Changes in waist circumference and mortality in middle-aged men and women. *PLoS ONE* **2010**, *5*, e13097. [CrossRef] [PubMed]

34. Stelmach-Mardas, M.; Mardas, M.; Warchoł, W.; Jamka, M.; Walkowiak, J. Successful maintenance of body weight reduction after individualized dietary counseling in obese subjects. *Sci. Rep.* **2014**, *4*, 6620. [CrossRef] [PubMed]

35. Phillips, C.M.; Perry, I.J. Lipoprotein particle subclass profiles among metabolically healthy and unhealthy obese and non-obese adults: Does size matter? *Atherosclerosis* **2015**, *242*, 399–406. [CrossRef] [PubMed]

36. Perreault, M.; Zulyniak, M.A.; Badoud, F.; Stephenson, S.; Badawi, A.; Buchholz, A.; Mutch, D.M. A distinct fatty acid profile underlies the reduced inflammatory state of metabolically healthy obese individuals. *PLoS ONE* **2014**, *9*, e88539. [CrossRef] [PubMed]

37. Jung, H.S.; Chang, Y.; Eun Yun, K.; Kim, C.W.; Choi, E.S.; Kwon, M.J.; Cho, J.; Zhang, Y.; Rampal, S.; Zhao, D.; et al. Impact of body mass index, metabolic health and weight change on incident diabetes in a Korean population. *Obesity* **2014**, *22*, 1880–1887. [CrossRef] [PubMed]

38. Karelis, A.D.; Messier, V.; Brochu, M.; Rabasa-Lhoret, R. Metabolically healthy but obese women: Effect of an energy-restricted diet. *Diabetologia* **2008**, *51*, 1752–1754. [CrossRef] [PubMed]

39. Karelis, A.D.; St-Pierre, D.H.; Conus, F.; Rabasa-Lhoret, R.; Poehlman, E.T. Metabolic and body composition factors in subgroups of obesity: What do we know? *J. Clin. Endocrinol. Metab.* **2004**, *89*, 2569–2575. [CrossRef] [PubMed]

40. Badoud, F.; Lam, K.P.; Perreault, M.; Zulyniak, M.A.; Britz-McKibbin, P.; Mutch, D.M. Metabolomics Reveals Metabolically Healthy and Unhealthy Obese Individuals Differ in their Response to a Caloric Challenge. *PLoS ONE* **2015**, *10*, e0134613. [CrossRef] [PubMed]

41. Stelmach-Mardas, M.; Mardas, M.; Walkowiak, J.; Boeing, H. Long-term weight status in regainers after weight loss by lifestyle intervention: Status and challenges. *Proc. Nutr. Soc.* **2014**, *73*, 509–518. [CrossRef] [PubMed]

42. Phillips, C.M.; Dillon, C.; Harrington, J.M.; McCarthy, V.J.C.; Kearney, P.M.; Fitzgerald, A.P.; Perry, I.J. Defining metabolically healthy obesity: Role of dietary and lifestyle factors. *PLoS ONE* **2013**, *8*, e76188. [CrossRef] [PubMed]

43. Camhi, S.M.; Katzmarzyk, P.T. Differences in body composition between metabolically healthy obese and metabolically abnormal obese adults. *Int. J. Obes.* **2014**, *38*, 1142–1145. [CrossRef] [PubMed]

44. Camhi, S.M.; Crouter, S.E.; Hayman, L.L.; Must, A.; Lichtenstein, A.H. Lifestyle Behaviors in Metabolically Healthy and Unhealthy Overweight and Obese Women: A Preliminary Study. *PLoS ONE* **2015**, *10*, e0138548. [CrossRef] [PubMed]

45. Calanna, S.; Piro, S.; di Pino, A.; Zagami, R.M.; Urbano, F.; Purrello, F.; Rabuazzo, A.M. Beta and alpha cell function in metabolically healthy but obese subjects: Relationship with entero-insular axis. *Obesity* **2014**, *21*, 320–325. [CrossRef] [PubMed]

46. Hankinson, A.L.; Daviglus, M.L.; van Horn, L. Diet composition and activity level of at risk and metabolically healthy obese American adults. *Obesity* **2013**, *21*, 637–643. [CrossRef] [PubMed]

47. Kimokoti, R.W.; Judd, S.E.; Shikany, J.M.; Newby, P.K. Food intake does not differ between obese women who are metabolically healthy or abnormal. *J. Nutr.* **2014**, *144*, 2018–2026. [CrossRef] [PubMed]

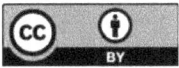

© 2016 by the authors. Licensee MDPI, Basel, Switzerland. This article is an open access article distributed under the terms and conditions of the Creative Commons Attribution (CC BY) license (http://creativecommons.org/licenses/by/4.0/).

nutrients

MDPI

Article

Eicosapentaenoic and Docosahexaenoic Acid-Enriched High Fat Diet Delays Skeletal Muscle Degradation in Mice

Nikul K. Soni [1],*, Alastair B. Ross [1], Nathalie Scheers [1], Otto I. Savolainen [1], Intawat Nookaew [2,3], Britt G. Gabrielsson [1] and Ann-Sofie Sandberg [1]

[1] Division of Food and Nutrition Science, Department of Biology and Biological Engineering, Chalmers University of Technology, Gothenburg SE-41296, Sweden; alastair.ross@chalmers.se (A.B.R.); nathalie.scheers@chalmers.se (N.S.); otto.savolainen@chalmers.se (O.I.S.); bggabr@gmail.com (B.G.G.); ann-sofie.sandberg@chalmers.se (A.-S.S.)

[2] Division of Systems and Synthetic Biology, Department of Biology and Biological Engineering, Chalmers University of Technology, Gothenburg SE-412 96, Sweden; intawat@chalmers.se

[3] Department of Biomedical Informatics, College of Medicine, University of Arkansas for Medical Sciences, Little Rock, AR 72204, USA

* Correspondence: soni@chalmers.se; Tel.: +46-31-772-3816

Received: 26 May 2016; Accepted: 25 August 2016; Published: 3 September 2016

Abstract: Low-grade chronic inflammatory conditions such as ageing, obesity and related metabolic disorders are associated with deterioration of skeletal muscle (SkM). Human studies have shown that marine fatty acids influence SkM function, though the underlying mechanisms of action are unknown. As a model of diet-induced obesity, we fed C57BL/6J mice either a high fat diet (HFD) with purified marine fatty acids eicosapentaenoic acid (EPA) and docosahexaenoic acid (DHA) (HFD-ED), a HFD with corn oil, or normal mouse chow for 8 weeks; and used transcriptomics to identify the molecular effects of EPA and DHA on SkM. Consumption of ED-enriched HFD modulated SkM metabolism through increased gene expression of mitochondrial β-oxidation and slow-fiber type genes compared with HFD-corn oil fed mice. Furthermore, HFD-ED intake increased nuclear localization of nuclear factor of activated T-cells (Nfatc4) protein, which controls fiber-type composition. This data suggests a role for EPA and DHA in mitigating some of the molecular responses due to a HFD in SkM. Overall, the results suggest that increased consumption of the marine fatty acids EPA and DHA may aid in the prevention of molecular processes that lead to muscle deterioration commonly associated with obesity-induced low-grade inflammation.

Keywords: eicosapentaenoic acid (EPA)/Docosahexaenoic acid (DHA); obesity; skeletal-muscle metabolism; mitochondrial β-oxidation; transcriptome

1. Introduction

The World Health Organization (WHO) estimates that chronic inflammatory conditions accounts for more than 17 million deaths every year [1]. Obesity is considered one of the main underlying factors for chronic inflammation and has almost doubled since 1980 and now over 1.4 billion adults worldwide are obese. Obesity, once considered a problem only in developed countries, is now also a major problem in low- and middle-income countries. Parallel to the increase in obesity, diseases associated with chronic inflammation such as cardiovascular diseases and type 2 diabetes are also rising [1]. One of the major concerns associated with low-grade inflammation is sarcopenia—loss of muscle mass. Generally, after the age of 50 the muscle mass reduces at a rate of up to 1%–2% annually, while fat mass increases [2,3]. At the same time, muscle strength drops at the rate of 1.5% annually between the age of 50 and 60 years and at the rate of 3% thereafter [4]. Obesity accelerates age-related muscle deterioration [5] exacerbating the risk for type 2 diabetes (T2D) by approximately 30% [6]. The negative feedback loop defined as the combination of excess weight-gain and reduced muscle mass, strength and performance is known as sarcopenic obesity [7]. Further suggestions of a role for inflammation in sarcopenia includes an association between increased TNF-α [8] and Il-6 [9] and decreased muscle mass and strength.

Skeletal muscle (SkM) constitutes about 40% of total body mass in adult lean men and is an adaptable tissue in response to changes in lifestyle such as diet and physical training [10,11]. SkM is one of the major sites of glucose metabolism, accounting for about 30% of postprandial glucose disposal [12]. This makes SkM a crucial organ for maintaining healthy glucose concentrations in the body, with loss of muscle mass also associated with increased type 2 diabetes risk. Changes to diet may impact on SkM and use of fish oil rich in the fatty acids eicosapentaenoic acid (EPA) and docosahexaenoic acid (DHA) have been proposed to improve SkM metabolism [13]. An intervention with marine fatty acids improved muscle mass and function in older adults [13] and animal studies suggest a role for marine fatty acids in SkM anabolism and increased protein synthesis [14,15]. In addition, marine fatty acids have anti-inflammatory activity in animals and humans [16], which may reduce the loss of inflammation-mediated SkM mass in older adults. Supplementation with EPA and DHA, the two main marine fatty acids, could be the basis for a simple, safe and low-cost solution for preventing and mitigating negative changes to SkM metabolism. For such a strategy to be credible, it is crucial to understand the underlying signaling mechanisms mediated by EPA and DHA on SkM.

Our previous intervention studies showed that mice fed high fat diets (HFDs) supplemented with herring improve muscle mass compared with mice fed HFD supplemented with beef [17,18]. In several randomized control trials in humans, marine fatty acids improve muscle volume, a surrogate marker for improved muscle performance [13,19,20]. In order to build on these results and determine if EPA and DHA, or other components in fatty fish, are responsible for improving muscle metabolism and to determine what the underlying mechanisms could be, we conducted a follow-up trial on earlier work with fatty fish [17,18]. Here we have used transcriptomics to explore how replacing a commonly used source of dietary fat, corn oil with purified EPA and DHA interacts with gastrocnemicus skeletal muscle (gSkM) gene expression, in order to investigate how EPA and DHA can affect muscle deterioration.

2. Materials and Methods

2.1. Animal Experiment

Six-week old male C57BL/6 J mice (Harlan BV, The Netherlands) were grouped 5–6 mice/cage, and were housed in a temperature and humidity-controlled environment with 12 h light/dark cycle for three weeks to acclimatize to the facility. At nine weeks of age, mice were switched from a normal mouse chow to one of three intervention diets: high fat diet with EPA and DHA (HFD-ED), a high fat diet with corn oil (HFD-corn oil) or the same mouse chow as during the acclimatization period (control group). Mice were maintained on these diets for 8-weeks (see Diets for details). After 8-weeks the animals were anesthetized by intraperitoneal injection of sodium pentobarbital (>60 mg/kg) and blood was collected from the heart followed by cervical dislocation. Plasma was obtained by centrifugation at 4 °C of EDTA whole blood (10 min; 10,000× *g*). The tissues were weighed and snap-frozen in liquid nitrogen immediately after dissection. Both, tissues and plasma were stored at −80 °C until further analysis. The animal experiments were approved by the Animal Ethics Committee at the University of Gothenburg (Dnr: 253-2009) [21].

2.2. Diets

The mice were fed a standard control chow during the 3-weeks acclimatization period. The mice did not differ in body weight at the start of the study (Table 1) and the body weights were measured weekly during the study. We removed two mice from the control group due to unsocial behavior, thus there were *n* = 9 mice in control and *n* = 12 mice in either HFD group. HFD were used to induce obesity in the mice. The two HFD used in the study differed only in their fatty acid composition. The reference

HFD was prepared with 5 weight/weight (w/w)% corn oil, while the treatment HFD was prepared with 2 w/w% purified EPA and DHA (EPAX AS Lysaker, Norway) plus 3 w/w% corn oil. The control diet provided 24 energy% (E%) as protein, 12 E% as fat and 65 E% as carbohydrates, whereas the two HFD contained 25 E% as protein, 32 E% as fat and 44 E% as carbohydrates (Table 2). The diets were prepared by Lantmännen AB (Kimstad, Sweden). Access to water and diet was ad libitum and the diets were changed three times per week throughout the study.

Table 1. Changes in Body Weight Composition and Plasma Lipid Composition.

Parameter	Control	HFD-ED	HFD-Corn oil
Total number of animals; n	9	12	12
Initial body weight (g)	27.5 ± 0.8	28.6 ± 0.8	24.3 ± 0.5
Final body weight (g)	31.4 ± 1	33.8 ± 0.8	36.2 ± 0.9
Change in body weight (g)	3.9 ± 0.5 [a]	5.2 ± 0.3 [a]	8.6 ± 0.5 [b]
plasma cholesterol (mmol/L)	5.6 ± 0.4	5.5 ± 0.4	5.2 ± 0.6
plasma triglyceride (mmol/L)	0.9 ± 0.1 [a,b]	1.1 ± 0.1 [a]	0.7 ± 0.1 [b]

The data are shown as mean $\pm$ SEM; different letters show significant different tested by ANOVA followed by Tukey's multiple comparison test. To calculate the changes in body weight (g), initial body weight values from individual animals was subtracted from the final body weight measurement.

Table 2. Diet Compositions Namely Control, HFD-ED and HFD-Corn Oil (CO) [21].

Ingredient (g/100 g Diet)		Control	HFD-ED	HFD-CO
Protein	Casein	22.2	25.6	25.6
Carbohydrates	Sucrose	5.0	10.0	10.0
	Corn starch	56.0	34.8	34.8
	Cellulose	5.0	5.8	5.8
Fat	Total	5.0	15.0	15.0
	Corn oil	2.5	3.0	5.0
	Coconut oil	2.5	10.0	10.0
	EPAX oils [a]	0	2.0	0
Minerals [b]		2.0	2.5	2.5
Miconutrients [c]		3.0	3.0	3.0
Choline bitartrate		1.6	2.0	2.0
Cholesterol		0	1.0	1.0
Methionine		0.2	0.3	0.3
Energy content (kJ/100 g)		1599	1752	1752
Protein E%		24	25	25
Carbohydrate E%		65	44	44
Fat E%		12	32	32
Fatty acid composition [d] (mg/g diet)	C10:0	0.20	1.47	1.33
	C12:0	2.37	7.58	7.72
	C14:0	1.54	4.58	4.78
	C16:0	1.90	3.44	3.59
	C18:0	0.68	2.26	2.49
	SFA	6.70	19.33	19.91
	C18:1n9	2.82	4.80	5.26
	MUFA	2.82	4.80	5.26
	C18:2n6	3.62	5.03	7.36
	C18:3n6	0.12	0.22	0.26
	n-6 PUFA	3.74	5.26	7.62
	C20:5n3 (EPA)	0.00	2.03	0.01
	C22:6n3 (DHA)	0.00	4.58	0.01
	n-3 PUFA	0.00	6.61	0.02

[a] EPAX 1050. EPAX 6015. [b] $CaCO_3$ (57.7%); KCl (19.9%); KH_2PO_4 (11.9%); $MgSO_4$ (10.4%). [c] Corn starch (98.22%); $Ca(IO_3)_2$ (0.0007%); $CoCO_3$ (0.064%); CuO (0.02%); $FeSO_4$ (0.5%); MnO_2 (0.035%); Na_2MoO_4 (0.001%); $NaSeO_3$ (0.0007%); ZnO (0.1%); Vitamin A (0.013%); B_2 (Riboflavin-5-phosphate sodium; 0.027%); B_3 (0.1%); B_5 (Ca Pantothenate; 0.057%); B_6 (0.023%); B_7 (0.0007%); B_9 (0.007%); B_{12} (0.00008%); D_3 (0.007%); E (0.25%); K (0.003%). [d] Analyses were performed in triplicate and data was obtained by Gas chromatography mass spectroscopy.

2.3. Muscle Composition

Gastrocnemicus skeletal muscles were dissected and weighed directly after sacrifice. Plasma total triglyceride and cholesterol was measured enzymatically with Konelab Autoanalyser version 2.0 at the Department of Clinical Chemistry, Sahlgrenska University Hospital, Gothenburg, Sweden. Clinical chemistry procedures have been previously described in detail [21].

2.4. RNA Isolation and Quality Assurance

Four mice, representative from each diet group on the basis of body weight, plasma triglyceride and plasma cholesterol levels were selected for RNA isolation and microarray analysis (Supplemental Table S1). Total RNA from gSkM was purified using the RNeasy® Plus Universal Mini kit (Qiagen Nordic, Sollentuna, Sweden). RNA samples were quantified spectrophotometrically (NanoDrop 2000c UV-Vis Spectrophotometer, Thermo Scientific, Wilmington, NC, USA) and the quality of the RNA was controlled by the ratio of 28S and 18S rRNA (RNA 6000 Nano LabChip for Agilent 2100 Bioanalyzer (Agilent Technologies, Santa Clara, CA, USA).

2.5. Western Blot Analysis

Nuclear and cytosolic extracts were prepared using NE-PER Nuclear and Cytoplasmic Extraction Reagents kit (78833, Thermo Fisher Scientific). Western blot analysis was performed as described earlier [22]. Briefly, the protein concentration was measured in duplicate using the Pierce BCA Protein Assay kit (Thermo Fisher Scientific) for equal protein loading to the SDS-PAGE. After transfer of the proteins to the membranes, the membranes were stained with 0.5% Ponceau S (Merck Chemicals, Darmstadt, Germany) to visualize the protein transfer. For the detection of specific proteins, the following primary antibodies were used: Rb-anti-m acetyl-CoA carboxylase (Acc; 3662; Cell Signaling Technology), Rb-anti-m phospho-acetyl-CoA carboxylase (P-Acc; Ser79, 3661; Cell Signaling Technology), Rb-anti-m troponin c1 (Tnnc1; sc-20642, Santa Cruz Biotechnology), Rb-anti-m Nuclear factor of activated T-cells (Nfatc4; sc-13036, Santa Cruz Biotechnology). The secondary antibodies were: HRP-conjugated Horse-anti-m IgG (7076; Cell Signaling Technology), Goat-anti-m IgG (sc-2020; Santa Cruz Biotechnology) and Rb-anti-m IgG (7074; Cell Signaling Technology). As loading control for each western blot, either glyceraldehyde 3-phosphate dehydrogenase (anti-Gapdh; sc-47724; Santa Cruz Biotechnology), or lamin (anti-lamin A/C, sc-6215; Santa Cruz Biotechnology) was used. Western blots for the protein Acc, P-Acc and Tnnc1 are in supplemental Figure S1.

2.6. Microarray—Data Acquisition and Analysis

RNA was labeled and hybridized to MouseWG-6_V2.0 Expression BeadChip (R3_11278593_A; Illumina, CA, USA) that contains 45,281 transcripts, at the SCIBLU Genomics core facility (Swegene Centre for Integrative Biology at Lund University, Sweden). The content of this BeadChip is derived from the National Center for Biotechnology Information Reference Sequence (NCBI RefSeq) database (Build 36, Release 22) [23], supplemented with probes from the Mouse Exonic Evidence Based Oligonucleotide (MEEBO) [24] set, as well as example protein-coding sequences from RIKEN FANTOM2 database [25]. The raw and normalized data is available in SOFT format at the Gene Expression Omnibus database under Accession Number GSE76361.

The Illumina bead array files were imported to GenomeStudio Gene Expression (GSGX) software 1.9.0. The un-normalized expression data (fluorescence intensities) were extracted for the mean intensity of arrays. R Studio software (Version 3.2.3, © 2015 RStudio, Inc., Boston, MA, USA) was used for microarray data analysis. The data was quantile normalized and variance-stabilizing transformation (VST) was performed using the default setting of *lumiExpresso* function from the lumi package [26]. The top 100 differentially expressed genes regulated by HFD-ED compared with HFD-corn oil are provided in supplemental Table S2. The Empirical Bayes method from the limma package was then applied to the signals to calculate moderated *t*- and *F*-statistics, log odds and differential expression for comparisons between the diets from skeletal muscle tissue [27]. The Generally Applicable Gene-Set/Pathway Analysis (GAGE) Bioconductor package was used for gene-set enrichment analysis (GSEA) for functional inference [28]. Before implementing the gage function, canonical signaling and metabolic pathways from the KEGG mouse database was prepared for better-defined results. For the microarray data, false discovery rate (FDR) adjusted p-values were calculated and FDR adjusted p-value < 0.05 was considered significant. The Pathview package was used to visualize the data, where the *pathview* function downloads KEGG graph data and renders a pathway map, based on experimental results [29].

2.7. Fatty Acid Analysis

Approximately 100 mg gSkM tissue was weighed, freeze-dried and extracted using the Folch total lipid extraction method [30]. Briefly, 5 mL chloroform–methanol (2:1 v/v) was added to the samples followed by sonication at 40 Hz for 30 min at RT (Branson 8510, Branson Ultrasonics Corp, CT, USA). One mL of physiological saline (0.9% NaCl) was mixed with the samples followed by brief vortexing and centrifugation for 5 min at 3000 rpm (1700× g), to separate the two phases. The organic lower phase was collected and the remaining aqueous phase was re-extracted with 1.5 mL chloroform. The two extracted phases were combined and evaporated under N_2 and re-dissolved in 1 mL isopropanol. All solvents were from Sigma-Aldrich, Sweden.

Solid phase extraction (SPE) method was used to separate lipid classes [31]. Internal phospholipid (C17:0) and triglyceride (C19:0) standards (Nu-Chek prep, Inc., Elysian, MN, USA) were added to the samples. Hexane conditioned aminopropyl SPE columns were loaded with 1 mL of extracted SkM lipid samples. Neutral lipids, free fatty acid and phospholipids were eluted with chloroform–isopropanol (2:1), diethylether-2% acetone and methanol, respectively and evaporated under N_2. Dried SPE fractions were methylated by overnight incubation with 1 mL 10% acetyl chloride in methanol and 1 mL toluene. After methylation, 0.3 mL water and 4 mL petroleum ether was added to the samples and the resulting two phases were separated by 3 min centrifugation at 3000× g. The upper phase was then removed, evaporated under N_2 and re-dissolved in 250 μL isooctane [32].

The fatty acid methyl esters (FAMEs) were analyzed by gas chromatography mass spectrometry (Focus GC, ISQ, Thermo Fischer Scientific, USA) using a ZB-WAX column (30 × 0.25 mm I.D., 0.25 μm) (Phenomenex, UK). One μl of sample was injected in splitless mode. The injector temperature was 240 and helium was used as the carrier gas with the flow of 1 mL/min. Oven temperature was as follows: 50 °C 1.5 min, ramped to 180 °C at 25 °C/min where held for 1 min, ramped to 220 °C at 10 °C/min, held for 1 min and ramped to 250 °C at 15 °C/min and held for 3 min. The transfer line was kept at 250 °C and ion source at 200 °C. Electron impact ionization (70 eV) was used and the FAMEs were detected by scanning a mass range from 50 to 650 m/z. An external FAME standard mix GLC 463 (Nu-Chek prep, Inc., Elysian, MN, USA) was used for identification of peaks in gSkM samples. Fatty acids were quantified against internal standards, summed and expressed as mg/g dry gSkM biomass and as a percentage of total lipid fractions.

2.8. Statistical Analysis of Western Blot and Fatty Acid Analyses

Differences in SkM western blot and fatty acid analyses were tested using ANOVA with Tukey's honest significant difference (Tukey-HSD) post-hoc test. Statistical significance between the protein groups was calculated with an unpaired 2-tailed Student's t-test. A p-value < 0.05 was considered statistically significant. Statistical calculations were performed using Microsoft® Excel® for Mac 2011 version 14.5.8 and R software (Version 3.2.3) under RStudio interface. All data are presented as mean ± SEM.

3. Results

3.1. Effect of EPA and DHA vs Corn Oil on gSkM Weight and Transcriptome

Delayed weight gain was observed in HFD-ED compared with HFD-corn oil fed animals (Table 1). Moreover, relative adiposity was lower in HFD-ED compared with HFD-corn oil fed mice [21]. Principle component analysis of the gSkM transcriptome did not detect any outliers in the data (Supplemental Figure S2a) indicating good analytical reproducibility. To visualize the global effects of different diets on gSkM, differential expression of the genes was performed on the following comparisons: HFD-ED versus control diet, HFD-corn oil versus control diet and HFD-ED versus HFD-corn oil. Venn diagrams show the number of differentially expressed genes (DEGs) corrected for multiple testing by Benjamini and Hochberg at *p*-value < 0.001 (supplemental Figure S2b). The total number of DEGs was 365, 129 and 383 for the comparison HFD-ED versus control diet, HFD-corn oil versus control diet and HFD-ED versus HFD-corn oil, respectively. Differential gene expression analysis found that the different fat composition of the two HFDs affected gene expression in gSkM differently when compared to the control group (Supplemental Figure S3).

3.2. gSkM Fatty Acid Composition

Neutral lipids: The total amount of neutral lipids was significantly higher in the mice fed HFD-corn oil compared to mice fed the other two study diets (Table 3). The concentration of fatty acid C12:0 was higher in HFD-corn oil fed animals compared with both HFD-ED and control diets (Table 3). C14:0 was higher in HFD-corn oil fed animals compared with control diet but there was no difference compared with HFD-ED fed animals. Fatty acids C16:0, C18:1 and C18:2 *n*-6 (linoleic acid) were higher in HFD-corn oil fed animals compared with mice fed HFD-ED or control diets, whereas no difference was observed between the control and HFD-ED fed animals. C22:6 *n*-3 (DHA) was higher in the HFD-ED fed animals compared to the control diet.

Free fatty acids: Free fatty acids (FFA) mainly comprised of saturated and monounsaturated fatty acids including C16:0, C19:0, C16:1 and C18:1 (Table 3). Apart from C12:0, which was higher in HFD-ED fed animals, the remaining FFAs were higher in HFD-corn oil fed animals compared with the other two diets. The concentration of C20:3 *n*-3 was higher in the HFD-corn oil fed animals compared with HFD-ED and the concentration did not differ compared with control diet. As expected, C22:6 *n*-3 concentrations were higher in the HFD-ED fed animals compared with HFD-corn oil. The total amount of FFAs in gSkM did not differ between the different groups.

Phospholipids: The concentration of C14:0 was significantly higher in the HFD-ED fed animals compared with the other two diets (Table 3). The amount of C18:1 was significantly lower in the HFD-ED fed animals compared with HFD-corn oil fed animals. The amount of C20:4 *n*-6 (arachidonic acid) was lower in HFD-ED fed animals compared with either HFD-corn oil or control diet fed animals. The amount of *n*-3 PUFA C20:5 *n*-3 (EPA) did not differ for any of the diets, with only very low concentrations measured, whereas the concentrations of C22:5 *n*-3 (DPA) and C22:6 *n*-3 (DHA) were significantly higher in the animals fed HFD-ED compared with animals fed HFD-corn oil but the expected increase in EPA was not found. The total phospholipid content was significantly lower in the HFD-ED fed animals compared with control diet fed animals but did not differ from that found in gSkM from the animals fed HFD-corn oil.

Table 3. The Fatty Acid Profiles of Different Lipid Fractions in Gastrocnemicus Skeletal Muscle.

Lipid Fraction	mg/g	mg/g	mg/g	% value	% value	% value
Neutral lipids	Control	HFD-ED	HFD-Corn oil	Control	HFD-ED	HFD-Corn oil
C12:0	0.12 ± 0.06 [a]	1.51 ± 0.42 [b]	2.87 ± 0.41 [c]	0.44 ± 0.18 [a]	3.93 ± 0.21 [b]	4.02 ± 0.33 [b]
C14:0	1.18 ± 0.24 [a]	3.15 ± 0.76	4.81 ± 0.49 [b]	4.35 ± 0.48 [a]	8.19 ± 0.52 [b]	6.74 ± 0.23 [c]
C16:0	8.11 ± 2.31 [a]	9.75 ± 2.28 [a]	19.01 ± 2.11 [b]	29.93 ± 1.78	25.35 ± 1.51	26.63 ± 2.34

Table 3. *Cont.*

Lipid Fraction	mg/g	mg/g	mg/g	% value	% value	% value
Neutral lipids	Control	HFD-ED	HFD-Corn oil	Control	HFD-ED	HFD-Corn oil
C18:0	0.55 ± 0.05	0.65 ± 0.05	0.68 ± 0.04	2.03 ± 0.48 [a]	1.69 ± 0.4 [a]	0.95 ± 0.09 [b]
C18:1	13.11 ± 3.05 [a]	14.86 ± 3.45 [a]	29.2 ± 2.19 [b]	48.38 ± 0.81 [a]	38.64 ± 1.06 [b]	40.91 ± 1.6 [b]
C18:2 *n6*	3.75 ± 0.78 [a]	7.29 ± 1.89 [a]	14.55 ± 1.25 [b]	13.84 ± 0.67 [a]	18.95 ± 0.9 [b]	20.38 ± 0.73 [b]
C18:3 *n3*	0.07 ± 0.04	0.07 ± 0.03	0.09 ± 0.02	0.26 ± 0.08	0.18 ± 0.04	0.13 ± 0.03
C20:3 *n6*	0.02 ± 0.01	0.01 ± 0 [a]	0.03 ± 0 [b]	0.07 ± 0.06	0.03 ± 0	0.04 ± 0
C22:5 *n3*	0.03 ± 0.01	0.06 ± 0.01	0 ± 0	0.11 ± 0.09	0.16 ± 0.01 [a]	0 ± 0 [b]
C22:6 *n3*	0.14 ± 0.02 [a]	1.1 ± 0.09 [b]	0.14 ± 0.02 [a]	0.52 ± 0.25 [a]	2.86 ± 0.68 [b]	0.2 ± 0.04 [a]
Total neutral lipids	27.1 ± 6.48 [a]	38.46 ± 8.89 [a]	71.38 ± 6.13 [b]			
Free fatty acids	Control	HFD-ED	HFD-Corn oil	Control	HFD-ED	HFD-Corn oil
C12:0	0.13 ± 0.04	0.16 ± 0.04 [a]	0.04 ± 0.01 [b]	6.6 ± 2.11	8.21 ± 2.26 [a]	1.61 ± 0.43 [b]
C16:0	0.52 ± 0.07 [a]	0.64 ± 0.02	0.78 ± 0.04 [b]	26.4 ± 3.14 [a]	32.82 ± 1.34 [b]	31.33 ± 2.03 [b]
C16:1	0.12 ± 0.03	0.09 ± 0.03	0.15 ± 0.05	6.09 ± 1.17	4.62 ± 1.3	6.02 ± 1.58
C18:1	1.07 ± 0.09	0.89 ± 0.07 [a]	1.29 ± 0.12 [b]	54.31 ± 4.03 [a]	45.64 ± 1.96 [b]	51.81 ± 1.68
C18:2 *n6*	0 ± 0 [a]	0 ± 0 [a]	0.11 ± 0.02 [b]	0 ± 0 [a]	0 ± 0 [a]	4.42 ± 0.46 [b]
C18:3 *n3*	0.09 ± 0	0.07 ± 0.01	0.07 ± 0.01	4.57 ± 0.64 [a]	3.59 ± 0.51	2.81 ± 0.27 [b]
C20:3 *n3*	0.04 ± 0 [a]	0 ± 0 [b]	0.04 ± 0.01 [a]	2.03 ± 0.27 [a]	0 ± 0 [b]	1.61 ± 0.24 [c]
C22:6 *n3*	0 ± 0 [a]	0.09 ± 0.03 [b]	0 ± 0 [a]	0 ± 0 [a]	4.62 ± 1.25 [b]	0 ± 0.14 [a]
Total free fatty acids	1.97 ± 0.17	1.95 ± 0.12	2.49 ± 0.21			
Phospholipids	Control	HFD-ED	HFD-Corn oil	Control	HFD-ED	HFD-Corn oil
C14:0	0.33 ± 0.02 [a]	0.83 ± 0.04 [b]	0.64 ± 0.07	2.17 ± 0.14 [a]	6.14 ± 0.28 [b]	4.7 ± 0.49 [c]
C16:0	5.06 ± 0.06 [a]	4.93 ± 0.09	4.73 ± 0.06 [b]	33.29 ± 0.76 [a]	36.49 ± 0.55 [b]	34.75 ± 1.37
C18:0	1.97 ± 0.33	2.65 ± 0.18	2.01 ± 0.26	12.96 ± 2.38	19.62 ± 1.41	14.77 ± 2.02
C18:1	3.67 ± 0.68 [a]	0.39 ± 0.26 [b]	2.07 ± 0.44 [a]	24.14 ± 3.71 [a]	2.89 ± 1.81 [b]	15.21 ± 3.12 [a]
C18:2 *n6*	1.73 ± 0.06 [a]	0.58 ± 0.09 [b]	2.13 ± 0.05 [c]	11.38 ± 0.28 [a]	4.29 ± 0.61 [b]	15.65 ± 0.6 [c]
C20:3 *n6*	0.05 ± 0 [a]	0 ± 0 [b]	0.06 ± 0.01 [a]	0.33 ± 0 [a]	0 ± 0 [b]	0.44 ± 0.04 [a]
C20:4 *n6*	0.57 ± 0.01 [a]	0.1 ± 0 [b]	0.55 ± 0.01 [a]	3.75 ± 0.12 [a]	0.74 ± 0.01 [b]	4.04 ± 0.28 [a]
C20:5 *n3*	0 ± 0	0.04 ± 0	0.02 ± 0.02	0 ± 0	0.3 ± 0.01	0.15 ± 0.15
C22:3 *n6*	0.54 ± 0.02 [a]	0.07 ± 0 [b]	0.26 ± 0.03 [c]	3.55 ± 0.18 [a]	0.52 ± 0.01 [b]	1.91 ± 0.23 [c]
C22:5 *n3*	0.05 ± 0 [a]	0.11 ± 0 [b]	0.06 ± 0.01 [a]	0.33 ± 0.02 [a]	0.81 ± 0.02 [b]	0.44 ± 0.05 [c]
C22:6 *n3*	1.23 ± 0.03 [a]	3.45 ± 0.06 [b]	1.07 ± 0.1 [a]	8.09 ± 0.3 [a]	25.54 ± 0.53 [b]	7.86 ± 0.73 [a]
Total phospholipids	15.2 ± 0.47 [a]	13.15 ± 0.34 [b]	13.61 ± 0.45 [b]			
Total Fat content	44.26 ± 6.99	53.56 ± 9	87.47 ± 6.45			

The fatty acid profiles from the mice fed, either control, HFD-corn oil or HFD-ED are shown as mean ± SEM and as a proportion of total fatty acid fraction; different letters show statistical difference tested by ANOVA followed by Tukey's multiple comparison test. For details see methods section.

3.3. Increased Mitochondrial B—Oxidation and Oxidative Phosphorylation in the Gskm of Mice Fed HFD-ED

Energy metabolism is a biochemical process to generate energy from nutrients via aerobic or anaerobic pathways. KEGG pathway analysis suggested that HFD-ED intake led to an increased regulation of energy metabolism relating to lipid metabolism, Krebs cycle and oxidative phosphorylation, leading to increased capacity for ATP production in gSkM compared with HFD-corn oil fed animals.

Eight gene transcripts were upregulated by HFD-ED compared with the HFD-corn oil fed mice (Figure 1a). Functionally, the enzymes in the β-oxidation pathway facilitate the breakdown of fatty acids to form acetyl-CoA, which enters the Krebs cycle. The upregulated gene products, which are responsible for transporting fatty acids into the mitochondria, were two carnitine palmitoyltransferases (*Cpt1a* and *Cpt2*). In addition, RNA transcription of genes responsible for the subsequent degradation of fatty acids within the mitochondrial matrix producing acetyl-CoA including short/medium chain acyl-CoA dehydrogenase (*Acadm*), long chain acyl-CoA dehydrogenase (*Acadl*), very long chain acyl-CoA dehydrogenase (*Acadvl*), acetyl-CoA acyl transferase 2 (*Acaa2*), enoyl-CoA delta isomerase 1 (*Eci1*) and aldehyde dehydrogenese (*Aldh2*), were upregulated by the HFD-ED diet.

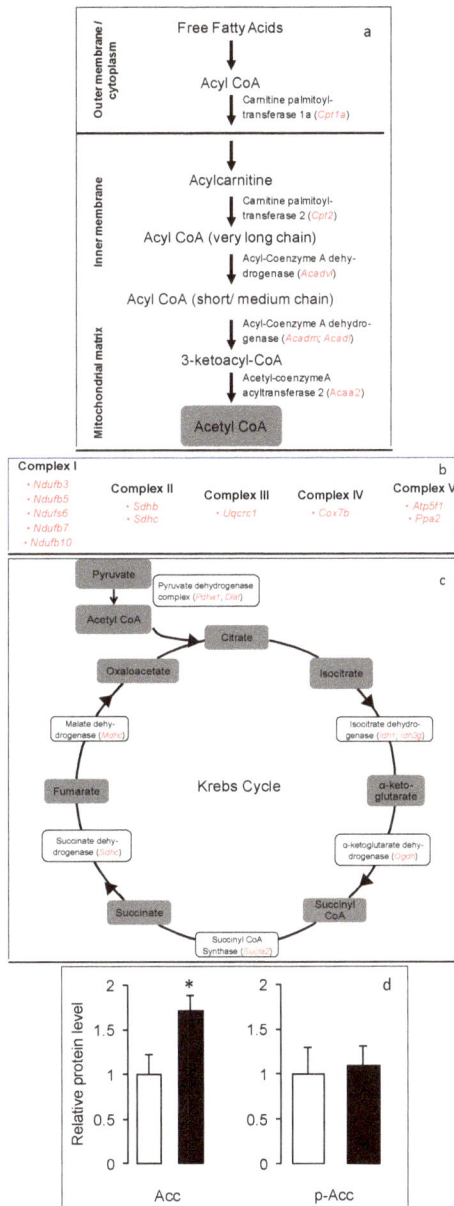

Figure 1. Pathway analysis of the gSkM transcriptome for the comparison of HFD-ED and HFD-corn oil fed mice. The illustration is based on the Kegg pathway database (http://www.genome.jp/kegg/pathway.html). (**a**) Fatty acid β-oxidation: Genes highlighted in red are upregulated in gSkM of mice fed HFD-ED compared with HFD-corn oil; (**b**) Electron transport chain: Genes highlighted in red are upregulated in gSkM of mice fed HFD-ED compared with HFD-corn oil; (**c**) Krebs Cycle: Genes highlighted in red are upregulated in gSkM of mice fed HFD-ED compared with HFD-corn oil; (**d**) Relative Acc protein levels in HFD-ED (white bars) fed mice was lower than HFD-corn oil (black bars) and there was no difference in the phosphorylation of Acc (p-Acc) protein after 8-weeks diet intervention. * Different at $p < 0.05$.

Pathway analyses showed a significant increase in the oxidative phosphorylation pathway in gSkM from the HFD-ED fed mice compared with HFD-corn oil animals (Figure 1b). Several genes involved in electron transport complex I-V were upregulated by HFD-ED fed mice compared with HFD-corn oil. Genes from the NADH dehydrogenase family that constitutes complex I (*Ndufa11*, *Ndufb3*, *Ndufb5*, *Ndufb7*, *Ndufb10* and *Ndufs6*); two succinate dehydrogenases (*Sdhb* and *Sdhc*) from complex II; ubiquinol-cytochrome c reductase core protein 1, cytochrome c oxidase subunit VIIb-Muscle and ATP synthase H+ transporting mitochondrial F0 complex subunit B1 (*Uqcrc1*, *Cox7b* and *Atp5f1*) constituting complex-III, IV and complex-V respectively, were upregulated.

HFD-ED upregulated the Krebs cycle in mice gSkM compared with HFD-corn oil (Figure 1c). The mitochondrial event consumes Acetyl-CoA producing NADH, $FADH_2$, GTP and the by-product CO_2. NADH and $FADH_2$ are in turn used by oxidative phosphorylation to generate ATP. Genes for key proteins in this metabolic pathway that were upregulated by EPA and DHA include pyruvate dehydrogenase E1 alpha 1 (*Pdha1*) and dihydrolipoamide S-acetyl transferase (*Dlat*), which converts pyruvate to Acetyl-CoA. HFD-ED upregulated several Krebs cycle genes including two kinds of isocitrate dehydrogenases (*Idh1* and *Idh3g*), oxoglutarate dehydrogenase (*Ogdh*), Succinate-CoA ligase GDP forming alpha subunit 2 (*Sucla2*), succinate dehydrogenase subunit a (*Sdha*) and malate dehydrogenase 2 (*Mdh2*), when compared with HFD-corn oil. There was no difference in the gene expression of *Acacb* (Acetyl-CoA carboxylase beta) but the total protein content of total acetyl-CoA carboxylase (Acc) was markedly lower in the gSkM of HFD-ED fed mice (Figure 1d). However, the phosphorylation levels of Acc did not differ in between the two HFDs (Figure 1d). This suggests increased internalization of fatty acids in mitochondria for potential β-oxidation in gSkM of HFD-ED fed mice rather than synthesis of fatty acids, as seems to be ongoing in HFD-corn oil animals.

3.4. Increased Expression of Muscle Contraction Pathway Genes in the Gskm of Mice Fed HFD-ED

Skeletal muscle fibers require stimulation from the neuromuscular junctions acting on the cholinergic nicotine receptor on the muscle cells to initiate contraction. These efferent cholinergic nerves are crucial for voluntary control of skeletal muscles. Gene expression of the cholinergic receptor nicotinic α polypeptide 1 (*Chrna1*), insulin growth factor receptor (*Igfr*) and two L-type voltage dependent Ca-channel genes (*Cacna1s* and *Cacnb2*), two calcium ATPases (*Atp1a1* and *Atp2a2*, a.k.a *Serca* 1 and 2, respectively), were upregulated by HFD-ED compared with HFD-corn oil fed mice (Figure 2a).

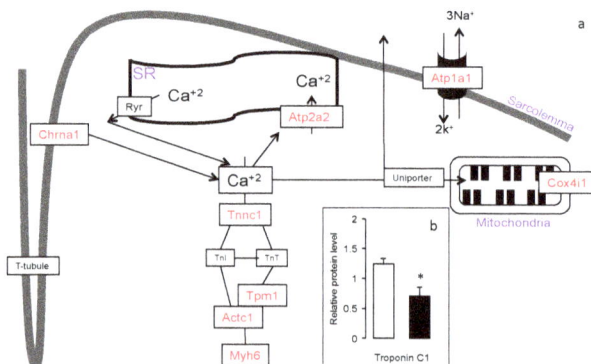

Figure 2. Pathway analysis of the gSkM transcriptome for the comparison HFD-ED versus HFD-corn oil fed mice. The illustration is based on the Kegg pathway database (http://www.genome.jp/kegg/pathway.html). (**a**) Nerve-Muscle contraction: Genes highlighted in red are upregulated in gSkM of mice fed HFD-ED compared with HFD-corn oil; (**b**) Relative Troponin C1 protein level in HFD-corn oil (black bars) fed mice was lower than HFD-ED (white bars). * Different at $p < 0.05$.

3.5. Increased Slow-Fiber-Specific Gene Expression Program in the Gskm of Mice Fed HFD-ED

The calcium mediated calcineurin-Nfat signaling cascade has been suggested to upregulate slow-fiber type gene expression. Differential gene expression of gSkM from the mice fed HFD-ED compared with HFD-corn oil suggested upregulation of several Nfat (*Nfatc1*; *Nfatc2*; *Nfatc4*) isoforms. The slow-fiber type genes troponin C1, cardiac/slow skeletal (*Tnnc1*), tropomyosin 1 alpha (*Tpm1*) and actin alpha 1 (*Actc1*) complex genes and crossbridge myosin heavy polypeptide isoforms (*Myh1*, *Myh2*, *Myh3*, *Myh6*, *Myh7*, *Myh8*) were upregulated in gSkM of HFD-ED fed mice compared with HFD-corn oil animals. Protein levels of *Tnnc1*, a biomarker for slow muscle fiber type, were higher in gSkM of HFD-ED fed mice compared with HFD-corn oil animals (Figure 2b). Furthermore, the gene product forming complex with *Nfatc2* and *Nfact4*, namely myogenin (*Myog*) and GATA Binding Protein 5 (*Gata5*) regulating the transcription of slow-fiber type gene expression was upregulated in the HFD-ED gSkM compared with HFD-corn oil. Nuclear localization of Nfat protein is essential for regulation of the slow-fiber-type gene expression. In the gSkM of HFD-ED fed mice, nuclear protein Nfat levels were significantly higher than HFD-corn oil fed animals (Figure 3). The master regulator of the calcineurin-Nfat signaling cascade, the regulator of calcineurin-2, *Rcan2*, was upregulated and its inhibitor glycogen synthase kinase 3β (*Gsk3β*) was downregulated in mice fed HFD-ED, compared with HFD-corn oil animals. Another transcriptional activator, suggested to be a direct target of marine fatty acids, peroxisome proliferator-activated receptor-γ coactivator 1α (*Ppargc1α*) was upregulated in gSkM of HFD-ED compared with HFD-corn oil fed mice.

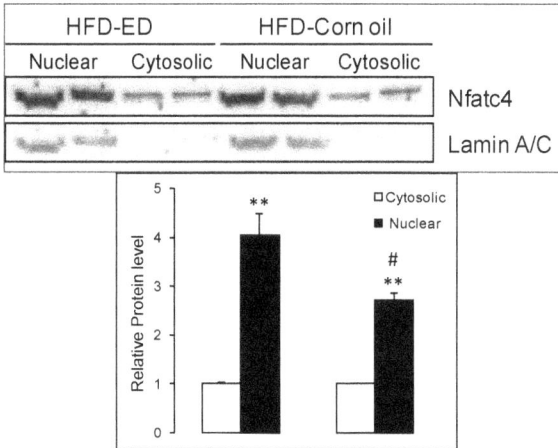

Figure 3. Representative Western blot is shown with LaminA/C loading control. Nuclear (black bars) and cytosolic (white bars) protein extract from the gSkM of HFD-ED (left-panel) and HFD-corn oil (right-panel) were analyzed by Western blot using antibodies for total anti-Nfatc4 antibody and the cytosolic protein levels in the HFD-ED was kept to 1. Different at ** $p < 0.05$ and # $p < 0.01$.

4. Discussion

In this study, we have shown that HFD-ED improves muscle metabolism and promotes a switch to slow-fiber type compared to HFD-corn oil. HFD-ED improves metabolism of fatty acids in gSkM by upregulating expression of genes coding for proteins involved in fatty acid β-oxidation, the Krebs cycle and oxidative phosphorylation. Lipid analysis shows that the HFD-ED fed animals had lower total fatty acid content compared to HFD-corn oil and control diet fed animals. Reduced ectopic fat accumulation in HFD-ED compared with HFD-corn oil fed animals suggests a physiological effect of EPA and DHA on muscle metabolic health. Higher expression of the genes involved in muscle contraction was found in gSkM of HFD-ED fed animals compared with HFD-corn oil fed animals. Western blot analysis showed reduced Acc protein levels in gSkM of HFD-ED fed animals compared with HFD-corn oil, confirming gene expression results. Acc is an inhibitor of fatty acid β-oxidation in mitochondria and the lower levels shows increase in mitochondrial fatty acid β-oxidation. In addition, increased Tnnc1 levels suggest increased muscle contraction in gSkM of HFD-ED fed animals compared with HFD-corn oil. Moreover, increased nuclear protein levels of the Nfatc4 isoform strongly suggests up-regulation of slow-fiber-type gene expression in gSkM of HFD-ED fed animals compared with HFD-corn oil fed animals (Figure 4).

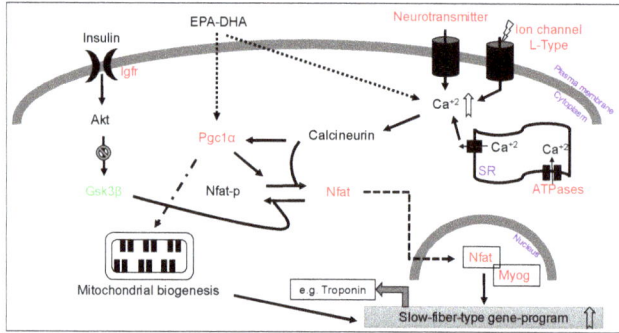

Figure 4. Schematic representation of the role of ED—enriched HFD on the gSkM transcriptome and modulation of ageing and/or obesity-induced sarcopenia in C57Bl/6J mice. Briefly, ED enriched HFD downregulates glucose synthase kinase 3 beta (*Gsk3β*) that phosphorylates nuclear factor of activated T cells (*Nfatc4*) and excludes it from entering into the nucleus. It also increases cytosolic calcium concentrations that in turn regulate calcineurin that then dephosphorylates Nfat allowing its localization in the nucleus. Upon localization, *Nfat* forms complex with myogenin (*Myog*) to turn on slow-fiber-type specific gene-program for e.g., Troponin C1. *Pgc1α*, a known master regulator of mitochondrial biogenesis was also seen upregulated by ED enriched HFD that could act upon multiple targets, one of which regulating dephosphorylation of *Nfatc4* isoforms and its further nuclear localization.

The gSkM neutral lipid and free fatty acid profiles reflect the higher amount of DHA in the feed of HFD-ED fed mice, though EPA was not detected in either fraction, in line with our previous findings in liver; that EPA was present in very low amounts, not in proportion to EPA in the diet [21]. There was no substantial proportional difference in gSkM fatty acid composition between the two HFD groups, even though HFD-corn oil fed mice had nearly twice the amount of total neutral lipids. This suggests that ED does not specifically upregulate any of the reactions related to β-oxidation and rather, leads to stimulation of β-oxidation in general, resulting in reduced total neutral lipids in SkM. Although there were several differences in the amount and proportion of free fatty acids and phospholipids, these differences were not quantitatively important aside from the increase DPA and DHA in mice fed HFD-ED but lower EPA in phospholipids fractions [33]. Notably C18:1 was substantially higher in HFD-corn oil fed mice compared with HFD-ED fed mice and this result was reversed for DHA. This could have implications for membrane fluidity within SkM and this may play a role in the observed transcriptome changes.

Previously we found that HFD-ED induced β-oxidation reduced liver fat compared to HFD-corn oil [21], similarly, reduced SkM fat can be due to the increase in β-oxidation and the lower amount of neutral lipids in HFD-ED fed mice. Reduced SkM mitochondrial fatty acid β-oxidation has been proposed as a key feature leading to insulin resistance [34,35] and high fat diets led to downregulation of the group of genes involved in oxidative phosphorylation in human SkM biopsies [36–38]. In the gSkM of the HFD-ED fed mice, the expression of rate limiting enzymes in fatty acid β-oxidation in mitochondria, *Cpt1* and *Cpt2* were upregulated compared with HFD-corn oil fed mice. Notably, the protein level of Acc was significantly reduced in gSkM of HFD-ED fed mice compared with HFD-corn oil. Acc regulates fatty acid metabolism by synthesizing malonyl-CoA (building blocks for new fatty acids) but suppresses mitochondrial β-oxidation by inhibiting fatty acid transporter *Cpt1*. Therefore, lower protein levels of Acc suggests entry of fatty acid into mitochondria via *Cpt1* transporter for mitochondrial β-oxidation in gSkM of HFD-ED fed mice compared with HFD-corn oil. A SkM specific isoform of *Acc* (*Acc2*) knockout mice were protected against fat-induced peripheral insulin resistance [39] whereas overexpression of *Cpt1* is sufficient to reduce insulin resistance [40]. Impairments in mitochondrial oxidative capacity in skeletal muscle have been seen in relation to a decrease in energy expenditure [35,41,42]. Thus, increased mitochondrial oxidative capacity in the gSkM of HFD-ED fed animals, supported by increased levels by *Cpt1* and decreased total protein levels of Acc may contribute to increased energy expenditure. Further work on a possible stimulation of energy expenditure by EPA and DHA, possibly via diet-induced thermogenesis is required.

Ageing and obesity may contribute to the decrease in the contractibility of skeletal muscle. Muscle contraction is regulated by intracellular calcium concentration via the thin filament regulatory proteins troponin and tropomyosin. In the absence of calcium, actin-myosin interaction and subsequently muscle contraction is inhibited. In the gSkM of HFD-ED, two ATPases, namely Na^+/K^+-ATPase transporting α2 polypeptide (*Atp1a2*; sodium pump) and ATPase Ca^{+2} transporting skeletal muscle slow switch 2 (*Atp2a2*; *Serca2a*) were upregulated compared with HFD-corn oil. A tissue specific knockout study shows that the sodium pump (*Atp1a2*) is required to prevent fatigue, and systematic analysis of Serca isoforms in calcium transport showed their importance for restoring muscle contractibility [43,44]. Protein levels of the oxidative fiber biomarker Troponin C1 were higher in gSkM of HFD-ED fed mice compared with HFD-corn oil, indicative of increased muscle contraction via control of intracellular calcium in mice fed HFD-ED. Together, these results suggest that HFD-ED contributes to increased calcium release into the sarcoplasm, compared with HFD-corn oil fed mice.

Calcineurin has been proposed to play a major role in the upregulation of slow-fiber-specific gene expression [45–47]. Earlier, it was found that inhibition of calcineurin by cyclosporin-A could result in an increased number of fast fibers in rat skeletal muscle [45]. Activated calcineurin phosphatase capacity is required for dephosphorylation of Nfat proteins, which then localize to the nucleus to initiate slow-fiber-specific gene expression [45,47]. Our data shows that the gSkM of HFD-ED fed animals has markedly higher nuclear levels of Nfat (Nfatc4 isoform) compared with HFD-corn oil, which could contribute to upregulation of the slow-fiber-specific gene expression upon nuclear localization. An earlier study showed abundant myogenin mRNA in slow oxidative muscles and this relationship followed phenotype transition caused by cross-innervation [48]. In HFD-ED fed mice, myogenin (P_{adj}-value = 0.06) tends to be higher compared with HFD-corn oil fed animals suggesting upregulation of genes for the slower muscle fiber phenotype. We also found that EPA and DHA increased gene expression of *Ppargc1α*, a master regulator of mitochondrial biogenesis leading to red type I fiber, also suggests genetic programing towards stimulating slower muscle fiber [49–52]. It is known that the products of peroxisomal β-oxidation are also targeted towards mitochondria for oxidation in skeletal muscle and therefore assist in complete lipid disposal [53]. Further support for an effect on muscle fiber type comes from stimulation of insulin growth factor 1 (*Igf*-1), which regulates the *Akt* pathway. Activation of *Akt* phosphorylates *Gsk3β* thereby inactivating it. *Gsk3β* phosphorylates *Nfat* and excluding its entry into the nucleus and subsequent DNA binding [54], which would down-regulate slow-fiber gene expression. In our study, *Gsk3β* was downregulated in the gSkM of HFD-ED compared with HFD-corn oil animals, indicating little Nfat phosphorylation and thus, conditions that would favor production of slow-fiber type. Resistance training, testosterone treatment, growth hormone, or dehydroepiandrosterone interventions have shown favorable effects in retaining muscle mass and function [19,55–58]. However, long-term use of growth hormone treatment can be harmful due to associated side effects, making this a poor choice for intervention against muscle loss. Our findings suggest a mechanistic basis for the human results and supports the case for further research on either

ED or fish oil supplements as potential molecules for the long-term prevention of sarcopenia. In this study we were unable to determine if muscle fiber type regulation is due to the effects of increased β-oxidation, or a direct effect of EPA or DHA on gene transcription.

Although the effects of EPA and DHA on gSkM gene expression are conclusive, due to the limited sample amount we have been unable to validate many of the possible physiological effects found from transcriptome analysis. Ideally, future work should study these effects across a wider range of SkM and perform histology to confirm the hypothesis on fiber-type regulation. Similarly, our results suggest an effect on many parameters related to energy metabolism, supported in part by finding a lower fat content in the gSkM of HFD-ED fed mice compared with HFD-corn oil. Future work will need to see if this effect extends to improved glucose disposal which could extend the findings to possible relevance for T2D. A role for regulation of calcium concentrations for signaling should also be tested using muscle cell models. Future work will also need to test if these pathways are still relatively upregulated with lower proportions of *n*-3 fatty acids and at lower amounts, to test if they are relevant at normal amounts of dietary fat.

These results clearly demonstrate the wide-ranging impact a difference in dietary fatty acid composition can have on SkM gene-transcription. It is unclear if ED regulates all of these gene targets simultaneously, or if some are a result of downstream interactions with initial ED targets. Given the clear sequential effects on energy metabolism from β-oxidation to oxidative phosphorylation, it appears likely that the observed upregulation of these processes is directly related to increased circulating EPA and DHA. Further studies on cell and rodent models of ageing and functional analysis of SkM are required to confirm these effects and the likely regulatory nodes for these mechanisms.

5. Conclusions

The skeletal muscle transcriptome from mice fed HFDs differing in fat composition for 8 weeks, showed marked differences in expression of genes coding for metabolic proteins. Our results suggest muscle-protective effects of EPA and DHA against catabolic degradation, possibly via stimulation of pathways that increase mitochondrial β-oxidation capacity and control calcium release for muscle contraction. These shifts in gene expression, even against a background of HFD are clearly favorable for hindering molecular progression towards muscle loss. With the limited availability of clinical treatments for preventing muscle loss, increased intake of fatty fish that are abundant in EPA and DHA, or supplementation with marine fatty acids could provide a safe and economic alternative to pharmaceutical interventions.

Supplementary Materials: The following are available online at www.mdpi.com/link, Figure S1: Protein lysate from the gSkM of HFD-ED and HFD-corn oil were analyzed by Western blot using antibodies for total Acc, p-Acc (Ser79) and total anti-Troponin C1. Gapdh was used as a loading control for the Western blot, Figure S2: (a) Principle Component Analysis (PCA) plot based on the normalized gene expression from the gSkM tissue fed control, HFD-ED and HFD-corn oil is plotted for assessing the quality of the datasets. No animals or any related data was excluded from further assessment. (b) Venn diagrams showing the number of differentially expressed genes (FDR adjusted *p*-value < 0.001) in each diet-comparison for gSkM tissue. HFD-ED compared with control diet and HFD-corn oil fed mice shows most transcriptional response to the diet. Key: ED = HFD-ED; CO = HFD-corn oil and CD = control diet, Figure S3: (a) Fatty acid β-oxidation pathway rendered by the pathview function from the Kegg pathway database. Genes highlighted in red are upregulated for the comparison HFD-ED vs. HFD-corn oil. (b) Krebs cycle pathway rendered by the pathview function from the Kegg pathway database. Genes highlighted in red are upregulated for the comparison HFD-ED vs. HFD-corn oil. (c) Oxidative phosphorylation pathway rendered by the pathview function from the Kegg pathway database. Genes highlighted in red are upregulated for the comparison HFD-ED vs. HFD-corn oil, Table S1: Table for the selection criteria for animals for microarray analysis. Animals marked in green were selected for microarray analysis, Table S2: The top 100 differentially regulated genes regulated by HFD-ED compared to HFD-corn oil fed mice, based on adjusted *p*-value.

Acknowledgments: The study was supported by grants from Stiftelsen Olle Engkvist, Byggmästare; The Swedish Research Council for Environment, Agricultural Sciences and Spatial Planning (222-2011-1322); the Region of Västra Götaland (VGR; RUN 612-0959-11) and the Swedish Research Council (VR project number 2013-4504). IN gracefully acknowledge Swedish Research Council (VR-2013-4504). We would like to acknowledge SCIBLU, Lund University for the labelling of RNA and hybridization to the Illumina microarrays chips, and CBI, University

Nutrients **2016**, *8*, 543

of Gothenburg, for the assistance with the animal experiments. We also acknowledge Chalmers Mass Spectrometry Infrastructure (CMSI), Chalmers University of Technology for their help with fatty acid profiling. We also gratefully acknowledge the kind gifts of the EPAX oils from EPAX AS, Norway (now FMC Corporation, USA).

Author Contributions: B.G., I.N., and A.S. designed the study. B.G. performed the animal experiments; B.G. and N.So. conducted the RNA isolation and microarray data collection. I.N. coordinated microarray experiment and analysis. N.So. and O.I.S. performed fatty acid analysis. N.So. performed statistical analyses and wrote the manuscript. A.B.R. and N.Sc. aided in the interpretation of the data and gave their input during the preparation of manuscript. All authors reviewed and approved the final version of manuscript.

Conflicts of Interest: The authors declare that they have no potential conflicts of interest.

References and Notes

1. World Health Organization. *Obesity and Overweight Fact Sheet N°311*; World Health Organization Media Centre: Geneva, Switzerland, 2015.
2. Lauretani, F.; Russo, C.R.; Bandinelli, S.; Bartali, B.; Cavazzini, C.; Di Iorio, A.; Corsi, A.M.; Rantanen, T.; Guralnik, J.M.; Ferrucci, L. Age-associated changes in skeletal muscles and their effect on mobility: An operational diagnosis of sarcopenia. *J. Appl. Physiol.* **2003**, *95*, 1851–1860. [CrossRef] [PubMed]
3. Candow, D.G.; Chilibeck, P.D. Differences in size, strength, and power of upper and lower body muscle groups in young and older men. *J. Gerontol.* **2005**, *60*, 148–156. [CrossRef]
4. Von Haehling, S.; Morley, J.E.; Anker, S.D. An overview of sarcopenia: Facts and numbers on prevalence and clinical impact. *J. Cachexia Sarcopenia Muscle* **2010**, *1*, 129–133. [CrossRef] [PubMed]
5. Rosenberg, I.H. Sarcopenia: Origins and clinical relevance. *J. Nutr.* **1997**, *127*, 990S–991S. [CrossRef] [PubMed]
6. Schmidt, M.; Johannesdottir, S.A.; Lemeshow, S.; Lash, T.L.; Ulrichsen, S.P.; Botker, H.E.; Sorensen, H.T. Obesity in young men, and individual and combined risks of type 2 diabetes, cardiovascular morbidity and death before 55 years of age: A danish 33-year follow-up study. *BMJ Open* **2013**, *3*. [CrossRef] [PubMed]
7. Roubenoff, R. Sarcopenic obesity: The confluence of two epidemics. *Obes. Res.* **2004**, *12*, 887–888. [CrossRef] [PubMed]
8. Schaap, L.A.; Pluijm, S.M.; Deeg, D.J.; Harris, T.B.; Kritchevsky, S.B.; Newman, A.B.; Colbert, L.H.; Pahor, M.; Rubin, S.M.; Tylavsky, F.A.; et al. Higher inflammatory marker levels in older persons: Associations with 5-year change in muscle mass and muscle strength. *J. Gerontol.* **2009**, *64*, 1183–1189. [CrossRef] [PubMed]
9. Visser, M.; Pahor, M.; Taaffe, D.R.; Goodpaster, B.H.; Simonsick, E.M.; Newman, A.B.; Nevitt, M.; Harris, T.B. Relationship of interleukin-6 and tumor necrosis factor-alpha with muscle mass and muscle strength in elderly men and women: The health abc study. *J. Gerontol.* **2002**, *57*, M326–M332. [CrossRef]
10. Zhao, X.; Wang, Z.; Zhang, J.; Hua, J.; He, W.; Zhu, S. Estimation of total body skeletal muscle mass in chinese adults: Prediction model by dual-energy X-ray absorptiometry. *PLoS ONE* **2013**, *8*. [CrossRef] [PubMed]
11. Kim, J.; Wang, Z.; Heymsfield, S.B.; Baumgartner, R.N.; Gallagher, D. Total-body skeletal muscle mass: Estimation by a new dual-energy X-ray absorptiometry method. *Am. J. Clin. Nutr.* **2002**, *76*, 378–383.
12. Meyer, C.; Dostou, J.M.; Welle, S.L.; Gerich, J.E. Role of human liver, kidney, and skeletal muscle in postprandial glucose homeostasis. *Am. J. Physiol. Endocrinol. Metab.* **2002**, *282*, 419–427. [CrossRef] [PubMed]
13. Smith, G.I.; Julliand, S.; Reeds, D.N.; Sinacore, D.R.; Klein, S.; Mittendorfer, B. Fish oil-derived *n*-3 pufa therapy increases muscle mass and function in healthy older adults. *Am. J. Clin. Nutr.* **2015**, *102*, 115–122. [CrossRef] [PubMed]
14. Alexander, J.W.; Saito, H.; Trocki, O.; Ogle, C.K. The importance of lipid type in the diet after burn injury. *Ann. Surg.* **1986**, *204*, 1–8. [CrossRef] [PubMed]
15. Gingras, A.A.; White, P.J.; Chouinard, P.Y.; Julien, P.; Davis, T.A.; Dombrowski, L.; Couture, Y.; Dubreuil, P.; Myre, A.; Bergeron, K.; et al. Long-chain omega-3 fatty acids regulate bovine whole-body protein metabolism by promoting muscle insulin signalling to the akt-mtor-s6k1 pathway and insulin sensitivity. *J. Physiol.* **2007**, *579*, 269–284. [CrossRef] [PubMed]
16. Fetterman, J.W., Jr.; Zdanowicz, M.M. Therapeutic potential of *n*-3 polyunsaturated fatty acids in disease. *Am. J Health Syst. Pharm.* **2009**, *66*, 1169–1179. [CrossRef] [PubMed]

17. Gabrielsson, B.G.; Wikstrom, J.; Jakubowicz, R.; Marmon, S.K.; Carlsson, N.G.; Jansson, N.; Gan, L.M.; Undeland, I.; Lonn, M.; Holmang, A.; et al. Dietary herring improves plasma lipid profiles and reduces atherosclerosis in obese low-density lipoprotein receptor-deficient mice. *Int. J. Mol. Med.* **2012**, *29*, 331–337. [CrossRef] [PubMed]
18. Nookaew, I.; Gabrielsson, B.G.; Holmang, A.; Sandberg, A.S.; Nielsen, J. Identifying molecular effects of diet through systems biology: Influence of herring diet on sterol metabolism and protein turnover in mice. *PLoS ONE* **2010**, *5*. [CrossRef] [PubMed]
19. Rodacki, C.L.; Rodacki, A.L.; Pereira, G.; Naliwaiko, K.; Coelho, I.; Pequito, D.; Fernandes, L.C. Fish-oil supplementation enhances the effects of strength training in elderly women. *Am. J. Clin. Nutr.* **2012**, *95*, 428–436. [CrossRef] [PubMed]
20. Smith, G.I.; Atherton, P.; Reeds, D.N.; Mohammed, B.S.; Rankin, D.; Rennie, M.J.; Mittendorfer, B. Dietary omega-3 fatty acid supplementation increases the rate of muscle protein synthesis in older adults: A randomized controlled trial. *Am. J. Clin. Nutr.* **2011**, *93*, 402–412. [CrossRef] [PubMed]
21. Soni, N.K.; Nookaew, I.; Sandberg, A.S.; Gabrielsson, B.G. Eicosapentaenoic and docosahexaenoic acid-enriched high fat diet delays the development of fatty liver in mice. *Lipids Health Dis.* **2015**, *14*. [CrossRef] [PubMed]
22. Amrutkar, M.; Cansby, E.; Nunez-Duran, E.; Piraz zi, C.; Stahlman, M.; Stenfeldt, E.; Smith, U.; Boren, J.; Mahlapuu, M. Protein kinase stk25 regulates hepatic lipid partitioning and progression of liver steatosis and nash. *FASEB J.* **2015**, *29*, 1564–1576. [CrossRef] [PubMed]
23. For More Information about ncbi refseq, Please Go to http://ftp.Ncbi.Nih.Gov/refseq/release/.
24. For More Information about meebo, Please Go to http://www.Arrays.Ucsf.Edu/archive/meebo.Html.
25. Functional Annotation of Mouse. Available online: http://fantom2.Gsc.Riken.Jp/ (accessed on 25 August 2016).
26. Du, P.; Kibbe, W.A.; Lin, S.M. Lumi: A pipeline for processing illumina microarray. *Bioinformatics* **2008**, *24*, 1547–1548. [CrossRef] [PubMed]
27. Ritchie, M.E.; Phipson, B.; Wu, D.; Hu, Y.; Law, C.W.; Shi, W.; Smyth, G.K. Limma powers differential expression analyses for RNA-sequencing and microarray studies. *Nucl. Acids Res.* **2015**, *43*. [CrossRef]
28. Luo, W.; Friedman, M.S.; Shedden, K.; Hankenson, K.D.; Woolf, P.J. Gage: Generally applicable gene set enrichment for pathway analysis. *BMC Bioinformatics* **2009**, *10*, 1–17. [CrossRef] [PubMed]
29. Luo, W.; Brouwer, C. Pathview: An R/Bioconductor package for pathway-based data integration and visualization. *Bioinformatics* **2013**, *29*. [CrossRef] [PubMed]
30. Folch, J.; Lees, M.; Stanley, G.H.S. A simple method for the isolation and purification of total lipids from animal tissues. *J. Biol. Chem.* **1957**, *226*, 497–509. [PubMed]
31. Kaluzny, M.A.; Duncan, L.A.; Merritt, M.V.; Epps, D.E. Rapid separation of lipid classes in high yield and purity using bonded phase columns. *J. Lipid Res.* **1985**, *26*, 135–140. [PubMed]
32. Lepage, G.; Roy, C.C. Improved recovery of fatty acid through direct transesterification without prior extraction or purification. *J. Lipid. Res.* **1984**, *25*, 1391–1396. [PubMed]
33. Tuazon, M.A.; Henderson, G.C. Fatty acid profile of skeletal muscle phospholipid is altered in mdx mice and is predictive of disease markers. *Metable* **2012**, *61*, 801–811. [CrossRef] [PubMed]
34. Lowell, B.B.; Shulman, G.I. Mitochondrial dysfunction and type 2 diabetes. *Science* **2005**, *307*, 384–387. [CrossRef] [PubMed]
35. Petersen, K.F.; Dufour, S.; Befroy, D.; Garcia, R.; Shulman, G.I. Impaired mitochondrial activity in the insulin-resistant offspring of patients with type 2 diabetes. *N. Engl. J. Med.* **2004**, *350*, 664–671. [CrossRef] [PubMed]
36. Patti, M.E.; Butte, A.J.; Crunkhorn, S.; Cusi, K.; Berria, R.; Kashyap, S.; Miyazaki, Y.; Kohane, I.; Costello, M.; Saccone, R.; et al. Coordinated reduction of genes of oxidative metabolism in humans with insulin resistance and diabetes: Potential role of pgc1 and nrf1. *Proc. Natl. Acad. Sci. USA* **2003**, *100*, 8466–8471. [CrossRef] [PubMed]
37. Sparks, L.M.; Xie, H.; Koza, R.A.; Mynatt, R.; Hulver, M.W.; Bray, G.A.; Smith, S.R. A high-fat diet coordinately downregulates genes required for mitochondrial oxidative phosphorylation in skeletal muscle. *Diabetes* **2005**, *54*, 1926–1933. [CrossRef] [PubMed]
38. Mootha, V.K.; Lindgren, C.M.; Eriksson, K.F.; Subramanian, A.; Sihag, S.; Lehar, J.; Puigserver, P.; Carlsson, E.; Ridderstrale, M.; Laurila, E.; et al. Pgc-1alpha-responsive genes involved in oxidative phosphorylation are coordinately downregulated in human diabetes. *Nat. Genet.* **2003**, *34*, 267–273. [CrossRef] [PubMed]

39. Choi, C.S.; Savage, D.B.; Abu-Elheiga, L.; Liu, Z.X.; Kim, S.; Kulkarni, A.; Distefano, A.; Hwang, Y.J.; Reznick, R.M.; Codella, R.; et al. Continuous fat oxidation in acetyl-coa carboxylase 2 knockout mice increases total energy expenditure, reduces fat mass, and improves insulin sensitivity. *Proc. Natl. Acad. Sci. USA* **2007**, *104*, 16480–16485. [CrossRef] [PubMed]

40. Bruce, C.R.; Hoy, A.J.; Turner, N.; Watt, M.J.; Allen, T.L.; Carpenter, K.; Cooney, G.J.; Febbraio, M.A.; Kraegen, E.W. Overexpression of carnitine palmitoyltransferase-1 in skeletal muscle is sufficient to enhance fatty acid oxidation and improve high-fat diet-induced insulin resistance. *Diabetes* **2009**, *58*, 550–558. [CrossRef] [PubMed]

41. Schwerzmann, K.; Hoppeler, H.; Kayar, S.R.; Weibel, E.R. Oxidative capacity of muscle and mitochondria: Correlation of physiological, biochemical, and morphometric characteristics. *Proc. Natl. Acad. Sci. USA* **1989**, *86*, 1583–1587. [CrossRef] [PubMed]

42. Petersen, K.F.; Befroy, D.; Dufour, S.; Dziura, J.; Ariyan, C.; Rothman, D.L.; DiPietro, L.; Cline, G.W.; Shulman, G.I. Mitochondrial dysfunction in the elderly: Possible role in insulin resistance. *Science* **2003**, *300*, 1140–1142. [CrossRef] [PubMed]

43. Periasamy, M.; Kalyanasundaram, A. Serca pump isoforms: Their role in calcium transport and disease. *Muscle Nerve* **2007**, *35*, 430–442. [CrossRef] [PubMed]

44. Radzyukevich, T.L.; Neumann, J.C.; Rindler, T.N.; Oshiro, N.; Goldhamer, D.J.; Lingrel, J.B.; Heiny, J.A. Tissue-specific role of the na,k-atpase alpha2 isozyme in skeletal muscle. *J. Biol. Chem.* **2013**, *288*, 1226–1237. [CrossRef] [PubMed]

45. Dunn, S.E.; Burns, J.L.; Michel, R.N. Calcineurin is required for skeletal muscle hypertrophy. *J. Biol. Chem.* **1999**, *274*, 21908–21912. [CrossRef] [PubMed]

46. Dunn, S.E.; Chin, E.R.; Michel, R.N. Matching of calcineurin activity to upstream effectors is critical for skeletal muscle fiber growth. *J. Cell. Biol.* **2000**, *151*, 663–672. [CrossRef] [PubMed]

47. Dunn, S.E.; Simard, A.R.; Bassel-Duby, R.; Williams, R.S.; Michel, R.N. Nerve activity-dependent modulation of calcineurin signaling in adult fast and slow skeletal muscle fibers. *J. Biol. Chem.* **2001**, *276*, 45243–45254. [CrossRef] [PubMed]

48. Hughes, S.M.; Taylor, J.M.; Tapscott, S.J.; Gurley, C.M.; Carter, W.J.; Peterson, C.A. Selective accumulation of myod and myogenin mrnas in fast and slow adult skeletal muscle is controlled by innervation and hormones. *Development* **1993**, *118*, 1137–1147.

49. Lin, J.; Wu, H.; Tarr, P.T.; Zhang, C.Y.; Wu, Z.; Boss, O.; Michael, L.F.; Puigserver, P.; Isotani, E.; Olson, E.N.; et al. Transcriptional co-activator pgc-1 alpha drives the formation of slow-twitch muscle fibres. *Nature* **2002**, *418*, 797–801. [CrossRef] [PubMed]

50. Vega, R.B.; Huss, J.M.; Kelly, D.P. The coactivator pgc-1 cooperates with peroxisome proliferator-activated receptor alpha in transcriptional control of nuclear genes encoding mitochondrial fatty acid oxidation enzymes. *Mol. Cell Biol.* **2000**, *20*, 1868–1876. [CrossRef] [PubMed]

51. Wu, Z.; Puigserver, P.; Andersson, U.; Zhang, C.; Adelmant, G.; Mootha, V.; Troy, A.; Cinti, S.; Lowell, B.; Scarpulla, R.C.; et al. Mechanisms controlling mitochondrial biogenesis and respiration through the thermogenic coactivator PGC-1. *Cell* **1999**, *98*, 115–124. [CrossRef]

52. Puigserver, P.; Wu, Z.; Park, C.W.; Graves, R.; Wright, M.; Spiegelman, B.M. A cold-inducible coactivator of nuclear receptors linked to adaptive thermogenesis. *Cell* **1998**, *92*, 829–839. [CrossRef]

53. Noland, R.C.; Woodlief, T.L.; Whitfield, B.R.; Manning, S.M.; Evans, J.R.; Dudek, R.W.; Lust, R.M.; Cortright, R.N. Peroxisomal-mitochondrial oxidation in a rodent model of obesity-associated insulin resistance. *Am. J. Physiol. Endocrinol. Metab.* **2007**, *293*, E986–E1001. [CrossRef] [PubMed]

54. Neal, J.W.; Clipstone, N.A. Glycogen synthase kinase-3 inhibits the DNA binding activity of NFATc. *J. Biol. Chem.* **2001**, *276*, 3666–3673. [CrossRef] [PubMed]

55. Baker, W.L.; Karan, S.; Kenny, A.M. Effect of dehydroepiandrosterone on muscle strength and physical function in older adults: A systematic review. *J. Am. Geriatr. Soc.* **2011**, *59*, 997–1002. [CrossRef] [PubMed]

56. Emmelot-Vonk, M.H.; Verhaar, H.J.; Pour, H.R.N.; Aleman, A.; Lock, T.M.; Bosch, J.L.; Grobbee, D.E.; van der Schouw, Y.T. Effect of testosterone supplementation on functional mobility, cognition, and other parameters in older men: A randomized controlled trial. *J. Am. Med. Assoc.* **2008**, *299*, 39–52. [CrossRef] [PubMed]

57. Giannoulis, M.G.; Sonksen, P.H.; Umpleby, M.; Breen, L.; Pentecost, C.; Whyte, M.; McMillan, C.V.; Bradley, C.; Martin, F.C. The effects of growth hormone and/or testosterone in healthy elderly men: A randomized controlled trial. *J. Clin. Endocrinol. Metab.* **2006**, *91*, 477–484. [CrossRef] [PubMed]

58. Kirwan, J.P.; Solomon, T.P.; Wojta, D.M.; Staten, M.A.; Holloszy, J.O. Effects of 7 days of exercise training on insulin sensitivity and responsiveness in type 2 diabetes mellitus. *Am. J. Physiol. Endocrinol. Metab.* **2009**, *297*, E151–E156. [CrossRef] [PubMed]

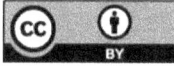

© 2016 by the authors. Licensee MDPI, Basel, Switzerland. This article is an open access article distributed under the terms and conditions of the Creative Commons Attribution (CC BY) license (http://creativecommons.org/licenses/by/4.0/).

MDPI AG

St. Alban-Anlage 66

4052 Basel, Switzerland

Tel. +41 61 683 77 34

Fax +41 61 302 89 18

http://www.mdpi.com

Nutrients Editorial Office

E-mail: nutrients@mdpi.com

http://www.mdpi.com/journal/nutrients

www.ingramcontent.com/pod-product-compliance
Lightning Source LLC
Chambersburg PA
CBHW051314020426
42333CB00028B/3333

* 9 7 8 3 0 3 8 4 2 6 8 6 8 *